TREATING TRAUMATIC STRESS
IN CHILDREN AND ADOLESCENTS

D1609625

Treating Traumatic Stress in Children and Adolescents

How to Foster Resilience through Attachment, Self-Regulation, and Competency

SECOND EDITION

Margaret E. Blaustein
Kristine M. Kinniburgh

THE GUILFORD PRESS
New York   London

Copyright © 2019 The Guilford Press
A Division of Guilford Publications, Inc.
370 Seventh Avenue, Suite 1200, New York, NY 10001
www.guilford.com

All rights reserved

Except as indicated, no part of this book may be reproduced, translated, stored in a retrieval
system, or transmitted, in any form or by any means, electronic, mechanical, photocopying,
microfilming, recording, or otherwise, without written permission from the publisher.

Printed in the United States of America

This book is printed on acid-free paper.

Last digit is print number: 9 8 7 6 5 4 3 2 1

LIMITED DUPLICATION LICENSE

These materials are intended for use only by qualified mental health professionals.

The publisher grants to individual purchasers of this book nonassignable permission to
reproduce all materials for which permission is specifically granted in a footnote. This license
is limited to you, the individual purchaser, for personal use or use with clients. This license
does not grant the right to reproduce these materials for resale, redistribution, electronic
display, or any other purposes (including but not limited to books, pamphlets, articles, video-
or audiotapes, blogs, file-sharing sites, Internet or intranet sites, and handouts or slides for
lectures, workshops, or webinars, whether or not a fee is charged). Permission to reproduce
these materials for these and any other purposes must be obtained in writing from the
Permissions Department of Guilford Publications.

The authors have checked with sources believed to be reliable in their efforts to provide
information that is complete and generally in accord with the standards of practice that are
accepted at the time of publication. However, in view of the possibility of human error or
changes in behavioral, mental health, or medical sciences, neither the authors, nor the editor and
publisher, nor any other party who has been involved in the preparation or publication of this
work warrants that the information contained herein is in every respect accurate or complete, and
they are not responsible for any errors or omissions or the results obtained from the use of such
information. Readers are encouraged to confirm the information contained in this book with
other sources.

Library of Congress Cataloging-in-Publication Data
Names: Blaustein, Margaret E., author. | Kinniburgh, Kristine M., author.
Title: Treating traumatic stress in children and adolescents : how to foster resilience through
    attachment, self-regulation, and competency / Margaret E. Blaustein and Kristine M.
    Kinniburgh.
Description: Second edition. | New York, NY : The Guilford Press, [2019] | Includes
    bibliographical references and index.
Identifiers: LCCN 2018031390| ISBN 9781462537044 (paperback : alk. paper)
Subjects: LCSH: Post-traumatic stress disorder in adolescence—Treatment. | Post-traumatic
    stress disorder in children—Treatment.
Classification: LCC RJ506.P55 B53 2019 | DDC 618.92/8521—dc23
LC record available at *https://lccn.loc.gov/2018031390*

For Lexi, Andrew, Jordan, and Shayna

You have been our most influential teachers.
You remind us daily about the dynamic nature of attachment,
the inherent struggles and joys of parenting, and the remarkable,
challenging, and ever-changing process of child development.
Being part of your growth has deepened our understanding
that no two children, and no two parents,
ever engage in this process the exact same way.

And for every child and every caregiver who has permitted us
to bear witness to their own unique developmental path,
our gratitude and respect for allowing us to join you
on the journey.

About the Authors

Margaret E. Blaustein, PhD, a practicing clinical psychologist, is Director of the Center for Trauma Training in Needham, Massachusetts. Her career has focused on the understanding and treatment of complex childhood trauma and its sequelae. Since 2004, Dr. Blaustein has worked with Kristine M. Kinniburgh on the development, implementation, and refinement of the Attachment, Regulation, and Competency (ARC) intervention approach. She has provided extensive training and consultation to providers in the United States and internationally.

Kristine M. Kinniburgh, LCSW, is Director of Children's Services for Justice Resource Institute Connecticut. In this role, she focuses primarily on ensuring that trauma-impacted individuals and their families receive quality care that emphasizes the promotion of resilient outcomes. Since 2004, Ms. Kinniburgh has worked with Margaret E. Blaustein on the development, implementation, and refinement of the ARC intervention approach. They are coauthors of the foster-parent curriculum *ARC Reflections* and the caregiver skill-building curriculum *ARC Grow.*

Preface

Why are we revising this book?

Since 2004, the development, implementation, and refinement of the Attachment, Regulation, and Competency (ARC) intervention approach has been the cornerstone of our work. From the beginning, we have viewed ARC as a continual work in progress that builds upon both expansions in empirical knowledge and lessons harvested from real-world practice. Just as our clients grow, so too do we grow and learn as clinicians, trainers, organizational consultants, and developers. In this new edition, we have incorporated that growth and that learning into our approach.

Over the near-decade since we completed the writing of the first edition of this text, we have had the rich experience that comes from collaborating with hundreds of systems, engaging with a wide range of providers, and learning from the growth process of the many youth and families these systems and providers serve. Through this work, we have continued to refine our understanding of how best to support youth and families who have experienced complex chronic trauma, and the systems that partner with them.

In our clinical practice—and in our own lives—we have a firm belief that crisis represents an opportunity to learn, grow, and develop resources that will support us in the next inevitable challenge. Together with our clients and colleagues, we have confronted countless moments of challenge in our work. In each of these moments, we have attempted to engage our curiosity, openness, and creativity to uncover the pathway toward hope and change. We recognize that the complexity of the work we do and the population we partner with necessitates our receptivity to open-ended learning and to our own change process. With this second edition, we hope to share the new lessons we have learned.

So, what has changed?

In the original framework, as delineated in the 2010 edition, ARC was described as a core-components model of intervention organized around three core domains—attachment, regulation, and competency—addressing 10 key targets of intervention. We described trauma experience integration as the summative goal of intervention, building upon the work done to address the remaining targets in the framework.

Although the core structure of the framework has remained consistent over time, based upon our continued understanding of good practice with this population, we have refined the nuances of the framework in a number of ways, as follows:

■ *Foundational strategies.* We have identified three foundational strategies relevant to all intervention components: engagement, education, and routines and rhythms. These are described in individual chapters toward the beginning of the book and are then addressed in an integrated manner within each intervention chapter.

■ *Refinement of the core ARC targets.* We have refocused the central ARC targets onto eight (rather than 10) core goals of intervention: three within attachment, two in regulation, and three in competency. We have also reexamined our understanding of each of these treatment targets. Two have changed in name (i.e., affect expression is now *relational connection*; consistent response is now *effective response*). Some targets have undergone significant shifts in conceptualization (most notably, the two renamed targets); all have been expanded and refined.

■ *Trauma experience integration.* We have expanded our understanding of trauma experience integration as this construct relates to complex trauma. We view trauma experience integration as a fluid process that occurs through targeted, attuned clinical practice with both child and caregiving systems. We conceptualize this process as one that is addressed throughout treatment via attention to the eight key treatment targets, rather than as a process that is separate from them. We describe our frame of trauma experience integration early in the book, we address it within each treatment chapter, and we return to it at the end of the book using a clinical case to illustrate one example of the fluid treatment process.

■ *Caregiver skill building.* We have more explicitly addressed the role of caregivers—whether primary or systems of care—in each of the core child-focused intervention targets.

■ *Systems applications.* In recognition of the growing use of this framework in less traditionally clinical systems of care, and by a range of providers, we have worked to expand the applicability of this book to the numerous providers and systems that work with youth and families.

Having immersed ourselves in this work for the past 15 years, we are clear that the learning process is a continuous one. Although readers who have been familiar with ARC since its beginnings will certainly recognize the original framework within these revisions, we hope that those readers will also recognize the ways in which this latest conceptualization enhances our practice. We imagine that another revision may well be needed in another decade's time. Until then, we will work to stay curious.

Acknowledgments

The development of the Attachment, Regulation, and Competency (ARC) treatment framework, and ultimately of this book, has been a process of the heart that has continued over a period of 15 years and has been influenced by the contributions, support, and wisdom of many different people.

During this time, one of our most influential learning grounds has been the Trauma Center in Brookline, Massachusetts, and the dedicated, passionate team with whom we have worked there. We are extremely appreciative of the support, collegiality, and contributions of our peers that we have received over the past number of years. Although we would love to thank each team member individually, we know that we would inevitably leave out one or two, so we thank all of our colleagues as a group. It has been a sincere honor and a great pleasure to work with all of you and to learn from your wisdom and dedication.

The ARC framework had its earliest roots in a model developed in collaboration with Alexandra Cook and Michele Henderson, and we appreciate their contributions to its initial conceptualization. Our early thinking about the nuances of culture was greatly enhanced by rich discussion with and feedback from Beau Stubblefield-Tave of the Cultural Imperative. Our thanks to Dawna Gabowitz, Erika Lally, and Jodie Wigren for providing feedback on drafts of the first edition of this book; to Wendy D'Andrea for her assistance with tracking down references; and again to Erika for sharing two of her drawings for use in our handouts. Our thanks to Janina Fisher for her generosity in allowing inclusion of one of her activities; to Katrin Neubacher, our amazing inaugural ARC postdoctoral fellow, for her support with the second edition of this book, including feedback on drafts, help with updating references and worksheets, and general all-around, behind-the-scenes excellence; and to Alice Connors-Kellgren, our second ARC fellow, for helping us continue to keep our projects running.

Our work applying the ARC framework both within our own community and across the United States has been supported in part by the National Child Traumatic Stress Network (NCTSN) and funded by the Substance Abuse and Mental Health Services Administration (SAMHSA). We have very much appreciated the opportunity the NCTSN has given us to team with systems locally as well as to collaborate with excellent colleagues from around the country who stretch our minds and expand our understanding of this work. We feel truly honored to be members of this innovative and passionate network of brilliant individuals who have dedicated their lives to addressing the realities of childhood traumatic stress.

Outside of the NCTSN, we have had the great pleasure of collaborating with gifted individuals in numerous agencies both in the United States and elsewhere. It has been no small astonishment to us to watch this number grow over time. Our collaborators have included residential schools, group homes, juvenile justice facilities, transitional living programs, day schools, community-based teams, PreK–12 school systems, home-visiting services, community mental health centers, child welfare systems, and many more. These programs serve a wide range of youth, including youth with different developmental abilities; youth who have been adjudicated in the system; youth who identify as lesbian, gay, bisexual, transgender, or queer (LGBTQ); youth who have been diagnosed with major mental health issues and with co-occurring substance use disorders; youth who have been trafficked; and youth who have spent the majority of their lives in the custody of systems and who are now entering into adulthood. To all of our collaborative partners, we hope you have no doubt of the degree to which we honor the opportunity you have given us to enter into your lives, to both support and learn from your work, and to contribute to the lives of the children and families you serve. We are humbled by your hard work, creativity, and dedication. We continue to learn a great deal from all of you, and we leave every collaborative project feeling richer than when we entered it.

As our work has expanded, it has grown well beyond the ability of any two individuals to sustain it. We have been privileged to work with a patient, humor-filled, passionate, and brilliant group of trainers from all over the globe, who enrich this framework with their own expertise and wealth of experience. Although this list is likely to grow, as of the writing of the acknowledgments, we thank our current group of lead ARC trainers: Joshua Arvidson, Beth Barto, Tracie Carlson, Jon Ebert, Heather Finn, Stacey Forrest, Jeremy Karpen, Valerie Krpata, Rachel Liebman, Kristin Mortenson, Tiffany Naste, Emily Neal, Katrin Neubacher, Kelly Pratt, Jana Pressley, Christina Russell, Tara Sagor, Liza Simon-Roper, Joseph Spinazzola, Kati Taunt, Julie Thayer, Natalie Turner, and Dana Wyss. Given that we have inevitably left someone off this list, we apologize in advance and state in our defense that it is very likely that either one of us would have eaten the marshmallow.

Our journey with the second edition of this book was perhaps even more of a leap than with the first. It involved many episodes of stepping in and stepping away, revising our thoughts, challenging our ideas, and edits upon edits upon edits. Several years past our initial deadline, we are extremely grateful to The Guilford Press and Executive Editor Kitty Moore for believing in this project and being so positive, and for hanging in there with us.

Our families have provided foundations and life lessons in the invaluable influence of support, love, humor, wisdom, and "hanging in" through the tough times.

From MEB—To my children, Jordan and Shayna, who were not there when I started this journey but who have made me ever-more grateful for it: You were the best choices I ever made and have been the greatest gifts and the greatest sources of joy and challenge of my life. You teach me and remind me every day that parenting is equal parts amazing and terrifying, that this rhythm of relationship we are in changes daily and often unexpectedly— but boy, is it worth learning the dance. Although it is clear to all of us that I will never achieve perfection, I promise always to strive to be the very best me I can for you.

To my parents, Donna and Arnold Blaustein, my thanks and my love for . . . well, everything, but among many other things, for the ways you have shown me, in everything you do, the immense capacity of human beings to make it through and transcend the inevitable curveballs that life throws our way, and to do so with grace, compassion, and humor.

To Rich, Keri, Josh, Megan, and Nicole—I feel so lucky to have you all in my life, and to watch and be part of your continued life journey. And to Vera Rosenbaum, who was here for the last edition and is here only in my heart for this one, my continued and everlasting thanks for the unconditional love and the many, many life lessons.

From KMK—My thanks and love to Todd for being my partner in everything, for your quiet strength and unfaltering patience, for being the amazing father that you are to our children, and above all for offering consistent love and support throughout this journey.

To my children, Lexi and Andrew, for being my teachers; for helping me to gain a deeper understanding of the concepts about which we write by challenging me to truly engage them, to feel them, to live them in my own life. Thanks to you, I have a deeper appreciation for the gift of parenthood in all of its glory and defeat. Each of you is truly unique and through your own journeys you have both shown me the amazing capacity that all children have for growth and for resilience. The experience of watching you grow has been the greatest joy of my life. To my mother, Maureen Jentoft, for being my model of consistency, strength, and unwavering, unconditional love and support. My journey has been guided by you, and I will always strive to make you proud.

From both of us—Our deepest thanks go to all of the children, adolescents, and families with whom we have worked. There is nothing we do in our work, and nothing in this book, that we didn't first learn from one of you.

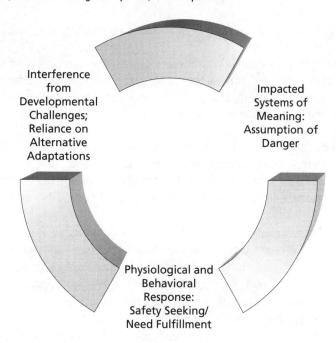

FIGURE 2.1. A three-part model for understanding child behaviors.

working animal vs. *companion*); and by personal experience (e.g., *frightening animal* vs. *beloved pet*). As described originally in the writings of Piaget, over the course of our development these systems of meaning grow and change through a process of *assimilation* (the interpretation of new information through existing mental structures) and *accommodation* (the expanding and shifting of mental structures to incorporate new information). These mental changes are not random: We build these schemas as an adaptive process, in response to input from our physical and social worlds, and working toward a goal of maintaining cognitive equilibrium. In this way, all children actively construct their understanding of the world (Piaget, 2003, 2008; Piaget, Garcia, Davidson, & Easley, 1991; Piaget & Inhelder, 1991).

The ways in which we make meaning are built upon, and strongly influence, our beliefs about our experiences. This tenet is at the heart of cognitive models of treatment, which operate on the assumption that various mental health disorders (e.g., depression) involve altered or maladaptive cognitions and assumptions (e.g., the tendency to catastrophize: "This is terrible"), and cognitive therapists work actively with clients to challenge them. It is also at the foundation of relational and client-centered models of psychotherapy, which emphasize the role of relationship in shifting clients' internal working models of self and other. It is widely accepted that our beliefs—conscious or not—influence our interpretations, our emotional responses, and our actions. Consider the following situation:

Jimmy is 11 years old, in the sixth grade. During an unannounced fire drill, his teacher stops the lesson and tells the students to line up quickly. The students rush to the door, and, as Jimmy lines up, he feels someone bump into him from behind—hard enough that he falls forward a step before he catches himself.

So . . . what exactly is the situation? Let us consider two possible scenarios:

> *Scenario A:* Jimmy catches himself with his arm against the door, avoiding bumping into the student in front of him. He turns to the student behind him, a new student named Mike whom he's never really spoken to, and says, "Hey, man, be careful—where's the fire?" Both students laugh, and Jimmy turns back to face the front of the line.

> *Scenario B:* Jimmy catches himself with his arm against the door and feels a surge of anger. He's convinced that someone shoved him on purpose—it seems like other students are always trying to start something. He turns and sees that the person behind him is that new kid, Mike, and he shoves him hard, saying, "Hey, man, you better watch out!"

In both scenarios, the available information is the same: A student is pushed from behind. The situation is ambiguous: The action could have been accidental, or it could have been purposeful. In the first scenario, the student assumes benign or neutral intent; in the second, the student assumes malicious intent. Clearly, these assumptions carry very different emotional charges and lead to different behavioral responses.

All of us hold assumptions that are formed by the collective pool of our experiences in the world, beginning with the internal working models of self and other we develop within our earliest attachment relationships (Bowlby, 1958). As in the above scenarios, these assumptions guide our interpretation of events, particularly when those events are ambiguous or uncertain: When in doubt, our previously developed systems of meaning guide us.

Beliefs that are built upon a foundation of danger may be particularly strong. If you have ever developed food poisoning after eating a particular food, you know that you never quite look at that food the same way again: Even if you logically know that not *all* clams are bad, the distress, discomfort, and fear elicited by that one bad experience is difficult to let go of. Similarly, although someone may have hundreds of experiences of safety as a driver or passenger in an automobile, it may take only one serious accident to build a belief that cars are inherently dangerous. Even when, on a *cognitive* level, you recognize your belief as illogical, your body may continue to react—on a *physiological* level, your belief in danger continues to hold. Thanks to evolution, our brains have a remarkable ability to use life experiences in the service of continued survival.

For children who have experienced repeated stress, chaos, danger, and harm in their relationships and their environments, these assumptions may be rigid and generalized. It is not that *one* individual is dangerous; *all* individuals are potentially dangerous. This generalized sensation of danger may be particularly prominent for children whose families and communities have experienced systemic injustices and racism, or who are identified as members of a stigmatized social group: For these children, individual exposures to trauma and stress may be embedded in and exacerbated by ongoing and/or intergenerational experiences of injustice and a deeply internalized felt sense of vulnerability and danger in the world.

The belief systems of children who have experienced trauma may include the following:

- "I'm not safe."
- "People want to hurt me."
- "People cannot be trusted."

- "The world is dangerous."
- "If I'm in danger, no one will help."
- "I'm not good enough/smart enough/worthy enough for people to care about me."
- "I'm not powerful."
- "It will never get better."

For children who have a basic and enduring belief that the world is dangerous, it is adaptive and protective to maintain a defensive stance, a constant vigilance for signs of danger. Unlike the clear and concrete cue of a food item in the case of food poisoning, or the car following a motor vehicle accident, when children have experienced multiple and chronic stressors, the cues of danger are widespread and may be overt or subtle. This is particularly true when trauma is experienced early in life because core systems of meaning—and the associated cues of danger—have their foundations in sensory, affective, and visceral experience, rather than in language. For instance, for a child who has been inadequately cared for, cues of danger may include delays in gratification, feelings of deprivation or need, increases in physiological arousal, or perceived rejection or abandonment. For a child who has experienced verbal abuse, cues may include signs of anger, control by others, loud noises, or raised voices. We refer to these cues as *triggers:* those signals that act as a sign of possible danger, based on historical traumatic experiences, and which lead to a set of emotional, physiological, and behavioral responses that arise in the service of survival and safety. Common triggers for children who have experienced developmental trauma include the following:

- Perception of a lack of power or control
- Unexpected change
- Moments of transition
- Feeling threatened or attacked
- Feeling vulnerable or frightened
- Feeling shame
- Feelings of deprivation or need
- Intimacy and positive attention

It is important to note the subjective nature of many of these triggers: Cues of danger are often not absolutes. Keep in mind the example of Jimmy, standing in line: Was he pushed by accident or on purpose? The "reality" of the situation is not what dictates his interpretation or response but rather his guiding assumptions. When these guiding assumptions are predicated on danger, it is the rare person who is not likely to err on the side of staying safe: in other words, to assume danger until proven otherwise.

Note also that beliefs and associations about these cues are frequently not held at a conscious or verbal level. As discussed above, our brains become increasingly efficient at the tasks they do most often; for a child exposed to frequent stress and violence, these tasks include the assessment and labeling of danger. Many of these associations were laid down long before language formed and/or were laid down on a visceral, physiological level. It is because of this nonconscious, nonverbal foundation that traumatic assumptions and associations are so entrenched and often so automatic.

Understanding and working with children's triggers and danger responses are discussed in depth in Chapter 8 (caregiver–child attunement) and Chapters 10 and 11 (identification and modulation).

Step 2: Physiological and Behavioral Responses— Safety-Seeking Behaviors and Need-Fulfillment Strategies

It is a central tenet of this framework that human behavior is not random: Our behavior and actions are largely functional or else arise to serve some function and continue because no more effective or sophisticated adaptation yet exists. Even the most seemingly "pathological" of children's behaviors may make sense, when understood in light of the purpose they serve for the child.

For children who have experienced chronic and early trauma, two salient factors have helped to shape their behavioral responses: (1) the presence or threat of danger, often on an ongoing basis; and/or (2) the absence of sufficient fulfillment of physical, emotional, relational, and environmental needs. As a result, in a highly simplistic manner, many of the behaviors seen in children in the face of cues of potential danger may be thought of as either (1) safety-seeking or danger-avoidance behaviors and/or (2) need-fulfillment strategies.

Safety-Seeking Behaviors

> While there are an infinite number of stressors that can cause a subjective sense of overwhelming stress and distress in a child, there are finite ways that the brain and the body . . . can respond to those stressors.
> —MICHAEL DE BELLIS (2001, p. 540)

Over the course of millions of years of evolution, the higher cortical structures of the human brain have developed, advanced, and become increasingly sophisticated. We are able to plan, delay responses, focus attention, integrate information from multiple senses, solve problems, generate novel solutions, form and retain complex memories over long periods of time, and integrate experience across time and place. The subcortical structures of the brain, however, are more primitive. These are the structures that, among other tasks, prioritize our survival. We differ little from other mammals in these structures, and their activation sets off a chain of responses that is hardwired.

Much of the time our behavior and actions are in the control of our higher cortical structures. We engage purposefully in our lives as we act upon the world. As we are doing so, our brain undergoes a constant process of absorbing, filtering, interpreting, and either acting upon or discarding information and input from the world around us. Information that is irrelevant is discarded; information relevant to our task may be acted upon or "filed."

When information is labeled as "dangerous," a rapid mobilization occurs in the body. The brain signals the release of neurotransmitters responsible for rapidly increasing arousal; as these are pumped throughout our bodies, our heart rates increase, our sensory systems become hyperalert to further cues of danger, and all nonessential tasks—that is, those not relevant to immediate survival—are disengaged. Among tasks considered nonessential in the face of immediate threat is complex thought. Why would this be the case? Consider the following example:

It is late evening, and you are walking down a curving side street toward your parked car. Tired after a busy day at work, you are paying little attention to your surroundings. The sidewalks are blocked by snow, but the road is clear, so you walk along the center of the road, knowing that the street is generally quiet. Suddenly, you hear a screech of tires, and you turn to see a car barreling down the road, directly toward you.

In this moment, which part of your brain do you want to have in charge? You can *think,* or you can *jump out of the way.* Most of us, of course, would rather jump first and think later.

In the face of danger, our *limbic systems*—the structures of the brain concerned with arousal and emotion—increase in activation, and our higher cortical structures, particularly the *prefrontal cortex*—the part of our brains that engage in executive functions—decreases in activation. In a split second, our bodies mobilize for action.

But what if the danger is not really danger? Let's say that, rather than continuing down the road toward you, the car in the example above speeds midway down the road and then suddenly turns right into a side alley. Objectively, you were never in danger: The driver had no intention of continuing down the road. Is your heart pounding any less?

The human danger response does not require actual, physical danger in order to be activated; it merely requires the *perception* of danger. Once your brain has labeled something as dangerous, regardless of "objective reality," your body will respond. In the previous section we discussed the often entrenched and generalized nature of children's "danger systems": For the child who has experienced ongoing chaos, violence, and stress, the array of signals that may be labeled as potentially dangerous is wide. As a result, the danger response may be activated often and indiscriminately, leaving the child at the mercy of frequent surges of arousal, rapid changes in physiology, and loss of access to higher cognitive structures. Although these changes are adaptive and perhaps lifesaving in the middle of the street with a car careeningtoward you, they are significantly less useful in the middle of math class or while interacting with peers.

Behaviorally, what does this danger response look like? There are four primary categories in which we classify the human danger response: we may *fight,* we may *flee,* we may *freeze, and/or we may submit.* The response in which we engage depends in large part on the nature of the threat. Fleeing, or escape, often offers our greatest chance of survival: In the presence of a large, unbeatable threat (such as a car), whenever possible, we attempt to escape. When flight is not possible, we may fight: An adult who is being assaulted, for instance, may attempt to fight off an attacker, hoping to eventually either subdue or flee from the threat. The two remaining danger responses, freezing and complying, are less often discussed but often the ones most available to children in moments of danger. Freezing is a defense used when neither fight nor flight is possible. It is the danger response most readily available to small animals trying to avoid attackin the jungle, and to small children trying to avoid attack by their much larger caregivers. The freeze response is a state of extreme vigilance and arousal, despite a physical stilling and lack of observable physical movement, and may be thought of as an attempt to remain unseen, unnoticed, and untargeted by the ready danger. Submit or comply is a strategy used to remain alive when an individual is actively under attack, and when flight is not possible and remaining unseen is no longer an option. The act of submission, often perceived by the individual as an act of helplessness and remembered in the aftermath with shame, is in fact a powerful strategy that attempts to appease and accommodate the attacker and that allows the individual to survive the experience of danger.

Although we use the terms *fight, flight, freeze,* and *submit,* actual behaviors used by children in the face of perceived threat or escalated arousal may vary. Examples follow of observable behaviors in children:

Fight: Externally directed physiological arousal

- Aggression
- Irritability/anger
- Trouble concentrating
- Hyperactivity or "silliness"

Flight: Withdrawal and escape

- Social isolation
- Avoidance of others; sitting alone in class or at recess
- Running away

Freeze: Stilling and hypervigilance

- Constricted emotional expression
- Stilling of behavior
- Observable vigilance toward the environment

Submit: Appeasing and accommodating others

- Overcompliance and denial of needs
- Shifts in behavior and relational strategy
- "Pleasing" behaviors ("You're so pretty"; "You're the best")
- Denial of affect or reaction

Need-Fulfillment Strategies

Immediate physical danger is rarely the only salient stressor shaping the behavior of the children with whom we work. A lack of predictable fulfillment of the range of human needs—physical, emotional, relational, and environmental—is often superimposed upon other stressors or is the formative stressor. Many factors impair caregivers' ability to provide for their children, including environmental stressors such as extreme poverty and homelessness, social stressors such as domestic and community violence, and individual factors such as substance use and mental health issues. In addition, many children have been affected by attachment losses and placement changes and disruptions.

In the "Tasks of Childhood" section of Chapter 1, we describe in detail the ways in which the child's development of competencies across a continuum of functions relies on the sensitive and consistent response of the caregiver. When this response is not available or is inconsistent, the young child will develop his or her own strategies to either maximize the possibility of response or to meet the need in other ways.

Consider the following example:

Susan is 4 years old and lives with her mother, a young, single parent who is experiencing significant depression. Susan's mother spends most of her time curled up on the sofa, watching television or sleeping. When Susan tries to get her mother's attention, her mother generally ignores or dismisses her. Sometimes her mother will hold her if Susan climbs up on top of her, but most of the time her mother pushes her off and tells her to go play. Susan doesn't like to be too far from her mother, though, because she worries that something bad will happen. When Susan feels worried or upset, her mother often doesn't notice, but if Susan starts to cry loudly and throw a tantrum, her mother will generally rouse herself enough to try to comfort her.

For Susan, the lack of attention and care from her depressed mother represents a danger and a significant stressor: Four-year-old children need external soothing, comfort, and care, and Susan is just entering the age when she is cognitively aware of this need. The only way for Susan to get her emotional needs met is to maximize the connection to her attachment figure by remaining as close as possible, and to communicate her needs loudly by tantrumming.

Imagine Susan 2 years in the future. She is in kindergarten, where many children are vying for attention from a single teacher. Susan is feeling sad one day and tries to climb onto her teacher's lap. Her teacher gives her a quick hug, then tells her to return to her seat. For Susan, this perceived rejection serves as a trigger, and she copes with the perceived danger—the lack of attention—in the way she has learned: by refusing to return to her seat and then escalating her demands into a tantrum. Her teacher's attempts to deescalate the situation by walking away only amplify the perceived danger, and Susan becomes increasingly dysregulated.

It is the rare clinician in this field who has not heard a child with a history of distressed attachment characterized as *manipulative, needy,* or *demanding.* Although these behaviors, on the surface, are unappealing, there is an alternative frame for them. A child who is *manipulative,* who tries to control the situation, the environment, and other people, is generally a child who is attempting to fill some need, and who has learned that adults cannot be relied upon to fill those needs independently.

Children from distressed early environments often show behaviors that may be categorized as attempts toward *need fulfillment.* Needs may substitute for one another; for instance, a child who craves attention and care but receives little of either may instead seek out physical objects or sensations, and a child who has been physically deprived may try to fulfill needs through emotional contact. Following are examples of common need-fulfilling behaviors among children who have had inadequate or inconsistent early care.

Emotional/relational needs

- Emotionally demanding behavior (whiny, interrupting, dramatic)
- Seeking negative attention or connection (acting out)
- Poor interpersonal boundaries (e.g., too much sharing)
- Attempts to control the environment; may be described as *lying* or *manipulative*

Physical needs

- Physical nurturance-seeking behavior (e.g., too much physical contact, poor physical boundaries, sexualized behaviors)
- Hoarding or stealing food, clothing, objects

Step 3: Interference from Developmental Deficits Due to Early Gaps in Care and Reliance on Alternative Adaptations

Thus far, our three-part model for understanding behavior points to the role of a *system of meaning* that assumes, and is vigilant toward, prevalent danger, and to *adaptive physiological and behavioral responses* in the face of these cues. The third step in our model highlights the role of developmental challenges stemming from inadequate or distressed early caregiving systems.

As described in detail previously, children who have experienced developmental trauma have invested much of their energy in survival, rather than in the development of competencies. As a result, they may be impacted across domains of development.

Regulatory and Emotional Development

Children who have experienced chronic trauma demonstrate core deficits in the capacity to regulate physiological and emotional experience. They may have difficulty understanding what they feel, where it comes from, how to cope with it, and/or how to express it. The ability to maintain a comfortable state of arousal is impacted such that children may fluctuate from hypo- to hyperaroused states, escalate or constrict rapidly, and/or disconnect from affect and experience. Whichever the case, splintered state shifts and a lack of coherence and connection across emotional states are the result.

Intrapersonal (Self) Development

Children's understanding and perception of self may be strongly impacted. From an early age, children may develop a negative self-concept and a reduced felt sense of competency. Agency is affected; children may feel a lack of power and control over their lives and actions, and they may be more likely to perceive actions as "failures" and to blame themselves, rather than external factors, for those failures. Over time, children will have greater difficulty forming a coherent identity and sense of self, with a lack of integration across experience, a fragmented understanding and manifestation of self and identity, and reduced or absent future orientation.

Interpersonal (Social) Development

Following on the challenges within their earliest connections, children often continue to struggle in interpersonal relationships. Challenges may exist with forming relationships or with maintaining them over time. Children may have (1) difficulty reading social cues, (2) overly rigid or diffuse physical and emotional boundaries, and (3) a basic lack of trust in, or an overdependency on, others. In the absence of healthy models of relationship, children may be vulnerable to further victimization or negative influence in their search for connection and attachment.

Cognitive Development

Trauma is toxic to the brain, and the neurocognitive development of children who have experienced chronic trauma may be impacted on a structural level, a biological level, and a functional level. Children may show early lags in receptive and expressive language, as well as difficulty with sustained attention and concentration. Over time, children show delays and impairments in executive functioning, including in planning, problem solving, organization, and delaying response. Altered states of consciousness and structural impacts may affect children's memory, resulting in impairment in the consolidation of experience (i.e., transfer from short-term to long-term storage) and a difficulty retrieving relevant information in current problem solving. Behaviorally, children may experience increased frustration in the face of challenging task performance, noncompliance with directions, and negative emotional response. Over time, children who have experienced trauma are at significantly higher risk for school disciplinary problems, grade retention, and dropping out.

Alterations in competencies in these domains will interact with, and layer on top of, the child's behaviors and emotions when confronted by signals of danger. In the face of the intense arousal and dysregulation brought on by these triggers, and in the absence of developmentally appropriate skills or external supports, the child is left with no choice but to rely on alternative adaptations—or a range of behaviors and strategies designed to help the child cope with internal and external experience. Common alternative adaptations include the following:

- Emotional numbing/constriction
- Withdrawal/avoidance of others
- Indiscriminate attachments
- Hypercontrol of the environment/rigidity
- Substance use/abuse
- Alterations in eating patterns
- Constricted or excessive sexual behaviors
- Self-injury
- Sensation-seeking behaviors
- Aggressive or other externalizing behaviors

Ironically, it is these alternative adaptations that frequently become the reason for a child's referral and the target of treatment. As a result, well-meaning clinicians invest efforts in treatment of the child's coping skills, rather than core areas of impact: the domains of developmental competency, the systems of meaning, and the lack of safety in the surrounding context.

Pulling the Model Together

Let us put the various components of the model together, as we consider Janae.

Janae's mother, a heroin addict, was unpredictable and often frightening. Her behavior changed rapidly: In one moment she might be barely responsive, in another she might be intrusive and emotional, and at certain times she would fly into sudden and volatile rages. Janae learned to be constantly watchful and vigilant. At a young age, Janae learned that her best survival strategy was to remain "invisible," particularly when her mother was in a rage; if she froze and did not move, she was less likely to become the target of her mother's anger.

At the age of 8 Janae was removed from her mother's home and placed in foster care. Her current foster parents describe her as "cold" and disinterested in forming a relationship with them. The home is a somewhat chaotic one, with five children in it, and Janae often appears reactive and irritable, frequently escaping to her room. She is protective of her belongings, and flew into a rage one day when she discovered one of her foster sisters looking through her clothing drawer. When reprimanded by her foster mother, she froze and then tried to run out of the house.

Janae is a child whose early experiences involved chaos, inadequate care, and sudden violence. The unpredictable nature of her mother's behaviors taught her to be constantly alert to cues of danger, and the mother's responses to her emotions and behaviors have led Janae to constrict and shut down her expressions and actions. Despite this apparent constriction, Janae's body operates at a baseline level of high arousal, due to the frequent activation of the danger response and the subsequent chronic dysregulation of her physiology.

Although there is a very wide range of cues that have become associated with danger for Janae, particularly salient ones are unpredictability and anger, especially from women. Janae is also fiercely protective of her space and her property, having been exposed to significant physical and emotional deprivation. In the face of these triggers, Janae's arousal escalates rapidly, and she fluctuates among the triad of danger responses, alternatively raging, escaping, and stilling. Her capacity to cope with her intense arousal is limited; failures within her early attachment system have impacted her ability to regulate her physiological and emotional experience, and the sudden surges in arousal leave her feeling overwhelmed. She has few reliable coping strategies and is unable to view others as potential resources. Her experience has taught her that other people are both untrustworthy and potentially dangerous, and she has little practice expressing her feelings or asking for help. In the absence of either reliable internal strategies or trustworthy external supports, she frequently acts out her distressed emotions with impulsive behaviors.

In Janae's story we see the impact of exposure to significant early stressors, including an unpredictable and often dangerous attachment system. Janae's systems of meaning are infused with danger and chaos, and she is left with little agency or control. Her physiological and emotional experiences are, in many ways, as dangerous as external events, as without adequate coping strategies, she is often at the mercy of internal experience. In a new, ostensibly safer caregiving system, her behaviors and actions are misinterpreted, and the misattunement of her caregivers confirms her beliefs about self and others, while forcing her to continue to rely on previously developed safety strategies.

Is Development Fixed?

It is without question that chronic early trauma exposures may seriously and significantly derail and alter children's developmental pathways. The harm that is done may last not just throughout the child's life, but on into the next generation, as stress, chaos, and adversity are passed down from parent to child (Noll, Trickett, Harris, & Putnam, 2009). Given the wealth of evidence suggesting the harmful nature of these exposures, then, the question arises as to whether developmental pathways can be altered. Can a child whose life has been steeped in danger and survival, who has known chaos, adversity, invalidation, and/

or indifference throughout his or her life—and perhaps, from before birth—find peace, health, and joy?

It is our unshakeable conviction, and that of many others in this field, that they can. The literature on resilience is a testament to this conviction, as are the lives of the many children and adults we have encountered in our practice. The potential for resilience is remarkable. We have met many individuals who have managed to harness some factor or factors—an internal quality, an external resource, pockets of strength and competency—and convert them into growth and health, when their histories and experiences should have predicted continued despair and challenge.

As our understanding about the impact of complex trauma grows, so too does our capacity to change outcomes. The factor that itself contributes to the toxic nature of trauma—the plasticity and adaptability of children's brains—is also the factor that highlights the possibility for positive change. We believe strongly that all children have both the capacity for, and the right to lead, joyful, healthy lives to the best of their abilities, and that the ultimate goal of the child clinician is *not* a reduction in pathology, but rather a targeting and building of the core developmental competencies, the systems of meaning, and the safe caregiving system that will allow the child to continue to build a positive future.

involving one-to-one treatment; rather, these youth and their families present in a range of settings, including schools, residential programs, shelters, and primary care services.

Increasingly, there is a recognition of the value of identifying core components of treatment, rather than emphasizing models of intervention that require strict or rigid adherence to sequenced practice elements and structures, and many existing approaches have incorporated flexibility into their models of intervention (Strand, Hansen, & Courtney, 2013). The ARC framework was specifically designed to incorporate a core-components model. ARC identifies key targets of intervention for youth who have been exposed to trauma and their caregiving systems. These targets were drawn from extensive review of the extant literature on the impact of complex trauma and attachment stress on developmental course, as well as factors leading to resilient outcomes within this population. We have significant clinical experience with this population in a range of settings, and principles selected for inclusion were reviewed with and modified by input from clinicians and other professionals working in the field. These principles have now been refined and adjusted through over a dozen years of application and evaluation in a wide range of service settings with a diverse population of children and families.

Translation of Clinical Principles across Settings (or, Bringing the Mountain to Muhammad)

Because youth may present for services in a range of settings, and in recognition of the importance of "whole-systems" intervention, we selected principles that translate across service settings. For instance, when applied in an outpatient setting, ARC principles can be integrated into individual treatment with a child, dyadic caregiver–child treatment, psychoeducation and skill-building interventions with caregivers, and/or child and caregiver groups. In a milieu setting, attachment principles can be integrated into whole-systems intervention, including staff training and milieu structure. Intervention targets can be built into therapeutic groups or applied in more "organic" ways (e.g., incorporation of regulation tools into classroom settings). To date, ARC principles have been successfully integrated in diverse types of programs, including outpatient treatment settings, residential schools, locked juvenile justice facilities, therapeutic foster care, youth drop-in centers, community-based settings and homeless shelters, as well as by a range of individual clinicians in community and private settings. Increasingly, ARC principles have been incorporated into settings not traditionally considered to be "clinical" (e.g., schools, day care, and primary care practices) as a way to support trauma-informed practice.

Staying True to the Inner Clinician (or, Keeping the Art in Treatment)

Every professional is different. Every client is different. Excellent treatment involves a combination of art and science. There are few providers who do not recognize the value of flexibility and the ability to "think on your feet." Good therapeutic work involves a careful assessment of client needs and strengths, recognition of key treatment goals, and the flexibility to approach those goals in a way that works best for a particular client at a particular point in time.

The ARC framework does not attempt to replace clinical wisdom or to supplant preferred provider techniques with a singular approach that presumes that one size fits all.

Rather, ARC identifies key goals for intervention, skills involved in reaching those goals, and a range of examples of ways to get there, with a recognition that many paths may lead successfully to the same destination. One of the best pieces of feedback we have heard is that the framework supports and organizes current clinical practice, rather than replacing it.

So What *Is* ARC?

The ARC framework is a components-based model that identifies three core domains of intervention for children and adolescents who have experienced trauma and their caregiving systems: attachment, regulation, and competency. Within those three domains, eight "building blocks" or core targets of intervention are identified. These intervention targets are applied in service of the final goal: trauma experience integration. All core targets are supported through attention to three foundational strategies: engagement, routines, and education. A visual representation of the model appears in Figure 3.1; also see in the table on page 38.

   Taken together, ARC may be thought of as a four-level framework, in which overarching goals (i.e., strengthening the caregiving system) are supported by addressing specific treatment targets (i.e., supporting parent–child attunement); which in turn are supported by addressing and building specific skills (i.e., cultivating maternal curiosity about child behaviors) through the use of a range of intervention techniques (i.e., engaging a parent in a structured daily detective activity about his or her child).

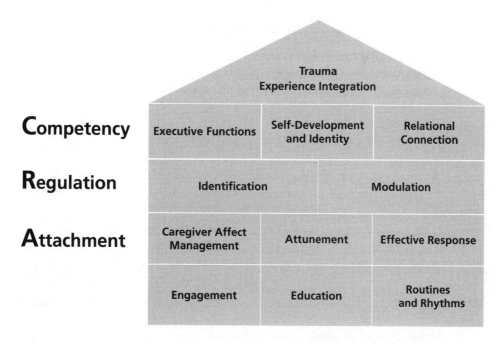

FIGURE 3.1. The Attachment, Self-Regulation, and Competency (ARC) framework. Graphic by Jeremy Karpen.

Outline of the Attachment, Regulation and Competency Framework

Broad domain	Core targets	Key subskills
Foundational strategies	Engagement	▪ Across treatment targets, explore and identify client stake and link to intervention practices.
	Education	▪ Across treatment targets, provide education about rationale and goal to caregivers and youth to enhance engagement and identify personal stake.
	Routines and Rhythms	▪ Use routines and structures to support key goals and to target challenging time periods. ▪ Incorporate routines into treatment process (i.e., session structure). ▪ Build daily rhythm by supporting routines in home and systemic settings. ▪ Build/explore/support rituals of child, family, and system.
Attachment	Caregiver Affect Management	▪ Provide psychoeducation about trauma, normalization, and validation. ▪ Identify challenging situations. ▪ Build self-monitoring skills. ▪ Enhance self-care and support resources.
	Attunement	▪ Provide parallel attunement to caregivers. ▪ Support caregiver active curiosity. ▪ Use reflection to mirror child's experience. ▪ Integrate attunement skills into support for youth self-regulation. ▪ Support fluidity/pleasure in dyadic engagement.
	Effective Response	▪ Proactively identify behaviors to target (increase/decrease). ▪ Use attunement skills to identify patterns of behavior. ▪ Use "go-to" strategies (meet needs, support regulation) to reduce and address identified behaviors. ▪ Identify, experiment with, and enhance other behavioral response strategies (problem solving, positive reinforcement, limit setting) that increase youth and environmental safety.
Regulation	Identification	▪ Identification in self: language for emotions and arousal. ▪ Identification in self: connection of emotions, body sensations, behavior, and cognition. ▪ Identification in self: contextualization of emotions and arousal to internal and external experience. ▪ Identification in others: accurately reading others' emotional expression.
	Modulation	▪ Build understanding of degrees of energy and feeling. ▪ Build understanding of comfortable and effective states. ▪ Explore arousal states and develop agency over tools. ▪ Support and facilitate strategies that successfully lead to state change.
Competency	Relational Connection	▪ Explore goals of connection; build comfort and safety in relationship. ▪ Identify/establish resources for safe connection. ▪ Build skills to support effective use of resources.
	Executive Functions	▪ Support active recognition of capacity to make choices. ▪ Build age-appropriate active evaluation of situations. ▪ Build child capacity to inhibit response. ▪ Build/support ability to generate and evaluate potential solutions.
	Self and Identity	▪ Help children identify personal attributes (unique self). ▪ Build internal resources and identification of positive aspects of self (positive self). ▪ Build a sense of self which integrates past and present experiences, and incorporates multiple aspects of self (cohesive self). ▪ Support capacity to imagine and work toward future goals/outcomes (future self).
Trauma experience integration		Work with children to actively explore, process, and integrate historical experiences into a coherent and comprehensive understanding of self in order to enhance children's capacity to effectively engage in present life.

ARC Foundational Strategies

Across domains and intervention targets, attention is paid to three key strategies that are integrated into all elements of treatment: (1) sustaining active attention to *engagement* by exploring and identifying stake of the child, caregiver, and/or system for all goals; (2) providing *education* at all levels of the system to build empowerment, understanding, and client/system stake; and (3) building mastery and safety through the use of *routines and rhythms*. These *foundational strategies* are described in more detail in Chapters 5 and 6.

Attachment

Across cultures, the caregiving system, in whatever way it is defined, serves as the foundational context for healthy development. A safe, healthy attachment system can buffer the impact of highly traumatic stressors (cf. Cohen & Mannarino, 2000); conversely, a stressed attachment system can, in itself, create significant risk (cf. Crittenden, 1995; Wakschlag & Hans, 1999).

Given our understanding of the role of attachment in child development, it seems crucial to target the surrounding caregiving system when working with children and families who have experienced trauma. We define the caregiving system broadly: Numerous youth who have experienced complex trauma have experienced a range of caregiving systems. These systems may include biological parents or relatives, foster or adoptive parents, school systems, residential programs, caseworkers, and the myriad professionals who interact with these children. As noted, we encourage the application of a whole-systems approach, with the guiding assumption that youth can be only as safe as their surrounding systems, and that until youth are safe, other aspects of development will continue to be sacrificed.

Our attachment building blocks target two primary factors: (1) the building of a "safe-enough," "healthy-enough" relationship between the child and his or her caregiving system, which requires felt safety within the system itself; and (2) the building of skills and a context that the caregiving system will use to support the child's healthy development.

The Attachment Building Blocks

CAREGIVER MANAGEMENT OF AFFECT

As is highlighted throughout the ARC framework, caregivers play a crucial role in child development. Furthermore, the ability of caregivers to support their children in the face of stressors is a key predictor of child outcomes. Caregivers' ability to provide needed support to their children is either circumscribed or expanded by caregivers' ability to effectively manage their own experiences. This section details the role of caregiver affect management in child outcomes, factors that impact caregivers' capacity to manage emotional experience, the crucial role of support for caregivers, and key skills to target in the caregiving system.

Key skills and areas of foci within this intervention target include (1) psychoeducation about the nature of trauma and normalization of caregiver response; (2) building of caregiver self-monitoring skills; (3) building of caregiver resources for addressing physiological and emotional experience; and (4) enhancing caregiver supports. Applications for family systems, milieu, and other caregiving systems, as well as clinician self-applications, are discussed.

ATTUNEMENT

Attunement is the capacity of caregivers to accurately read children's cues and respond appropriately. There are two primary errors that adults make in reading children's cues: We either miss the cues altogether or we react to overt behaviors, rather than "reading" the emotional message or need underlying the behavior. Children who have experienced significant early trauma may have a particularly difficult time communicating feelings, wants, and needs effectively. This second intervention target emphasizes the particular importance of accurate attunement in the caregiving system of children who have experienced complex trauma.

Key skills and areas of foci within this intervention target include (1) parallel attunement to the caregiving system, to support caregivers in feeling seen and understood; (2) engaging caregiver curiosity about children's communication strategies; (3) building caregiver capacity to reflect, mirror, and respond effectively to children's communications; (4) using attunement strategies purposefully to support youth regulation; and (5) building fluidity and pleasure in caregiver–child interactions.

EFFECTIVE RESPONSE

Although research on parenting practices emphasizes that there is no one "right way" to parent a child, studies highlight the importance of consistent and safe responses to child behaviors: Children do better when they have a clear understanding of rules and when there is a degree of predictability in adult and environmental response. Successfully parenting a child who has experienced significant trauma, however, has many complications. Children who have experienced considerable chaos may exert rigid control in an attempt to gain some sense of safety, and they may resist or resent imposed rules. Behaviors that appear to be oppositional or defiant may instead communicate anxiety, vulnerability, or overwhelm. Typical parenting practices may trigger strong responses in children with dysregulated emotions. Caregivers may be reluctant to impose consequences on children who have been badly hurt, or they may be overly restrictive in an attempt to keep their children safe. Many caregivers have themselves experienced significant trauma in their own families of origin, and may have no ready model of safe parenting available.

This section highlights key intervention targets for building effective caregiver response. Here we emphasize the importance of understanding the function and pattern of child behaviors in the context of *need fulfillment* and *regulation*, and of managing understandable adult affect in the face of challenging youth behaviors, so that responses to behavior are proactive rather than reactive. Behavioral techniques (e.g., limit setting, the use of positive reinforcement and praise) are framed as experiments to be applied thoughtfully and in combination with an understanding of the "why" of behaviors, and not just the "what." Caregiver felt success in implementing techniques is viewed as essential, and strategies are provided to increase caregiver mastery.

Regulation

As detailed throughout the introductory chapters, developmental trauma has a significant impact on the child's ability to regulate physiological, emotional, behavioral, and cognitive experience. Children are affected by failures of the attachment system (our earliest context for learning the lessons of regulation of the self), by the impact of significant stress on regulatory systems, and by the combination of the two. As a result, we work with children who have significantly dysregulated internal experience and limited ability to understand, tolerate, and manage that experience.

The regulation building blocks target children's awareness and understanding of internal experience, and their ability to modulate and shift that experience effectively.

The Regulation Building Blocks

IDENTIFICATION

Children who experience early trauma often learn to disconnect from their emotional and physical experience. In the context of a caregiving system that does not provide adequate reflection of and language for emotional states, and/or in the presence of frequent experiences of overwhelming arousal and affect, many children have challenges with differentiating emotions ("I just feel bad"), little or no awareness of physical and emotional states ("I don't know how I feel"), and little or no understanding of the connection between emotions or physiological states and the experiences that elicit them ("I don't know why I feel that way"). In order to regulate emotional and physiological experiences in a healthy way, children must first have some awareness and understanding of internal states.

This intervention target highlights a number of skills and points of intervention. Treatment goals include building a vocabulary for emotions and physical states, providing education about the human alarm response and trauma triggers, and normalizing the experience of mixed emotions. Children are taught to be "feelings detectives." Provided exercises and information highlight skill building in children's ability to identify emotions and bodily states in self and other; to connect emotions to body sensations, thoughts, and behavior; and to understand the links between feelings and internal and external factors.

MODULATION

Complex trauma takes a significant toll on children's capacity to effectively regulate physiological and emotional experience. Overwhelming and chronic stress exposes children to chronically high and dysregulated arousal levels. Caregiving systems, which normatively serve as a buffer and external regulator, may be themselves impaired, leaving the young child alone to struggle with extreme emotional and physiological experience. Most children develop adaptations to help them manage their experience, but these adaptations may themselves leave children vulnerable to ongoing challenges.

This intervention target highlights those skills necessary to help children learn to maintain optimal levels of arousal and to expand their "comfort zone" to be able to tolerate a range of emotional experience. Specific targeted skills include (1) building an understanding of degrees of feelings, and (2) building facility with tolerating and moving through arousal states by using strategies that comfortably and effectively increase and decrease arousal. Clinicians are encouraged to develop "toolboxes" with youth by teaching specific skills and strategies directed toward the energy of the emotion, and to engage supports and resources to help youth engage with and utilize identified tools.

Competency

Ultimately, our goal for the children and families with which we work is the building of resources, both internal and external, that allow for ongoing healthy development and positive functioning across domains of competency, including social connections, community involvement, and academic engagement. These intervention targets highlight the importance of children achieving felt mastery and success; receiving the tools to continue functioning as active constructors of their lives; and developing and consolidating a positive and coherent sense of self. Although the building of developmental competency is often relegated to the category of "supportive therapy" or adjunctive treatment when discussing trauma-focused therapy, we view the building of competency as a core component of treatment for children exposed to early developmental trauma.

The Competency Building Blocks

RELATIONAL CONNECTION

The capacity to tolerate, build, and sustain connection with others is a key predictor of resilient outcomes over time. When there is no comfort in sharing aspects of the self, people are unable to create intimate human relationships, or, often, to get basic needs met. Many children who experience trauma struggle with the ability to safely and effectively communicate internal experience, build connection, or tolerate relationship. Early attempts to connect may have been met by anger, rejection, or indifference. Children learn quickly that connecting may make them vulnerable, and they learn to avoid or disconnect from relationships to increase felt safety. Other children may desperately connect in an attempt to get needs met, leaving them vulnerable to experiences of rejection or exploitation. Over time, without effective modeling and experience in relationship building, youth exposed to trauma may be increasingly impaired in their understanding of how to engage and sustain safe relationships.

The primary goal of this intervention target is to provide children with skills that help them effectively and safely build connections with others in order to meet emotional or practical needs. Specific targeted skills include (1) exploration of the goals of connection as well as historical experiences in relationship, (2) identification of safe connection resources, (3) creation of opportunities for connection and communication, and (4) supporting communication through skill building.

EXECUTIVE FUNCTIONS

Among the most important tasks for a young child is the development of a sense of agency: the knowledge that he or she has the ability to make an impact on the world. Agency develops as we *try,* we *do,* and we *choose.* To some degree, a sense of agency relies on adequately operating executive function skills: those cognitive skills held in the prefrontal cortex that allow us to exert control over our actions by delaying response, anticipating consequences, evaluating outcomes, and actively making decisions. For children exposed to chronic trauma, regular engagement of the "alarm mode" of their brains may lead to inadequate development of prefrontal control skills. Research demonstrates impaired executive function abilities in this population, as compared with same-age peers (Beers & De Bellis, 2002;

Mezzacappa, Kindlon, & Earls, 2001). Research on resilient youth highlights the role of problem-solving skills in positive outcomes: Not surprisingly, youth who are able to make choices effectively and are active players in their own lives do better than those who are not (Cicchetti et al., 1993; Werner & Smith, 2001).

This intervention target emphasizes the development of executive function skills, including the ability to actively evaluate situations, inhibit response, and make thoughtful decisions. A contrast is made between *acting* and *reacting,* and the skills in this section focus on building youth awareness of *choice.* This chapter highlights the importance of integrating previously addressed skills, including identification (awareness of internal experience) and modulation (managing arousal), and the key role of timing. Included in this section is information on ways to integrate caregivers into efforts to support their children's executive functions, as this skill set is a highly scaffolded one throughout development.

SELF DEVELOPMENT AND IDENTITY

Growth of a coherent and positive sense of self normatively occurs over the course of development: Young children gradually internalize the typical responses of others and the environment; latency-age children incorporate experiences across domains and begin to integrate values, opinions, and other attributes; and adolescents actively explore and construct the self, developing an increasingly complex and nuanced sense of identity, including an awareness of future possibilities. Young children exposed to chronic trauma often internalize negative experiences and self-values. Their internal experience may be fragmented and state-dependent. For many children impacted by trauma, there is no sense of future, only a number of disconnected "nows."

In this section, intervention targets four aspects of self and identity: (1) The *unique self* involves an exploration and celebration of personal attributes, including likes and dislikes, values, opinions, family norms, and culture. (2) The *positive self* involves the building of internal resources and identification of strengths and successes. (3) The *coherent self* emphasizes examination of self across multiple aspects of experience: self before and after trauma, self with biological parents versus adoptive, self as displayed versus self on the inside, and so forth. (4) The *future self* involves a building of the child's capacity to imagine the self in the future and to explore possibilities.

Trauma Experience Integration

As conceptualized in ARC, trauma experience integration for youth who have experienced complex trauma is something that happens continuously throughout the course of treatment, through both simultaneous and sequential processes. Trauma-affected youth (and caregivers) often shift rapidly across emotional and physiological states: at times, overwhelmed by states of arousal; at times, able to pause and reflect on experience; and at other times, able to engage in purposeful action. These states are strongly influenced by the individual's experience of danger (both real and perceived), and treatment must adapt and shift according to client needs and presentation. Because of these shifting states, the attunement of the provider (i.e., the ability to accurately read and respond to child or caregiver needs) is an essential element of treatment.

ARC defines "trauma experience integration" as the sequential development of the capacity to first *survive and tolerate* moments of overwhelming distress and arousal brought on by both real and perceived experiences of danger in the world; to build an ability to *engage curiosity and reflect upon those states*; and ultimately to be able to *engage developmental capacities* in service of purposeful action in the present moment. This goal is addressed sequentially throughout treatment, by gradually increasing tolerance for affect and supporting child and adult curiosity. It is also addressed simultaneously, as children and adults shift across states (e.g., from overwhelm to curiosity and then back again).

We identify three key child and/or caregiver states that drive intervention choices, and three corresponding overarching goals. *Note that we view all ARC targets as relevant to all states and goals.* Identified fluid states and goals include:

1. **Distress tolerance and regulation:** Engaged when youth and/or caregivers present in states of overwhelmed affect and physiology, intervention focuses on present-moment distress tolerance. A key emphasis is building tools and resources to support child or caregiver ability to cope with current experience.

2. **Curiosity and reflection:** When caregivers and/or children are reasonably calm and able to engage resources, intervention can address important reflective capacities. In this state, intervention can focus on supporting youth and families with their ability to recognize and understand triggers, behavioral responses, and patterns that emerge in relation to internal/external contexts.

3. **Engaging in purposeful action:** As children and/or caregivers are increasingly able to understand and provide language to their experience; to develop a narrative that connects past, present, and future; and to harness internal and external resources in moments of distress, intervention can emphasize purposeful engagement of developmental resources in the present moment.

These states and related treatment process are described in greater depth in Chapter 4. Throughout the book, we address intervention considerations for each of the eight core ARC targets as may be applied in each client state in support the integration of traumatic experiences. In Chapter 15, we return to trauma experience integration and highlight the ways that treatment in all stages acts in service of this crucial integration process.

ARC Intervention Section Guide

Following a great deal of early feedback from the clinicians and other professionals with whom we worked while developing the ARC framework, we have designed the ARC intervention sections to be as user-friendly as possible. Each "building block" or core target chapter is organized around the following sections.

Main Idea and Key Subskills

At the start of each chapter, we include a simple description of our overarching goal for each target, followed by the identified subskills described for working toward that goal.

Key Concepts

This is the "why" section. These concepts provide the rationale for the intervention principle as well as important teaching points for caregivers.

 Therapist Toolbox

This is the "to-do" section; it has four components:

 What's the Stake?

This section encourages providers to consider issues of engagement (for the child, for the caregiver, for the system) for each key target. We offer information about potential barriers to engagement as well as strategies for exploring with caregivers and children the rationale for incorporating work on specific treatment targets into the therapeutic process. The overarching goal is to work to actively team with children/teens and their caregivers in identifying goals and to utilize strategies that support connection, control, collaboration, choice, and voice throughout the work.

 Behind the Scenes

This section describes ways to incorporate the principle into therapy sessions and/or milieu–systemic interactions, important points to remember, and overarching principles.

 Teach to Caregivers

Important points of education for caregivers as well as specific strategies to build the intervention principle are described here. For the attachment domain, this section focuses on techniques for building safety in the caregiving environment. For the regulation and competency domains, this section discusses ways in which caregivers can support their children's skill acquisition. This section also provides a guide for individual and group interventions with caregivers as well as for staff training within a system.

 Tools

Often presented in menu format, these tools are specific activities individual and group therapists may incorporate into their sessions. Activities are presented as examples, and clinicians are reminded that creativity is often an essential part of the therapeutic process. Therapists are encouraged to expand on and individualize these examples to fit their clients.

Developmental Considerations

In this section particular applications and considerations are discussed for three developmental stages: early childhood, middle childhood, and adolescence. The reader is encouraged to consider, for instance, how attachment principles remain relevant in later adolescence, yet are distinct from these principles as applied in earlier childhood. Given the impact

46 I. OVERVIEW

of trauma on development, readers are encouraged, when planning intervention strategies, to think in terms of developmental stage rather than chronological age.

🏠 Applications

As a flexible framework, ARC is based on principles that translate across intervention settings. This section provides examples of applications of each principle within individual dyadic, group, and milieu–systemic interventions.

◯ Trauma Experience Integration: State-Based Skills Application

In this section we describe various means of addressing core targets according to client state and following our identified fluid-phasic model of trauma experience integration.

🌐 Real-World Therapy

Therapy occurs in the "real world." This section discusses the realistic pitfalls and considerations when working on this principle with real kids and families.

🔊 Routines and Rhythms

Throughout the text, we denote examples of ways to structure activities or use routines in service of goals with this icon.

Cultural Considerations

In the first edition of this book, we used an icon to denote cultural considerations. Our intention was to highlight the importance of the provider understanding children, families, and systems in the context of the many overlapping influences on their lives. As a treatment framework that emphasizes the essential ingredient of provider attunement and formulation, our stance has been to encourage every provider and every system we collaborate with to reflect about their own multidimensional cultural influences, as well as those of the clients with whom they are working, and to consider the role of these influences in client presentation and needs, and provider and system intervention approach. We define culture broadly; it may include self- or societal-defined categories such as race, ethnicity, language, country or culture of origin, gender or gender identity, sexual identity and orientation, community affiliation, or religion. Culture may also include nuances such as the neighborhood in which clients grow up, the particular traditions of the family of origin, or the particulars of the client's generation or current society. As has been pointed out to us, everyone lives in multiple cultures simultaneously (B. Stubblefield-Tave, personal communication, May 18, 2006).

In the current edition of this book, we have made the decision to remove the cultural considerations icon. Through the process of collaboration with a rich and diverse group of systems and individuals, we have been challenged to consider the ways we have addressed the nuances of culture in our framework, and the many ways in which we continue to need to grow. We are increasingly aware that consideration of the complex and often intersecting influences of embedded context—for every client, for every provider, and for every system—must be an interwoven component of the work, and for that reason we have chosen to integrate these considerations throughout the text.

ARC Resources

In the back of this book are numerous resources: educational handouts, clinical worksheets, and expanded examples of individual and group activities. These resources are organized by type and by targeted domain and are often referenced within specific intervention sections. We offer these resources as examples of ways to target specific areas, but we also encourage those who are reading this book to be creative: Often the best interventions are those we come up with in the moment or in context, targeted to the specific child, group, or family with which we are working.

Using the ARC Framework: Potential Strategies for Implementation

As a flexible framework, rather than a structured protocol, practitioners may question (as we often do, when working with complex children and families) where to begin. "I like the framework," we've heard, "but how do I *do* ARC?"

Partly as a response to this question, the intervention sections that follow each contain an "Applications" subsection that describes considerations for implementing the principle in individual treatment, group, and milieu–systems settings. This section highlights, for instance, ways to apply the "Caregiver Affect Management" principle when working with an individual parent versus with the staff in an agency. For the range of practitioners who may be utilizing this resource, we encourage you to consider the following as possible ways of using framework principles, skills, and key concepts.

Integration into Outpatient Therapy

The principles and building blocks of ARC have become, for us and for many of the outpatient clinicians with whom we work, our guide to building individual treatment goals and plans. By examining client and family/system presentation within the context of the eight building blocks, we can develop concrete treatment goals within each domain.

For instance, if our assessment points to a child with sudden angry outbursts and a caregiver who becomes overwhelmed in the face of these, our treatment goals may include (1) building caregiver tolerance for child affect through development of his or her own coping skills and supports (Caregiver Affect Management); (2) building the caregiver's understanding of the reason for the outbursts through psychoeducation in trauma and developmental expression of emotion (Attunement); (3) building child ability to "read" cues of distress in his or her body and understand where they come from (Identification); (4) building child coping strategies for managing distress (Modulation, supported by Attunement); and (5) building child ability to use the caregiver or other resources as a support (Relational Connection, again supported by Attunement).

Other ARC building blocks may intertwine in the above goals. For instance, identifying the best strategy to use and ways to plan for potentially stressful situations may involve problem-solving skills (Executive Functions), and targeting the child's feelings of accomplishment in his or her ability to manage internal and behavioral experience may build felt efficacy (Self and Identity Development). Increasing felt predictability around identified "trigger points" may decrease arousal (Routines used in service of Modulation), and helping caregivers learn to "pick their moment" in supporting regulation versus limit setting will target parenting strategies (Effective Response). The Session Fidelity Checklist/Tracking Tool (in Appendix A) may be useful in tracking which ARC principles, and subskills are addressed within a given session; we have often recommended that clinicians begin with simply tracking, prior to making significant changes. Tracking our "choice points" in session often helps us understand and define what we are targeting with clients—and perhaps what we are missing.

The intervention sections contain many examples of ways to integrate principles into individual, dyadic, and/or familial treatment sessions. We encourage practitioners to consider both formal exercises as well as informal "tuning in"—in conversation, in play, and in interaction. We also encourage consideration of ways to structure the session so that it integrates these principles in practice. For instance, consider ways to build a consistent session routine: to integrate modulation activities into opening and closing portions of each session, to regularly "check in" at start and/or end of each session to build affect identification and expression skills, to integrate competency-building activities, and so on.

Group Treatment

The principles contained within the Regulation and Competency sections translate easily into group activities. Many of the exercises provided as examples in the intervention section menus can be used in group formats, and additional activities are described in Appendix C. We encourage practitioners to consider the population with which they are working, including (among other factors) developmental stage, intervention setting, cultural context, treatment focus, and intergroup safety in selecting and developing activities for use in treatment groups. We have worked with a number of programs that have developed groups using ARC principles and have been impressed with the variation we have seen in groups' formats, structures, and foci, while still integrating key ARC principles. In addition to considering specific ARC principles as treatment targets, we encourage consideration of the role of routine and rhythm when structuring groups for children, adolescents, or caregivers.

Caregiver Support and Education

The Attachment principles specifically target caregiver education, skill building, and support. In addition, every intervention section contains key concepts, developmental considerations, and "teach-to-caregivers" information. This material may provide a guide for development of caregiver education sessions (either one on one or in groups) and/or caregiver workshops. Included in Appendix B are many caregiver educational handouts and worksheets; some may be of use in your own work with caregivers. Consider these to be a guide; our experience is that written information is helpful for some, but not all, caregivers. Consider other ways to build awareness of the same principles, whether in targeted

Part II

The Integration
of Traumatic Experiences

4

Trauma Experience Integration

What Is Trauma Experience Integration?

Many thoughtful models of trauma-focused treatment address "trauma processing," or the exploration and integration of traumatic memories and associated affects, cognitions, sensory experiences, and behavioral responses within the larger narrative of self. The definition of *trauma processing* is a more challenging one for children who have experienced multiple, prolonged stressful exposures, than for those who have experienced single or well-defined events. For a child whose life has involved, for instance, chronic early neglect, unpredictable caregiving associated with parental mental illness or substance abuse, repeated acts of violence, separation from a biological parent, multiple out-of-home placements and attachment disruptions, and revictimization due to difficulty negotiating relationships, it is difficult to define the starting and endpoints for focal trauma processing. A term that many use, and that feels to us more fitting for children who have experienced complex trauma, is *trauma experience integration*; this term is intended to encompass the range of ways that children exposed to more complex trauma may process traumatic experiences.

For purposes of this framework, we define two related but distinct types of trauma experience integration that may be relevant for children who have experienced more chronic trauma exposures, each of which is explored in more detail in the sections that follow. In describing these, consider the accompanying examples.

1. *The Integration of Fragmented Self-States and Associated Early Experiences.* Identifying and reflecting upon current fragmented aspects of self-functioning (including emotions, actions or inability to act, interpersonal relational styles, cognition, physiological states, and embedded models of self and other) and linking these to the subjective themes (e.g., shame, helplessness, rage, attachment loss, vulnerability) relevant to the repeated experiences of early childhood.

Emma's aunt, who is her legal guardian, has picked her up from school and is driving her to an appointment. Emma, 13, begins to tell her aunt a story about something that happened at school that day. Her aunt is focused on the road, and midway through the story, fails to respond to a question Emma asked. Emma becomes enraged, yelling and calling her aunt an expletive. When the aunt begins to set a limit ("Calm down! I'm trying to drive") Emma shouts, "Stop yelling at me!" She then unlocks the car door and begins to open it, threatening to jump out even though the car is still in motion.

In this example, Emma's behavior clearly stems from more than the present moment. Without needing to explicate her history, we can see the impacts of themes of perceived rejection, associated shame, loss of control, and potential danger. In the face of these cues, Emma shifts self-states: From being relatively in control and sharing a positive experience, she shifts into rage, increased arousal, danger avoidance, and preemptive rejection. These reactions are elicited by the present moment, but they are driven by the past.

2. *Processing of Specific Events.* Building a narrative around the emotions, actions or inability to act, interpersonal relational styles, cognitions, and physiological states, along with embedded models of self and other, evoked in relation to specific past memories of trauma or overwhelming stress, and incorporating or shifting these into a more coherent, realistic, and broader narrative of self and other.

Emma's memories of her biological father are hazy. Although she knows he sexually abused her when she was young, her explicit memories feel "foggy" and mixed up. She has a hard time distinguishing one memory from the next, but when she thinks about him, she always pictures the tattoo on the right side of his chest, remembers the feel of his stubble against her stomach, and begins to feel panicky and out of breath. She tries really hard not to think about him, but on a recent date a boy tried to kiss her, and she suddenly felt like she couldn't breathe and her body had turned cold, as if she were frozen. Before she could stop it, she saw the image of her dad's tattoo, and felt like she couldn't move.

Emma's memories of her mother are clearer, and she feels angry and confused when she thinks about their relationship. Her mother was unpredictable. Most of the time it felt like she was checked out, just not really available, but sometimes she got really emotional, either violent and rageful or weepy and dramatic, and on rare occasions she was affectionate. Emma likes to think about her mother only in small pieces and finds it easier to remember the things she's mad about than the things she misses.

Processing of experience for complex trauma often includes the development of a coherent story of self, across time and place, and is a key part of self and identity work. Development of self-narratives, including narratives around discrete traumatic events, is described in Chapter 14. A number of treatment models have thoughtfully and carefully addressed the process of developing trauma narratives, and so we primarily focus in this chapter on our understanding of the broader goals, targets, and process of trauma experience integration over the course of treatment, as applies to populations who have experienced complex developmental trauma.

How Trauma Influences Self-States

As described in previous chapters, children who have experienced complex developmental trauma have been exposed to recurring, chronic stressors that activate the parts of their brain responsible for survival. As with any recurring pattern, when children experience repeated and similar sources of stressful input over time, their brains develop increasingly efficient patterns of response to help them cope with and manage these stressors. These patterns of response can be behavioral (e.g., taking action or stilling), affective (e.g., surges of rage, shame, and/or fear), cognitive (e.g., shifts in cognitive focus, specific meaning making around cues or experiences), physiological (e.g., increase or decrease in arousal, muscular tension), and/or relational (e.g., shifts in patterns of approach or avoidance). Embedded within those patterns is a system of meaning regarding *self, other,* and *self-in-relation-to-other*—that is, distinct attachment patterns and meaning making about self and relationships. These often include dichotomous beliefs about other people that may be grounded in themes such as safety, trust, and acceptance (e.g., safe vs. unsafe, accepting vs. rejecting, trustworthy vs. likely to betray). These beliefs are often associated with meaning making about the self and involve feelings of self-worth versus feelings of shame and damage. Although these states are frequently disconnected from previous experience in the child's conscious awareness, they are driven by that experience.

These patterns of response have developed to serve some function—in the brain of the child, at essence, the function is survival—and as such they are often rigid and largely automatic when elicited by pertinent cues. Furthermore, these patterns may be encapsulated and fragmented, or dissociated, from other self-states, such that many different functional patterns are elicited in the child by the range of cues, or themes, related to past experience.

Prominent *themes* associated with developmental trauma, referred to alternatively in other sections of this book as "triggers" or cues of potential danger, include (but are certainly not limited to) shame, loss, vulnerability, deprivation, helplessness/loss of control, isolation, mistrust/betrayal, injustice, attachment disruption, and invasion/violation of boundaries (emotional, relational, and physical). As described in Chapter 2, detection of and response to these themes does not require their actual presence, merely the *perception* of their presence. In other words, if a child's brain decides that rejection exists, then the pattern of self that developed for self-protection in the face of rejection will emerge—regardless of whether the rejection was objectively present and intended, or not.

The Goal: Trauma Experience Integration

From our perspective, the ultimate goal of treatment for children who have been exposed to chronic, complex early traumatic experiences is to build their capacity to harness internal and external resources in service of effective and fulfilling navigation of their life, across domains of functioning, as they define and meet self-identified personal goals. Past experiences often interfere with and override children's capacity to engage purposely in present life. Their current reactions are primarily driven by the overwhelming biological mandate of safety seeking, elicited by perceptions of harm and lack of need fulfillment in their environment.

For the many children who are like Emma, past experiences influence present reactions in a way that is not fully contextualized in the moment. By continuing to be guided by fragmented self-states that emerge in response to feelings of danger, shame, rage, helplessness, and loss, and to be impacted by specific memories and associated intense experiences, these children are unable to engage in their lives in purposeful, goal-oriented, and fulfilling ways.

As described in Chapter 4 and referenced throughout this book, we view trauma experience integration as an integrative goal that is addressed repeatedly throughout treatment via application of the core ARC targets, with the specific approach varying by current client (child and/or caregiver) state. The child or caregiver often moves from moments of survival and distress tolerance, into moments of curiosity and reflection, and often back again, gaining skill and capacity in harnessing internal and/or external resources that increasingly allow self-and-other attunement and ultimately engaged action.

The Role of Attachment

Integration of traumatic experiences requires the capacity to observe and be curious about actions, thoughts, feelings, physiological states, and embedded models of self and other that play out in the present in relation to historical experiences. *Reflection* and *attunement* (described in detail in Chapter 8) play a key role in this crucial process of trauma experience integration. Many children's lives have involved a *lack* of reflection or *biased/inaccurate reflections*. Because children act out distress with often apparently contradictory behaviors, there continues to be both internal and external misattunement. An important goal, therefore, is to cultivate and support a more accurate and empathic internal and external mirror for children's experience.

The holder of the "reflective lens" (i.e., the curious observer) is likely to shift developmentally: For younger children, and for all clients early in this process, it is likely that the initial holder of this lens will be external: a caregiver, whether professional or primary. Over time, particularly for older children and adolescents, the goal is to increasingly build the capacity for self-reflective processes and for accurate self-attunement. As such, we view trauma experience integration as a process that is embedded within the caregiving/attachment system.

The challenge, of course, is that just as the child's ability to be curious and to reflect requires a generally regulated state, so too does curious observation (i.e., attunement) by the caregiver (see Chapter 7 for *caregiver affect management*). The caregiver's survival state (i.e., intense distress) can and often does interfere with the ability to read children's behaviors, needs, and adaptations accurately. In turn, caregiver responses can often inadvertently increase the child's felt sense of danger, thereby expanding the child's need to engage in survival actions. It is for this reason that throughout treatment, we emphasize the key role of the caregiving system (whether primary, resource, milieu, or provider) in the process of supporting youth who have experienced trauma, and the parallel need for the provider or family support system to attune to and support the caregiver and approach intervention in a paced manner.

It is important to emphasize that adult affect is relevant not just for the role it plays in influencing caregiver responses to youth behavior, but also for its role in the caregiver's own experience. Trauma experience integration in the children with whom we work and for whom we care requires that the caregiver bear witness. Whether the techniques we use are verbal or nonverbal; focus on narrative, expressive strategies, movement, or play; whether we are in the role of therapist, counselor, case manager, or primary caregiver—accurate reflection and attunement necessitate our witnessing of often unbearable pain and the recognition that humans are capable of terribly distressing acts.

Bearing witness is rarely a completely disconnected process. Although most professionals learn the skills to maintain a reasonably comfortable objectivity and distance, empathic work requires, to some degree, the capacity to resonate with and respond to the affect, relational dynamics, thoughts, systems of meaning, and physiological energy of our clients. Just as attachment is a dyadic, rather than a one-sided, process, therapeutic work happens in the context of a relationship, and these relational connections have an impact on both the child client and the helping professional.

The understandable affect of the caregiver can misdirect us in this work. For instance, when applying this point to ourselves as providers, we need to be aware that our own affect may lead us to prematurely close topic areas that the child needs to explore, because of our own anxiety or discomfort with material; to open up other topic areas for which the child is not yet ready because of our own "need to know"; and to carry our work (and its associated sequelae) with us beyond our treatment space. These possibilities make it particularly important for clinicians to monitor, modulate, and seek support for their own affective responses. A number of written resources on this topic may be useful (e.g., Pearlman & Saakvitne, 1995; Saakvitne, Gamble, Pearlman, & Lev, 2000).

The Foundation: Understanding Child and Caregiver Patterns

Integration of traumatic experiences requires the building of a reflective process (in the child, in the caregiver, in the system) that includes an observation of and curiosity about the patterns of behavior, self- and other-perceptions, thoughts, feelings, and physiological states that emerge in daily life and that may be driven by past experience. As noted previously, this reflective process frequently begins as an externally directed one, with a goal, as developmentally appropriate, of building both the child's and the caregiver's own curiosity and self-reflective capacity. For a provider or system to successfully support the child's or family's reflection, our work must first start with our own attuned understanding of child and family patterns.

The starting point of clinical practice, as first described in Chapter 3, therefore involves the development of formulation: working to understand the child (and/or caregiver) within the context of his or her life, and the necessary adaptations that have developed in response. This starting place may be broadly understood as the provider's purposeful application of Attunement. Our early and ongoing assessment involves proactively tuning into and identifying the range of self-states and coping patterns shown by children, caregivers, and family systems. Go beyond diagnosis to build a trauma-informed conceptualization of behaviors and responses. For instance, imagine that you are working in a residential program with an adolescent boy who has an extensive history of physical abuse by an adult male caregiver. We could imagine that themes involving issues of trust, respect, and control versus mistrust, disrespect, helplessness, and vulnerability would be relevant. Keeping these themes in mind, observe the teen within the milieu. The client's history suggests that he may be particularly triggered by, and leery of, authority figures, especially males. In what way do his behaviors and interactions with adults and with peers suggest adaptations that make sense? For instance, is he reactive to limit setting? Quick to engage in a power struggle? Withdrawn when challenged by authority? Identify key patterns and themes, along with functional associated patterns of self, so that rather than focusing purely on diagnostic presentation (e.g.,

"This teen has oppositional defiant disorder"), the response to difficult behaviors is, "Yes, that makes sense."

Assessing and Understanding Child and Caregiver States and Matching These to Treatment: The Dynamic Process of Intervention

As we begin to develop attuned understanding of children and caregivers, our ongoing process should include tuning into and observing specific patterns as they occur, and adjusting our understanding of child and caregiver needs and adaptations according to those observed patterns. These patterns are likely to shift markedly according to child and/or caregiver state: as key triggers elicit fragmented self-states, the child or caregiver may shift rapidly from a calm, reflective state to an overwhelmed, angry, or withdrawn one—all in service of survival.

Throughout our work, as described in each treatment target section of this book, we approach the core targets in varying ways depending upon child, adolescent, and/or caregiver state. For instance, caregiver affect management might focus on identifying external resources and validation of caregiver experiences for the parent who is overwhelmed and visibly anxious (State 1); and it might focus on understanding personal triggers and identifying targeted internal resources and strategies for the parent who is in a state in which she is able to be reflective (State 2). For this reason, provider attunement to the shifting states and capacities of the child or adult client will guide treatment choices. Here, we briefly describe these states and overarching goals and considerations, keeping in mind that presentation and capacities will vary greatly across clients, and therefore the individual's response to an attempted intervention is likely to be your strongest guide.

State 1: Distressed and Overwhelmed

This state is often a pervasive one at the start of treatment, as client distress is often the precipitant that leads to the referral for services. For many children and their caregivers, this state will continue to predominate throughout treatment, particularly in more acute treatment settings. Even in less acute settings, though, or in non-mental-health settings (e.g., schools or after-school programs), fragmented states of distress are often the most prominent indicator of a trauma-related response, and lead to behaviors that feel the most challenging to the adult caregivers involved with the child. Because chronic developmental trauma is typically associated with long-lasting stressors that are layered and multifaceted, and therefore with many entrenched survival patterns and danger cues, it is common for trauma-impacted youth and adults to move in and out of these states of overwhelm throughout the course of treatment.

In states of overwhelm, the child and/or the caregiver may present on either end of the arousal scale: constricted and shut down or highly aroused and reactive. The provider or caregiver may observe out-of-control behaviors, withdrawal, lack of affect or escalated affect, and signs of heightened arousal such as rapid speech or physiological disorganization (restless movement, feet tapping, fingers moving). The child or caregiver may be engaging in self-regulatory strategies such as self-injury, substance use, or primitive gross motor movements (e.g., rocking). Relational patterns may change: for instance, the typically engaged child may present as disconnected or clingy. These fragmented states of overwhelm are often marked by a shift in functioning, although children and caregivers who are experiencing significant stress and who have limited internal or external resources may remain in these states of overwhelm for lengthy periods of time. These self-protective states are often misperceived by others (e.g., as defiance, as manipulation, as rejection), and responses to behaviors that fail to take into account the child or caregiver's need—for instance, for control or safety—may inadvertently escalate the situation. Child and caregiver states can easily exacerbate each other; the overwhelmed parent can quickly escalate an anxious child's response, and an overwhelmed and distressed child can, in turn, quickly escalate his or her caregiver's reaction.

> Following the incident in the car, Emma has been closed up in her room all afternoon. When her aunt knocks to tell her that dinner is ready, Emma mutters that she is not hungry. Her aunt opens the door and sees Emma curled up on her bed, hugging a stuffed animal. Emma refuses to make eye contact, rejecting her aunt's attempts at conversation with one-word responses. Her aunt feels increasingly angry at the perceived disrespect, finally shouting, "I can't believe you're acting like this when you're the one who almost got us killed today! You want to act like a baby, fine—you can just go to bed now, without anything to eat if you're not hungry." Emma feels sudden panic break through her previously numb state and jumps up off her bed, rushing at her aunt, who is standing in the doorway, and pushing her, shouting, "I hate you!"

STATE 1 OVERARCHING GOAL: DISTRESS TOLERANCE AND REGULATION

When working with youth and caregivers who are in current states of overwhelm, our primary goal is to support their ability to tolerate distress and to navigate the present situation in as effective a way as possible. Whereas for some youth or families, current states of overwhelm may represent fragmented self-states and associated patterns of behavior triggered by perceived dangers, as in the case of Emma, above, in many cases the child or family will be responding to very real ongoing experiences of stress and adversity. Our role as providers—whether clinicians or other systems of care—in these moments is typically to observe, mirror, and validate the child or caregiver's experience, provide opportunities for external regulation supports or coregulation, work to build internal capacities, help to stabilize the most challenging behaviors and patterns of connection, and engage in and build upon strengths.

State 2: Adequately Regulated and Able to Reflect

Overwhelmed states typically cycle with calmer states, even in highly stressed children and caregivers. In these moments, children and/or caregivers typically have some capacity to reflect upon and be curious about their own experiences as well as, for caregivers, that of their children. The ability to sustain curiosity depends strongly on content (what the individual is thinking about); on distress tolerance (how well the individual can manage his or her response to the content); and on external resources and supports (how safe the individual feels in the context of the current environment). For instance, a highly stressed adolescent who is currently in a calm state and is meeting with a relatively new provider with whom there is minimal relationship may be able to sustain curiosity concerning the concrete behaviors or areas of strength about which the provider inquires (e.g., "I'm curious what your favorite things to do with your friends are when you're feeling OK?" or "What are three ways I'm going to know if you're starting to feel frustrated with me?"), but may quickly shift to overwhelmed and shut down if asked to reflect on more distressing content (e.g., "I wonder how being in a lot of different homes has made you feel about meeting new people?").

Because reflective capacity shifts according to content, internal resources, and external resources, the process of engaging child and/or caregiver curiosity is fluid and typically deepens over time, with increased predictability of safety, more reliable coping strategies, and stronger relationships. Observing a shift in the child or caregiver from calm and reflective to states of overwhelm (constriction and/or hyperarousal) is an important cue that the provider should potentially shift focus back to regulation. This focus may incorporate curiosity and awareness of the *need* to regulate—for instance: "I'm noticing that while we were talking, your behavior suddenly got really big again. Do you think we should take a break and do something to help your body feel comfortable again? What are you noticing?" In this manner, although the focus returns to supporting regulation, reflective curiosity continues to be engaged.

STATE 2 OVERARCHING GOAL: CURIOSITY AND REFLECTION

Children and caregivers who are reasonably grounded and present, who are able to engage in reflective activities—whether verbal, expressive, or symbolic—and sustain connection to them without shutting down or becoming overwhelmed are typically able to do the work of *attunement:* that is, awareness of and curiosity about self and other. The capacity for this skill is strongest when the child or caregiver has adequate internal resources or feels reasonably safe and connected to the provider or system of care—which can, in turn, act as an external modulator in times of distress.

In moments when the child is curious and reflective, the provider or treatment system can support the child in recognizing and understanding his or her own patterns of behavior, triggers, needs, and behavioral adaptations. This work can support the child in tuning in to internal sensations and physical and emotional needs in the moment, and in connecting this growing awareness to ways that the child navigates his or her world. The curious, regulated child is increasingly able to engage executive function skills (with support, and outside of moments of distress) to understand choices, to consider possibilities, to identify goals, and to anticipate needs. Typically, this work is strongly grounded in reflection upon and curiosity about the child's various "lenses": for self and identity, for relationships, and for the larger world.

In moments when a caregiver is able to engage reflection and curiosity, the work can shift from affect *tolerance* ("How can we help you survive and cope with this challenging child behavior?") to curiosity and understanding ("How can we work on understanding *why* this behavior is happening, why your own reaction is occurring, and how you might be able to respond to and address both of those things?") The overarching goal of this work is to support the caregiving system in accurately seeing, understanding, and cultivating the tools that will allow effective response to child behaviors, as well as cultivating the capacity to reflect upon and understand the caregiver's own patterns of response.

State 3: Reflective, Adequately Resourced, and Able to Connect Past, Present, and Future

As the child and/or caregiver builds internal and external resources that are increasingly reliable, and develops a greater awareness and understanding of his or her own relational, regulatory, emotional, and environmental needs and the patterns of these needs over time, the capacity to anticipate, experiment with, and apply in-the-moment strategies for successfully navigating daily experience expands. Children and caregivers who are able to engage in this work are typically able to demonstrate a capacity to tolerate even intense distress or challenging situations without becoming overwhelmed—or alternatively, when overwhelmed, are able to recognize this state and access resources and supports. They are able to understand the links among past, present, and future experience; have some empathic understanding of their own (or their child's) patterns of behavior and their origins; and have an investment or stake in shifting current danger-based adaptations.

The ability to sustain reflection and connection to resources is likely to be variable, shifting according to the impact of cumulative and/or particularly intense stressors. However, it is likely that as the child or caregiver who has achieved this state experiences increasing and sustained felt success over time, the ability to engage and apply developmental capacities will continue to grow, as mastery and competency generally cultivate further mastery.

STATE 3 OVERARCHING GOAL: ENGAGING PURPOSEFUL ACTION

The core goal of intervention in this state—and the ultimate goal of trauma treatment—is to support children and their caregiving systems in cultivating the ability to purposefully engage action in the moment, in service of their own identified goals. Quite simply, our goal is to cultivate those skills that allow children, adolescents, and caregivers to live their lives in the present, in a manner that moves beyond survival and that rests on a foundation of empowerment and joy.

Present action can mean many things. It can mean an adolescent recognizing the signs that she is being triggered (a surge of arousal, an urge to withdraw) and engaging a strategy that settles arousal, allows her to access resources, and gives her the time and space to regroup and attune to the source of her response. It may mean anticipating a challenging situation—a difficult conversation with a teacher or a visit with a sibling—and engaging coping strategies before, during, and after the situation that allow successful connection or communication. It may mean recognizing that your child's opposition is a sign of anxiety, and rather than reacting angrily, taking a breath, remaining calmly supportive, and using the behavioral response strategies that have been practiced and found to be effective.

Engaging in present action in an ongoing way typically requires a combination of capacities and resources. Present action requires environmental safety and the availability of adequate external supports, because the absence of safety requires that the child and/or caregiver continue to respond in service of survival. It requires an array of developmentally appropriate internal capacities: for instance, the ability to recognize feelings, to communicate to others, or to accept supports. It requires a stake in the effort: a belief that it matters to understand, address, and shift behaviors and emotions, and an investment in doing so. It requires knowledge and self-compassion: an empathic, attuned understanding of self and/

or other that acknowledges that behavior occurs for a reason, and that our past is one of the many factors that influences and shapes our present. And it requires agency: a belief that we have the capacity to act upon our present and to shape our future.

In the remainder of this book, we discuss in detail (1) the three foundational strategies we identify as essential to this work; (2) the eight core targets of intervention; and (3) the ways that we use these intervention targets across settings, provider type, and context in support of trauma experience integration. Each chapter includes a section describing the various ways we might address those targets dynamically, according to child and/or caregiver state. In Chapter 15, we return to the topic of trauma experience integration and revisit Emma, introduced previously.

Part III

Laying the Foundation

5

Foundational Strategies

Engagement and Education

Over the course of our work with the range of providers who support trauma-impacted children and families, one of the most frequently identified challenges we have heard is that of *engagement:* "This all sounds good," we hear, "But I can't get the mom to even get out of the car!" Mentors describe teenagers who are shut down and refuse eye contact, clinicians describe parents who fail to return phone calls, and systems describe staff that participate half-heartedly in training and are skeptical of system efforts toward trauma-informed care.

Over the course of literally thousands of hours of consulting to many professionals, agencies, and systems of care as well as in our own clinical practices, it has become very clear to us that for any trauma-focused intervention framework to be successful, it must consider issues of engagement. Specifically, we need to consider not just *what the intervention goal is* or what the *best-validated therapeutic technique* is, but *why this goal matters to this child, this family, or this provider/system,* and whether the *method is valid to the individual.* A crucial part of engagement, from our perspective, lies in the transparent, purposeful, and routine incorporation of *education* and information into the intervention process, and so we combine these two key foundational strategies in the current chapter.

What Is *Engagement*?

Engagement is often thought of in terms of simple presence: If a client is showing up for treatment (or a staff member for work), he or she is considered to be "engaged." Realistically, of course, engagement is about much more than just showing up. Engagement may be defined as the level of investment, participation, and felt stake of the child, caregiver, or provider in the process in which he or she is taking part. It is about active participation and collaboration, and it involves belief as well as action.

There are several crucial factors required for children, caregivers, or providers to be invested in a process. These include the following:

■ They have to believe that the intention of the process (i.e., the goal) matters, is valuable, and is relevant to their own goals and values.

■ They must feel that that the process itself (i.e., the therapeutic technique or approach) is a valid one.

■ They must believe that the process is a match for their own preferences, comfort level, and capacities.

■ In the case of an intervention, they must feel that the provider or system is equally invested.

These factors highlight several key aspects of engagement relevant to service provision using ARC as a framework:

■ *First, any provider using this framework must be attuned to the individual and collective goals of the child, family, and surrounding system.* Attunement allows providers to gain answers to these questions: What is it that each player wants right now? What is he or she hoping for in the future? Why is this goal relevant to his or her life? It is important to keep in mind that the *child's* goals, for instance, may differ from the *caregiver's* goals, or that in a system, the direct care staff's values and philosophy may differ from that of his or her supervisor or administrator. These goals may shift and change over time, and so this attunement must be dynamic. Engagement in treatment at all levels requires a stake in the process, and that stake must be explored in an ongoing manner.

■ *Second, the approach to treatment or service provision must be tailored, to some degree, to the needs, preferences, and capacities of the service recipient.* A child who struggles with language may be most comfortable with expressive or sensorimotor approaches; an adolescent who is constricted may require explicit permission to enter a residential program's activities at his or her own pace; a caregiver who is guarded with providers she perceives as authoritative or judgmental may engage eagerly with a parent partner. We believe strongly that there are many, many different valid, meaningful, and relevant ways to approach goals and achieve similar outcomes, and that our most successful treatments are those that attend to the preferences and needs of those who are receiving the services.

■ *Third, an understanding of the rationale for an intervention, an approach, or a process is a key part of stake.* For there to be "buy-in" from a child, family member, or provider, the individual must understand *why* this intervention may support his or her own goals. For instance: A teacher may want a child to stop acting out in school. A parent may want to receive fewer phone calls. A child may want other kids to stop picking on him. All of these goals may hinge on several core underlying strategies: for instance, helping the child manage feelings of distress and overwhelm **(Modulation)**; increasing the school's understanding of why the child is engaging in the behaviors **(Attunement)**; proactively identifying supportive ways for the school to respond to dysregulation **(Effective Response)**; and building the child's available support resources in the school **(Relational Connection)**. In turn, these goals rest on an understanding of *why it makes sense* that the child feels so dysregulated and overwhelmed at school, and has a hard time asking for help or using age-appropriate coping strategies. Because of this, *education* is a crucial underpinning of engagement and is identified as a foundational strategy for all treatment goals.

■ *Fourth, attention to relationship is at the heart of successful trauma-informed service provision*. The ARC framework was developed specifically for the population of individuals whose lives have been shaped, to greater or lesser degrees, by experiences of adversity, stress, and violence, most often in the context of human relationships. It is not just that the children and adults we work with have experienced harm; it is that they so often have experienced harm at the hands of others, whether intentionally or not. It is not surprising, then, that failures of relationship have played a key role in shaping current adaptations (of the child, of the caregiver), and that engagement in relationship is often a significant barrier to successful treatment. To invest and collaborate in an intervention process, the individual must believe that the person with whom they are collaborating is reasonably respectful, safe, supportive, and invested in a similar outcome.

Whom Are We Engaging?

One of the great challenges of working with children and families is the necessity of engaging with many different people and systems simultaneously. Because children do not exist in a vacuum, and because our goal, in large part, incorporates direct targeting of the child's surrounding world, treatment of a child often requires that providers build good-enough relationships with the child, with the child's primary caregivers, with other involved providers (e.g., a mentor or parent partner), and with other service systems (e.g., schools or child welfare). When children move through placements, such as from one foster home to another or from group care back to a primary caregiver, these relationships must often be rebuilt and recultivated over time.

And What about Us?

Engagement is not something that is simply about the "other"; it is bidirectional, and it is as important for the provider to feel invested as the individual. For this reason, providers working with children and families impacted by trauma must consider similar questions as those raised above for children and families. For example:

- "Do I feel that the goal or intervention target I am addressing matters? Is what we are doing meaningful?"
- "Am I using an approach that I think will be effective? Do I believe in what I am doing?"
- "Am I comfortable using this approach? Do I feel confident and capable using this strategy, in this situation, with this child/caregiver?"
- "Do I feel invested in this person, and do I feel that he or she is connected to me?"

As with children and families, the provider's own knowledge, preferences, and reflective awareness are crucial. We must believe in what we are doing, and we must question and challenge our own strategies and approaches when they no longer seem effective. And perhaps most importantly, we must also believe in the child or caregiver with whom we are working, and we must monitor, seek to understand, and be willing to address our own assumptions, biases, or anxieties.

What May Impact Engagement in Services?

Although engagement is often described as if it were a static construct ("This person is/is not engaged"), it is in fact dynamic and ongoing. For all of us, there may be times when we are deeply invested in a process, and times when something or a combination of factors—life stress, competing interests, barriers to participation—shift our capacity or our interest, and our investment wanes.

In clinical practice, there has long been a presumption that "client investment" is an obligation that rests solely on the client, and that "failures of participation" are largely reflective of the individual's own weaknesses, defenses, or lack of readiness. This presumption assumes that services are equally accessible, welcomed and welcoming, and feasible for all people. It is clear, though, that numerous considerations impact the capacity of the individual to engage in services (Ingoldsby, 2010).

A number of factors may influence engagement, particularly at the start of treatment, and should be considered and proactively addressed:

- **Perception of need:** For a child, caregiver, or provider to invest in an intervention process, there must be a belief that the intervention is helpful for achieving desired goals. Often, this perception varies by individual (e.g., a child may want to see a therapist, but his father believes that the hassle of coming in outweighs the benefits). Early in the work, it is crucial that the provider work with the child, the caregiver, and/or the provider system to identify *what matters* to each person entering into the process, and to provide education about why the intervention approach may support that goal.

- **Frame of "the problem":** Engagement is maximized when the provider and the service recipient hold a similar frame. A parent who believes that her child is oppositional and needs "to learn to behave better and listen," for instance, may be reluctant to engage in a treatment that emphasizes the role of the caregiver in child behavior and focuses on strategies that may differ in approach and philosophy from what she is currently doing. A provider who sees a teen as conduct-disordered will have difficulty engaging a family who views their son's anger as a justifiable response to his life experiences. Exploration of similarities and differences in perception and frame, and attunement to the perceptions and belief systems of the client, are crucial.

- **Capacity to overcome concrete or logistical barriers:** Investment in an ongoing treatment often requires the individual or family to negotiate numerous potential barriers: for instance, a grandmother bringing her 7-year-old grandson to treatment may need to rearrange her work schedule, arrange care for her youngest grandchild, arrange alternative after-school arrangements for an older grandchild, navigate public transportation on a weekly basis, and arrange finances to support all of this. These barriers may be significant; indeed, for many families they are overwhelming and prohibitive. From the start of an intervention process, it is crucial that the provider explore, identify, and help a family troubleshoot these very real barriers that interfere with available supports and services.

- **Psychological resources:** As meaningful as the concrete barriers to intervention that a family may face are the psychological barriers: the ways in which the child, the family, or the surrounding system is impacted by stress and distress. A parent experiencing intense depression, for instance, may need to harness significantly more energy to overcome even minor barriers; for this parent, just getting out of the house may feel overwhelming.

Degree of psychological resource at any given point in time will impact access to services, ongoing attendance, and ability to participate in a meaningful way. It is important that providers attend to the range of services and supports a family might need, with an understanding that what it requires for any individual or system to effectively engage will be different, and that these needs are likely to vary over time. As we discuss in Chapter 9 (Effective Response), an important starting point in addressing a child's behavior is to ask the question, "How do I understand *why* this behavior is happening?" Similarly, if a child or a caregiver is struggling with engagement or if this fluctuates over time, it is crucial that we try to understand the reasons why.

■ **Feeling a sense of connection to the provider:** Human relationships are complex, and the development of safety in relationship hinges on numerous factors. Consider the positive relationships in your own life and the ways you would describe them. It is likely that your descriptors include factors such as safety, respect, mutuality, trust, reliability, and fun; that you feel seen and understood; that you feel comfortable and able to be yourself. Now consider the demands we place—whether explicit or implicit—on those who enter into relationship with us in our role as professionals or as caregivers. We ask our clients to be vulnerable, to share personal experience often in the absence of mutuality; to agree to shift their behaviors, responses, and sometimes belief systems at our suggestion; and to place their faith and trust in us in the absence of "proof" that we are right, safe, or trustworthy. It is a high demand, and when it is not met, we are vulnerable to pushing back and blaming the recipient. It is essential that providers are clear about their role as co-constructors of relationship, and that we push ourselves to be aware, self-reflective, open to criticism and feedback, and flexible in our approach.

The experience of trauma in children/adolescents and their caregiver systems carries an extra layer of challenge in its influence on their engagement in treatment and in relationships with providers and systems.

■ **Relational stance:** Many of the children and families who engage with our service systems have experienced stress and distress in relationship. They may enter into relationship with providers using a self-protective stance—a guardedness that for many children and caregivers has been critical to survival over time. Conversely, they may struggle with boundaries, desperate to find someone who can help them, who can make them feel better, give them the answers, or take the pain away. In the absence of (impossible) provider perfection, the child or caregiver may feel betrayed or let down.

■ **Negative experiences with service systems:** Many families we work with have had numerous prior experiences with service systems—some positive, but others, less so. Families may report historical experiences of feeling disrespected, blamed, or misunderstood. Youth and/or their families may be mandated into service, leading to feelings of powerlessness and anger and placing the provider or system in the role of "adversary." Particularly for youth or caregivers who have experienced systematic injustices as a function of race, ethnicity, religion, social identity, or other categorical aspects of self, entry into a relationship with a provider may feel intensely vulnerable. This may be especially true when the provider is perceived as different on some or all of these dimensions.

■ **Ongoing experiences of adversity:** For far too many of the youth and families we work with, trauma is not simply a historical experience; it is an ongoing reality of their daily life in their homes, in their communities, in their schools, and in their larger worlds. There may be periods and pockets of safety that allow them to access and make use of supports, followed by times of stress that require withdrawal; or conversely an intense demand for services in times of crisis followed by "disappearance" when life evens out. Understanding the rhythms of the child or family's life, designing service approaches that can match the needs of highly stressed families, and understanding the ebb and flow of intervention in these circumstances without personalizing the perceived message to the provider is important for partnering successfully with stress-impacted youth and their families.

Addressing Engagement in Practice

The engagement process is an ongoing one that must be attended to at every stage of service provision and with every interaction. It is for this reason that all treatment chapters of this book include a section entitled "What's the Stake?" In this section, we encourage providers to consider the ways that each treatment target may be relevant to the child or caregiver's life, and ways to be curious about, collaborate on, and adjust treatment approaches. Here, we offer some broad suggestions both for entering into relationship and for cultivating engagement over time.

Setting the Stage: Early Engagement Strategies

Setting the Stage for Caregiver Engagement

Many of the caregivers with whom we have worked struggle with challenges related to their own historical experiences and/or multiple life stressors in addition to the stress of caring for a child with complex trauma. They may have had experience with multiple providers, organizations, and treatment modalities, and may have been told that their child has multiple diagnoses that require multiple medications. Finally, some have involvement with child protection and have been required to come to treatment. For all of the reasons listed, caregiver engagement can be a significant challenge.

Building a relationship is a process that begins from the moment of first contact with an individual. It is easy, at the point of a child or family's entry into a system, to get caught up in logistical demands (paperwork, consent forms, evaluation and treatment plans that may need to be filled out, the rules and requirements) and to lose sight of the *person*. First impressions matter and it is always our intention to set the stage for a collaborative relationship that is mutually agreed upon between the provider and the caregiver. In the following material we outline steps that we believe can be helpful in fostering collaboration at the start of a relationship.

1. Describe your program (or individual) mission and philosophy and ask about the client's goals and values. What are the program's core values? What are your beliefs about the (therapeutic/protective/educational, etc.) process? How do your goals and values map on to the goals, values, and needs of the presenting family?

2. Describe your treatment approach. For instance, we might describe ARC as follows: "ARC is a framework for working with children and families that recognizes the impact of

adverse life experiences on specific areas of functioning, and holds a belief that addressing these areas can support kids and families in healing. Three of the things we pay the most attention to are supporting relationships, helping with managing and understanding feelings and behavior, and helping kids build areas of competency." How you describe your approach should be tailored to the needs of the individual and the provider. Encourage caregivers to ask questions. For instance, a provider might say: "A lot of parents ask me things like how I help their kids with feelings, and what that has to do with getting them to behave better. I'm wondering if you have any questions like that, that are specific to what you're hoping will happen in our work together?"

3. Discuss caregiver involvement. The ARC approach considers caregiver involvement to be essential to successful outcomes. In our treatment approach, we work as a team, with caregivers as crucial members of that team. There are many things that impact caregiver involvement. It can be helpful to identify these challenges up front to normalize the situation for the caregiver and to anticipate roadblocks that are likely to emerge. We recommend the establishment of a caregiver involvement "contract" at the outset of treatment. The contract is a collaborative process that identifies a plan for your work. For example: Will you have individual appointments with the caregiver? How often? By phone or in person? Will the caregiver be incorporated into the child's session? At what point in the session would you like the caregiver to join? What is the caregiver's role? Some of these questions may be answered over time, and possibly new ones added, but it is helpful to give examples of each of these at the outset, and to be clear that you and the family will continue to revise the plan as needed.

4. Establish a frame of transparency, education, and collaboration. We view education as one of the foundational components of trauma-informed treatment, and the role of education in the treatment process should be emphasized from the start. Normalization of both adult and child responses to trauma, extreme stress, and parenting in general will act as a foundation for further education. Keep in mind that education is bidirectional: Highlight the role of primary caregivers as experts in their children and their families. Identified "problems" should be seen as targets or goals requiring collaboration, rather than problems for the provider to "fix." An interaction integrating all of these elements might go as follows:

MOTHER: It's just been hard. She's just up and down all the time, and I can never predict what she's going to do or how she's going to react. Like that time I was telling you about, when she just started screaming at me and then ran out the door. I almost had a heart attack, chasing after her, thinking she's going to get killed by a car.

THERAPIST: Boy, that sounds incredibly stressful for you. I can hear how overwhelming it's been. No matter how much you know as a mom, it's just so hard to know what to do in those moments when the behaviors and feelings get so big.

MOTHER: I never feel like I know what I'm doing anymore.

THERAPIST: I bet it feels like that sometimes, but you know, it sounds like you actually know your daughter really, really well. And as hard as things have been, a lot of what you're describing to me kind of makes sense. You and your daughter have been through a pretty rocky period since her dad was arrested last year, and most kids—and even most adults—who go through the kinds of things you two have are going to struggle with big feelings and sometimes big behaviors. Part of our work is going to be figuring out what sets off those big feelings, and what she needs. We can definitely talk more about that, and about what you're hoping will happen, and how to help you survive until we get there, okay?

5. Attune to caregiver wants and needs. A key part of early relationship building is ensuring that the caregiver's voice is in the room. Work to understand the caregiver's reasons for seeking services (if applicable) and his or her concrete goals ("What will it look like when things are "better"?); the caregiver's perception of good-enough treatment/educational/provider, "fit" and his or her understanding of the service process; and the family's past experience with treatment/provider systems.

6. Engage participation in identifying caregiver and/or family strengths. It is common early in our relationship with a family to focus on "the problems," particularly as these issues (a) have led families to engage in or be referred for services in the first place; and (b) are often the point of destabilization or concern for the family as well. However, a sole focus on "the problem" reifies the message that the child, the caregiver, or the family is itself problematic or "bad"— a message that many of the families with which we work have heard repeatedly, and from multiple systems. To reiterate: It is crucial that providers engage participants around identifying family strengths. What is working for this family? What is going well? What do family members feel proud of? What gives them strength? In what situations do they feel confident and capable? In what ways do they have fun? Both for our own engagement with family members and for their felt connection to us, it is crucial that we see them—and that they know that they are seen—as more than just a problem.

Setting the Stage for Youth Engagement

Early in our work with children and adolescents, a primary task is to establish relationship. As with caregivers, in the absence of a good-enough relationship, our intervention approaches will have limited impact. In the following material, we describe foundational strategies for engaging children and adolescents in the therapeutic process. These strategies are very similar to those we recommend for adults.

1. Describe the service process. Any new process, particularly for children who have experienced trauma, may provoke anxiety. Knowing what to expect is an important part of creating an initial sense of safety for youth. At the start of a service process, it is important to give children age-appropriate information about what the service process will entail, and to answer any questions they may have. For instance: How often will you see each other? How long will you meet for? In a day or milieu program, what will the schedule be like? What is the child expected to do? What if the child does not want to do what you want him or her to do? Provide basic information, anticipate areas of concern, and encourage and provide explicit permission for the child to ask questions at any point.

2. Engage the child's participation around his or her goals. When a child is referred for services, it is not uncommon for the caregiver to have goals, the child welfare provider to have goals, the teacher to have goals, the provider to have goals, and so on—but we often lose sight of what the goals of the *child* might be. At the beginning of service provision for

a child, be clear about why he or she was referred or mandated into services, but also ask about what the *child* wants. For instance: "So, I know your probation officer said that one of the conditions for your getting out of your program is to come to therapy every week, and that he really wants you to work on what he's calling 'anger issues.' I'm wondering, though, if there are things in your life that you really want, or how you even feel about coming in here?" It is crucial that throughout our work, we pay attention to the child's stake in the process and to accept and *not* personalize the range of ways a child may react to and feel about us.

3. Be interested in the whole child. Many of the children with whom we work come to us having been sent a message that they *are* problems. We have been told, "I have anger issues," "I make too much trouble for my mom," "I'm stupid," "I do bad things." Ideally, none of us—in our roles as providers, educators, protectors, mentors—are working with *problems*. What we are working with is *children,* and an important entry into engagement is to be clear that we are interested in the whole child, even if in our role, we at times need to focus on those areas of life that are more challenging or problematic.

4. Communicate a belief in the child's capacity for success. Two of the most important qualities in those of us who work with trauma-impacted populations are the belief that there is potential in every individual, and the capacity to see that potential in those with whom we are working. This does not mean entering into the work unrealistically. Many of the providers with whom we have worked are often in the incredibly challenging position of making decisions for the safety or health of children (based on their own behaviors or needs, or those of their primary caregivers) that acknowledge both the wish for "success," while holding the reality of current risk. However, our entry point must be one that believes and communicates that growth, health, and joy are possible. When a child says, "Forget it, I'm never going to be able to do this stuff!" we want to see and hear what he or she has said, but also hold the possibilities: "I know it's so hard to keep working at something when it feels impossible, and I can see that you're feeling really frustrated. But I've known a lot of kids, and I'm getting to know you, and I have to say, I really believe that we're going to get to the point where you know that you can handle this."

5. Establish the foundation for co-creating structure and routines. In the next chapter, we talk in detail about our third foundational strategy: the use of routines and structures. From our perspective, routines and structures create rhythmic, predictable ways to support engagement in a process, to build felt safety, and to increase mastery over time. These achievements are particularly important in the therapeutic process, and actively talking about this area and collaborating with youth on building acceptable routines for our work together is crucial early on.

6. Establish a frame for transparent and collaborative intervention. Particularly for youth, service provision across settings often takes place within a clear hierarchy: the providers or adults *do,* and the youth are *done to.* This approach often inadvertently reifies a number of the qualities of trauma itself, including disempowerment and loss of agency or choice. For service provision to qualify as trauma-informed, it must be transparent, collaborative, and offer opportunities for youth voice and choice. For instance, consider the following exchange.

THERAPIST: So, I've been thinking about what you said about it feeling like your mom is really reactive to you and doesn't trust you. It sounds like that's made things pretty hard at home, and you mostly try to stay away now. Does that sound about right?

TEEN: Yeah, pretty much.

THERAPIST: Is that something you wish were different?

TEEN: Sure, but honestly, I don't think it's gonna change. It's just kind of how she is now.

THERAPIST: You might be right, but I think we can't know it until we try. I have a few ideas about how we might help you and your mom get to know each other a little bit better, but I want to talk them through with you first. Honestly, I don't know that any of it will be super-comfortable for you, so I want you to really think through what will work for you, and what will just feel like too much, okay?

In this interaction, the provider is highlighting an identified goal of the child, linking the goal to potential strategies, engaging around the child's preferences, and actively encouraging the child's input. Note that this approach is an important way to scaffold executive function skills, as will be discussed in Chapter 13.

7. Integrate education, linking trauma and targeted skills. As a trauma-focused intervention, understanding the link between historical and current traumatic experiences and the child's adaptations and behaviors is a core foundation to effectively approaching service provision. In everything that we do, we incorporate an understanding that *behavior makes sense:* There is a reason, for instance, that the child is shutting down, or overwhelmed in school, or angry all the time, or giddy and silly at inappropriate times, or engaging in high-risk behaviors. A key part of engagement for every treatment target that we address is an understanding of *why* those targets are relevant for children and adolescents who have experienced trauma (in general), and why they are relevant for *this child,* in particular. Each treatment chapter of this book incorporates education as a foundational aspect of building children's stake in, and understanding of, treatment goals.

Engagement Over Time: Ongoing Considerations

The issue of engagement is far too complicated to be summed up in a simple set of steps; for this reason, we try to address it in every chapter, and we encourage providers to consider it in every interaction and for every part of the process. Broadly, there are questions that we think may be helpful in supporting the provider or system to repeatedly evaluate, address, and build connection and stake with the families with whom they are working.

Specifically, we encourage providers to consider the following.

1. How are my own attachment skills being applied in the context of this relationship and in support of skill development? Am I managing my own affect? Am I working to attune to this child/this caregiver/this system? Are my approaches and responses effective?
2. What is the stake in the process at this point? Why does this concept/goal/treatment target matter in this child's life? In this caregiver's life? Why do I think this goal is important?

3. How will this child/family/system define success around this target/in general? Are we recognizing the successes that are already happening? Is what we are working toward realistic? What is needed now/in future to support everyone involved in achieving and feeling moments of success?

4. What barriers are present right now? What do I anticipate might get in the way of what we are working on? What does the child/caregiver/system anticipate might get in the way? How might we get in front of, rather than react to, those barriers?

The Role of Education

In the preceding sections, we repeatedly reference the importance of education. We view education as a powerful "leveler of the field" in clinical practice. Having an understanding of *why* something might be happening is rarely the sole solution to addressing it, but is an important part of the process and can be powerful in shifting our lenses about ourselves or others.

Consider a relatively common early childhood scenario: A young toddler is attempting to pull a toy across the floor, but the toy keeps tipping over. Halfway across the room, the toddler drops to the floor, wails, and begins to kick his feet up and down. Most parents will recognize this behavior as both a response to and an expression of a moment of frustration, and though caregiver responses may differ according to parenting approaches, it is likely that the parent's response will in some way incorporate an understanding of why the child is acting this way.

Imagine now, though, that you are someone who has no idea what this child is doing. For the sake of argument, imagine that you have dropped onto this planet with little understanding that small people are qualitatively different from large people, that toddlers scream and cry when frustrated, and that this behavior is both a communication strategy ("I'm upset!") and a plea for help ("Make my toy work!" or "Help me feel better!"). Without that information or understanding, you might be frightened, angry, overwhelmed, or disgusted, and your responses are likely to be far less effective than they might have been.

Although this example is simplistic in many ways, the reality is that the behaviors, experiences, internal states, and interactions of individuals whose lives have been shaped by trauma and adversity can be and feel intensely complicated, confusing, and overwhelming. As human beings, we seek to understand our experiences—to provide labels, definitions, or explanations that fit with our understanding of the world. Far too often for trauma-impacted youth and families, these explanations center on deficits of self ("There is something wrong with me"), of others ("My kid has something broken inside him"), and of our relationships ("My mom hates me"). The integration of information about a range of relevant topics— trauma, normative development, attachment, relationships, resilience, and more—is crucial to our own perspectives as providers and to the empowering perspectives of the child and family members with whom we are working. For this reason, each of our treatment chapters includes education in the "Key Concepts" sections, as well as in separate "Teach to Caregivers" and "Teach to Kids" sections.

Throughout the work, we encourage providers to embody and cultivate an atmosphere of *curiosity:* a focus not just on *what,* but on *why* and *why it makes sense.* Be curious about and with children, their caregivers, and provider teams.

6

Foundational Strategies

Routines and Rhythms

The Foundational Role
of Routine and Rhythm in Trauma Treatment

The ARC framework views the creation of *rhythm* as a foundational and cross-cutting strategy in trauma treatment. Rhythm is attended to and created in multiple ways: through the use of predictable *structures* in treatment and in daily life; through the integration of *routines* into the lives of children, families, and systems; and through curiosity about and attention to *rituals* that create connection to community. These rhythmic processes are used in service of two primary goals:

1. To support felt safety and modulation through the establishment of predictability.
2. To reinforce key goals and support skills acquisition through the use of facilitating structures.

The Role of Routine and Rhythm in Normative Development

In normative development, routines are typically generated and organized first by the attachment system: Caregivers structure their young children's lives in a way that builds rhythm and predictability through responsive schedules of feeding, interaction, and sleep. By young childhood, children begin to internalize a reliance on structure and predictability: Most people have known a 4-year-old who wants to watch the same movie repeatedly, or a 6-year-old who corrects your actions because "That's not the way Mommy does it." This predictability helps young children learn about and organize their worlds.

As development continues, the young child's focal reliance on structure often relaxes into a subtler appreciation of rhythm in daily life. Most people's lives are guided, to some degree, by routinized experience. We wake at certain times, sleep at certain times, and have familiar routines that are so built into our day as to be invisible.

We often notice our routines only in their absence: when our typical morning schedule, for instance, is disrupted by unexpected demands. Most people can relate to the unsettled feeling that comes with the loss of an expected daily routine. Even though most of us do not have days that are structured and planned out minute to minute, the subtle routines in which we engage are grounding.

What Happens with Trauma?

For the children with whom we work, this "unsettledness" has often been part and parcel of their daily experience—lack of predictability has been the rule, rather than the exception. Many traumatic experiences take place in a context of internal and/or external chaos and loss of control. In the aftermath of trauma, moments of unpredictability may then become powerful triggers, or cues, of possible danger.

Parents, clinicians, educators, and others involved in the lives of children who have experienced trauma often describe children's strong reactions to change, difficulty with transitions, and rigid attempts to control themselves, others, and the world around them. These efforts at control may be viewed as a strategy for managing the anxiety of unpredictability: As long as a child does not know what is coming next, and in a world in which danger is always a possibility, the child must remain vigilant and rigid.

The Foundational Role of Rhythm in Treatment

Building rhythm in the life of a child who has historically experienced chaos requires a purposeful shifting of focus to increase the presence of these invisible, yet predictable, routines. Routines and rhythm may be attended to in the context of specific treatment targets and structures in relationships, in the therapeutic process, and in home and milieu settings.

When working to build routine and rhythm, it is important to consider the goal: Establishment of routines is *not* about structure for the sake of structure; rather, it is about supporting children, families, and systems in establishing predictability *in the service of modulation and felt safety*. Given this larger goal, it is important to strike a balance between structure and flexibility. As with all targets and skills within this framework, we encourage caregivers and providers to consider the question: "What is it that you are trying to help the child achieve?" If enforcing a routine consistently increases, rather than decreases, distress and arousal, perhaps it is time to consider shifting the routine. Similarly, if flexibility on the caregiver's part seems to increase controlling strategies by the child, it may be important to consider increasing structure. Use attunement skills to observe the intersection between routine, structure, and child functioning over time.

Use of Structure to Support Skill Acquisition

In the remainder of this book, we describe eight core targets of intervention along with key subskills and examples of ways to address these targets in various settings and with a range of populations. Many of these examples incorporate routines and structures: rhythmic, predictable ways to support children and caregivers in engaging in new skills. Our use of these examples is purposeful: Although we believe that there are many ways to approach any given target of intervention, the integration of rhythm and structure into any process is likely to support felt comfort, safety, and mastery.

Repetition plays a critical role in learning and brain development. In normative development the role of repetition in learning can be observed multiple times throughout a child's day. For instance, very young children often use play to develop mastery over fine and gross motor tasks and problem solving (e.g., using blocks to build a tower, completing puzzles, flipping the pages of a favorite book, sorting objects). Preferred play materials are often engaged with over and over again until mastery is achieved. As children grow older, they may engage in imaginary play related to fantasy or to real-life contexts such as "playing school." They often replay the same themes until a new challenge emerges.

Similarly, rhythm and structure are often foundational components of learning in school settings, from basic rhythmic phrases ("*i* before *e,* except after *c*") to the use of songs to help young children learn the alphabet and numbers, to the much more complicated patterns of numbers, language, and concepts learned in high school and college—patterns that we often recall best in rote (*rhythmic*) form ("$a^2 + b^2 = c^2$"; "kingdom, phylum, class, order, family, genus, species"). These rhythms help organize complex information and provide a foundation for the more challenging engagement with ideas that follows basic mastery of information.

Across settings, routines provide children with opportunities to practice needed developmental skills. Consider the mother who reads the same story to her child each night. This simple bedtime routine, in addition to supporting connection and transition, also fosters a variety of skills such as speech and language, anticipation, problem solving, and social interaction. Whereas the mother may be tired of reading that story, the child never tires because he or she is mastering a new skill and experiencing an inner sense of competence.

Throughout the book, we encourage readers to consider ways to incorporate structure and predictability in their attention to the identified key targets. For instance, how might the reflection and mirroring that are key aspects of *attunement* be systematically learned and practiced by caregivers? How might *identification skills* be built into a child's daily routine? In what ways might support for *executive functions* be incorporated into a milieu's practice of processing daily incidents? Many of the routines and structures given as examples in this book are intended to facilitate learning, mastery, and perceived competence—which may, over time, help to decrease feelings of shame and vulnerability.

In addition to building rhythm in attending to key targets, routine and rhythm are themselves an important way of fostering felt safety, modulation, and predictability into daily experience. In the remainder of this chapter, we describe goals and methods of incorporating various rhythms into clinical work, home, and milieu daily routines, and the specific role of routine in supporting modulation.

Integration of Routines into Treatment, Home and Milieu Life

Therapy Routines

Individual Therapy Routines

A primary goal in working with children who have experienced trauma is to support regulation of experience. Routines are often modulating (returning children to a comfortable level of arousal) in part because they enhance predictability and in part because child-specific routines often naturally support rhythm and/or regulation. If you observe children in their school settings, particularly very young children, you may notice many routines that actively support regulation. For instance, many preschool settings begin the day with circle time. During circle time books may be read, songs may be sung, and often a daily agenda reviewed. The goal is often to modulate the energy created by transition and free play to prepare for higher-order learning. With older children, "specials" such as music, gym, and art are often (in resourced schools) woven into the day. These activities also have regulation potential. It can be helpful to think about how to replicate these strategies within a therapeutic context. Consider the following example:

> Tanya is a 7-year-old girl who lives with her maternal grandmother with whom she was placed after experiencing years of exposure to neglect and parental substance abuse. When she transitioned into a new therapeutic setting, she struggled to engage and would often present with very high levels of arousal moving from one activity to another, while ignoring the provider who was trying to engage her. It was suggested that the therapist work on a therapy "check-in routine" that involved singing a hello song similar to songs that may be sung in circle time in preschool settings. Tanya responded with curiosity when her therapist began singing at the start of the session, and she sat and listened with interest. She focused only on the provider and was able to join in before the song ended.

In this example, it appeared that the song provided support for modulation of arousal and allowed Tanya to settle and engage in a manner that she had not been able to prior to this session. In addition, it provided a foundation for interpersonal engagement and joint attention.

Therapy routines create a structure and context for the therapeutic work. When we discuss routines with other clinicians, we often hear hesitation or concern about what may be perceived as introducing "rigidity" into the clinical work. Many clinicians, from a variety of theoretical and training backgrounds, have made rich use of child-centered methods (play, talk, sand tray, etc.) that emphasize following the lead of the child client. These clinicians have raised questions about whether integrating routines will diminish the fertile work found in spontaneous engagement with client material. Our perspective is that the two are not mutually exclusive, and that in fact, while not naming them as such, most clinicians will find their work guided, to some degree, by invisible routines and rituals. Indeed, routines often provide the subtle "surrounding structure" of sessions, but can be flexibly determined to account for the differing styles of our practice. Particularly with children who struggle with safety in relationships, we encourage clinicians to observe the subtle patterns that define their therapy process, and, as indicated, to "try out" simple additions to their therapy routines. Finally, it may be useful to bring those subtle patterns and invisible routines to the attention of our clients so that they can be active participants in the process of determining their own preferred rhythms.

There are many factors to consider as you establish or reestablish the context for your therapeutic relationship. Consider the following areas.

THERAPY STRUCTURE AND VALUES

- **Timing and therapeutic space.** Be aware of time—try not to start or end late. Punctuality builds boundaries and predictability around the treatment session. Consistency of the therapy room space itself may be an important "invisible" factor; when possible, use the same location. If this is not possible, it often helps to have consistent portable materials (e.g., the child's therapy folder, toy bag).

◆ **Transitions.** *We know that transitions can be triggering for children who experience trauma. The more predictable the transition, the safer children will feel. Consider the following areas.*

  ● Location: This is a concrete facet of the transition into the therapy room (e.g., the child who always wants to start at the art table).

  ● Time cues: When needed, use time cues. Some examples include in-session schedules, a timer to concretely break up session activities, and reminder cues when limited time remains in session.

  ● Regulation support: Consider modulation activities at the start and end of a session to manage surges of arousal that may be triggered by transition into and out of session time.

  ● Transitional objects: Trauma-impacted children and youth may be particularly sensitive to periods of disconnection or separation from the caregiver and, at times, from the provider. Consider the use of transitional objects (from home, brought into session; and/or from session, brought to home), dyadic periods of interaction at start and end, modulation activities, and the like.

■ **Values/rules.** Identifying some basic therapy rules or values may be an important part of establishing felt safety. We often suggest rules that target the following:

  ◆ **Basic safety.** For example, "When you have big feelings, we use words as 'tools' to let each other know that, rather than our hands or feet." Or, for an older youth, "When you have big feelings, I would prefer that you let me know that directly and with a tone and words that I can really hear and understand."

  ◆ **Control.** It may important to help children understand that they have control over therapy topics and their own personal boundaries: for example, "It's okay for you to say that you don't want to talk about something that I bring up."

  ◆ **Relational safety and boundaries.** It is helpful to talk with children about their right to give feedback to the therapist if they are feeling uncomfortable: "If I say something that you don't like, it's okay to tell me that it bothered you."

  ◆ **Physical boundaries.** Particularly for children whose experience has included physical boundary violations, it is important to be clear about physical space and contact rules. Although these are likely to vary by setting and by provider and client preferences, open discussion is important. For instance, a provider might say: "We have a rule here that grownups are not allowed to give kids hugs, since that's something that's just for special people like your mom or grandma. But one thing we can definitely do is high-fives—any time you're feeling like you want a high-five, just let me know!" Children should also know that they have the right to arrange themselves and their location (in space, in relation to providers, etc.) in a way that feels comfortable.

  ◆ **Communication about distress or need to pause.** We suggest that you offer children and caregivers opportunities to move in and out of distressing content. One common strategy used in this framework is to create a "pause sign." The pause sign can be a visual image of a stop sign, a television remote pause button, or any image identified by the child and caregiver to represent pause. The need to pause can also be signaled by a gesture or verbal cue. If this is implemented with a child and his or her caregiver, it is possible for each to have his or her own pause sign. The therapist should explain the pause sign early in treatment and discuss its implementation. Often the therapist, as well as the child and caregiver, can activate a pause. Generally speaking, the pause is followed by a modulation activity to support increased internal comfort.

Group Therapy Routines

As with individual therapy, group processes are often most successful when an element of routine and predictability is incorporated into the session structure. Many groups offer predictability in the organic coherence over time that is associated with group themes. Beyond the coherence provided by content, we encourage group leaders and curriculum developers to consider the important role of routine in structuring group sessions. As with individual sessions, consider the role of opening check-ins or icebreakers, modulation activities, and internal structure. In creating routines, consider the content focus of the group: For example, in a group focusing on coping skills, opening exercises might include a modulation activity or an affect identification check-in; in a group focusing on identity, opening activities might include an icebreaker question related to the self; and in a group focused on interpersonal relationships, dyadic or group cooperative activities might begin the session.

Groups vary widely depending on their nature (structured, content-focused, process-oriented, psychoeducational, etc.). All groups, however, share the common element of having a beginning, a middle, and an end. We encourage group leaders to consider either subtle or overt strategies to mark these transitions as a way to facilitate children's (or caregivers') capacity to successfully enter into, and transition out of, groups. Consider also the balance between activities that rely on active versus passive engagement with material, between higher- and lower-energy activities, and between independent and cooperative engagement. Strategize about ways to create and incorporate routine that helps group members be most successful (in modulating, engaging, building safety, etc.). It may be easier, for instance, for a child to follow a natural "bell-curve" progression of lower to higher to lower energy over the course of a group, then to move rapidly among low-, then high-, then low-, then high-energy activities. Early in a group, it is important to be flexible and to tune in to specific group needs. A structure that worked well for one group, for instance, may be more challenging with a different group. Be willing to adjust or enhance structure, as needed, to respond to the particular needs of individual group members or group dynamics.

Additional Considerations: Routines in Treatment

- Consider developmental and individual needs. We have found that younger children often prefer greater structure (and explicit naming of this structure), whereas older children and adolescents prefer subtler or "invisible" routines. However, every child is different. Allow children to contribute to the creation of therapy routines.

■ Therapy routines can be as simple as what happens on the walk between the waiting room and the therapy room, using an age-appropriate check-in to start every session, and creating a predictable transition at the end. See the table, "Examples of Individual Therapy Routine" (p. 85), for examples. Some children will need the entire session to be structured; others will need greater flexibility.

■ Young children who have a high need for control are likely initially to appear resistant to therapy routines. It is our experience, however, that routines are ultimately comforting. By providing predictability in the therapy setting, children are able to achieve a sense of safety and control because they know what to expect. Don't assume that a child who complains about your routine truly hates it. Consider the following example.

> Tamika, 5 years old, regularly complained about the "feelings check-in" built into the start of her weekly therapy session. Each week, she would arrive for session, sit at the small table in the room, and ask, "Do we need to do those stupid faces today?" The clinician would respond in the affirmative, Tamika would complete the check-in about her feelings and experiences that day, and then the two would transition to the symbolic play that Tamika loved, or to other activities.
>
> One day, the clinician entered the room with Tamika and immediately began to address an issue to which Tamika's mother had alerted her in an earlier phone conversation. After about a minute, the clinician noticed that Tamika was shifting in her chair and appeared tearful. When asked by the clinician whether something was wrong, Tamika burst out, "We didn't do those stupid faces!"

In this example, the clinician received a reminder of why we engage in routines: Even the ones that are "hated" on the surface offer predictability. Although we invariably have times when routines change or are disrupted, explicit naming of these disruptions, whether in advance (e.g., "Next week we're going to do something a little bit different") or in the moment (e.g., "I know we usually have free play right now, but there's something we need to talk about. Let's talk first, and then we can have free play right after, okay?") may be important in reducing distress.

The following table provides examples of ways to structure therapy sessions. Keep in mind that routines can be overt or subtle (e.g., a check-in can be very concrete and structured, or it can be as simple as, "So, how'd the week go?").

The relative balance and ordering of each of these therapy session routine elements will necessarily vary for every child. Some children may engage in structured activities for much of the session; others will have limited tolerance (or less need) for structured activities, and will need more extensive "open" time. Be flexible; every routine is child-specific.

Pay attention to the child's need for control when creating routines. For instance, while there may be an expectation that each session has a "therapist choice" and a "kid choice" time, the clinician may consider allowing the child to choose which comes first. To minimize power struggles, be sure to specify how long each will last and provide cues before transitioning.

Consider ways to incorporate caregivers into therapy routines. For instance, consider involving caregivers into a dyadic check-in, or inviting them in for a closing "therapy summary."

Examples of Individual Therapy Routines

Opening check-in	Feeling faces ☺ ☺ ☹	Point to face(s) on poster or handout that are closest to current feeling. Draw a picture of "feeling(s) for today."
	Ball toss	Roll or toss a ball back and forth and take turns telling one new thing that happened since previous session.
	Today's news	Have child name one good and one not-so-good thing that happened today; draw a picture or talk about it.
	Thumbs up/ sideways/down	Pick one event from the past week: Was it thumbs up (positive), thumbs sideways (neutral), or thumbs down (negative)? Why?
	Energy check	Use thermometers, numbers, or other scales to check in on energy. Where is the child's energy at right now?
Modulation activity		Use age-appropriate modulation activities at the start and end of each session. Consider the child's needs. For instance, a high-energy child may need activities that help her expend her energy and then focus (e.g., balancing peacock feathers, jumping up and down at higher, then lower, energy levels); a lower-energy or withdrawn child may need a mutual engagement activity such as throwing a ball back and forth. Most children prefer to have some choice—allow the child to pick from among two or more activities. Check energy level before and after the modulating activity: Has it gone up or down? How can the child tell? (See the "Modulation" section for further discussion of this concept.) Modulation activities may be individual (i.e., just the child and provider) or dyadic / familial (incorporating caregivers).
Structured activity ("therapist choice")		Include a structured or focal task in each session. Draw from attachment, regulation, and competency domains, and consider individual child needs and goals. Activities can be brief or comprehensive and often extend across sessions.
Free time ("kid choice")		"Kid choice," or open time, is an important part of therapy sessions. During open, unstructured time adolescents often engage in conversation, young children engage in rich symbolic play, and/or children of any age engage in activities that help them naturally modulate and balance the more challenging work of therapy (don't discount the importance of board games for helping children engage in the rest of "therapy work"!).
Closing check-out (note that closing routine often parallels opening)	Feeling faces	What face (on the poster or handout) is closest *now* to child's feelings? What has changed?
	Ball toss	Roll/toss ball back and forth; have child and therapist each pick one thing that child and therapist *liked* or *disliked* about therapy today.
	News wrap-up	Keep a running list: Of what did child feel proud in therapy today?
	Thumbs up/ down	What was the child's favorite or least favorite thing from today's session?
	Energy check	Where is the child's energy now? Is it the same or different from the start of session?
Modulation activity		Based on where the child's energy is now, build a closing modulation activity into session. Consider incorporating caregivers, as appropriate, into closing routines.
Clean-up	Contain it!	Clean-up is an important part of the session as well as a closing ritual for purposes of containment. Always actively involve the child in putting away therapy materials.

Home and Milieu Routines

The rhythms of daily life are, in themselves, often supportive of many of the key targets described in this book. For instance, morning and bedtime routines may support caregiver–child *attunement* and *relational connection,* and help children *modulate* and manage the transition to sleep; predictable daily schedules may help with anticipation and delayed gratification, important foundations of *executive functions*; and predictable family rituals may help to build a child's sense of *self* and *identity*.

In tuning in to home and milieu routines, we consider the ways that routines may support all of these key targets.

Where and When: Opportunities to Build In Routine

Work with caregivers to gradually increase rhythm and predictability in daily life. Remember to be selective and to work with the caregiver(s) and child to identify trouble spots; a good question in thinking about where rhythm may be needed is simply, "Which part(s) of your day feel most dysregulated or chaotic, and when do things feel like they go well?" See the following table for examples of common routine targets.

Morning	The morning transition is often difficult for everyone, but particularly for highly stressed, chaotic households or for busy systems. Support caregiving systems in creating consistent and realistic morning routines. Consider check-in approaches discussed in the preceding section as well as goal setting or planning for the day.
Mealtimes	Meals are often a forum for communication and a place for family "together time." In systems, meals provide an opportunity for less structured peer interaction and conversation. Mealtimes can support the development of social skills, turn taking, manners, and interest in others' activities. Work with families or systems to come together for meals that are part of a daily routine as often as possible. ■ Food choice is a common area in which children exert their need for control. Work with caregivers to avoid power struggles. Find a middle ground between too much flexibility and too much control. For instance, provide a predictable alternative (e.g., child can eat family meal or eat a peanut butter and jelly sandwich).
Play	Play is a child's natural means of expression. Caregivers should be encouraged to play with their children, and time should be allocated during the week for "family play" as well as solitary and peer-to-peer play. Although often mistakenly considered less important than chores, homework, or other task-oriented components of experience, play is a vital part of healthy development. In addition, play also provides a forum for socialization and skill building. ■ "Together time" should *not* be tied to rewards or consequences (e.g., "If you don't clean your room, you don't get to spend time with Mom"). For children with histories of neglect and abandonment, in particular, such a statement can be triggering. ■ Work with caregivers to build one-on-one time with each child in the family as well as to schedule full family times.
Chores	Performing chores helps to foster a sense of responsibility and self-efficacy. Of course, chores should be age-appropriate, but it is okay for even very young children to have expectations regarding their areas of responsibility. Such an approach conveys the idea that all family or community members are integral to the successful functioning of the system, and that the child makes an important contribution. Work with caregivers to develop child-appropriate and realistic daily expectations.
Homework	School achievement/success is an important area of competency for children. Caregivers can contribute by emphasizing the importance of homework, providing an appropriate environment to support homework completion, being available to provide help or encouragement, and emphasizing effort over success. Work with caregivers and children to identify child and family needs.

Family or community together time	It is important to build into daily routines a time for caregivers and children (or in a milieu, community members) to come together, formally or informally, to share experience. For instance, some families may consider holding a weekly "family meeting" to share significant events; it may be incorporated into mealtime, bedtime, etc. Regardless of the forum, it is important that there be opportunities for family or community members to share their experiences on a routine basis.
Safety routines	Young children are often exposed to information about safety routines or emergency response. It can be helpful to develop a plan for safety in the home. Plans may include familial response to contact with a perpetrator of violence, unexpected events (e.g., fire) or risk behaviors.

In building and addressing routines, a key overarching goal is to support modulation and felt safety. Although routines themselves may be naturally modulating, there are ways to more directly address modulation through a focus on *daily rhythm* as well as through *explicit inclusion of modulation strategies* in the daily schedule:

- **Daily rhythm.** Many children struggle to manage arousal effectively over the course of the day. In structuring the daily schedule, it is important to consider the child's "energy needs." For instance, limit highly arousing activities near bedtime; consider adding focusing activities (e.g., rehearsal/discussion of daily schedule, mindfulness exercises) prior to the start of the school day or other structured time periods; and build in activities that let the child expend energy when transitioning out of those times.

- **Explicit inclusion of modulation strategies.** Following is a table with some suggested activities to support ongoing modulation. Each of these is discussed again in Chapter 11 (Modulation):

Routines That Support Daily Rhythm and Modulation

Strategies	Examples of activities
Opportunities for connection/ attachment support	- Schedule routine time together (mealtimes, movie nights, play time, homework help). - Cook a meal together. - Do a project together. - Help the child with chores. - Teach a new skill (or have the child teach you).
Sensory strategies	- Sound: listening to music, using headphones or noise machines to drown out noise - Touch: hugs, weighted blankets, soft pillows, stuffed animals, cool stones, things to fiddle with, chewable jewelry - Smell: lotions, scent of cooking food, air fresheners - Taste: sharing a favorite food - Sight: pictures of safe people or favorite places, minimizing visual stimulation
Gross motor activities	- Small trampolines - Opportunities to run/jump/play - Exercise balls, yoga balls - Balance beams - After-school dance party
Activities that are naturally modulating	- Play (solo, joint) - Sports - Expressive arts, dance, theater - Yoga - Reading - Listening to music - Crafts

■ **Modulation routines** to target triggers or "challenge points." We have seen many families and systems experience positive outcomes by building specific modulation strategies (e.g., relaxation or yoga groups, deep breathing, jumping jacks) into key moments—transitions, mealtimes, and bedtime—of the daily routine. By preemptively including strategies that target the child's arousal level, rather than solely using strategies in reaction to dysregulation, the child may increasingly be able to maintain effective arousal levels. This automaticity is particularly important because it is very difficult for any of us to learn and use new skills during moments of dysregulation. The more opportunities children (and their caregivers) have to practice strategies, the more likely they will internalize them and use them in the moments that they need them the most. Consider the following example.

> Elena, a 9-year-old girl adopted from an orphanage in Romania at the age of 3, presented as full of energy. Her parents described her as "perpetually in motion," and she became both easily excited and easily distressed by daily experiences. She had particular difficulty settling into focused activities such as classroom time and homework. Her parents had reported that a number of strategies seemed helpful when Elena was upset, such as giving her a blanket to wrap around herself and playing soft music. They also reported that "speed dancing" (dancing to fast music in a cleared-out room in the house, an activity Elena enjoyed) seemed to help her expend energy when she became overly excited and started to get out of control. The parents began to build these activities into Elena's daily routine in an effort to help her modulate her arousal: In the morning, before leaving for school, they had "cuddle time" with the blanket and soft music; they worked with her school to allow Elena to engage in similar strategies in the nurse's office, both midday and "as needed" when upset; and they added "speed dancing" time into her after-school schedule. After a month, they reported that these strategies seemed to help Elena's daily modulation; in particular, they reported that she seemed less easily upset by minor stressors during the school day and better able to transition home in the afternoon.

In this example, the routine developed was a child-specific (i.e., individualized) one. However, many routines operate on a larger level by necessity—whether family- or systemwide. Although this broad application can support modulation, it can also challenge a trauma-impacted child. Whereas routines often form an umbrella under which many individuals function (e.g., within a milieu system or a family), it is important to account for individual needs to the degree possible. For instance, although all residents within a milieu may typically be expected to transition from school to a community activity, a particular resident may need 20 minutes of "downtime" following the highly stimulating school day before she can participate successfully in group activities. Similarly, whereas older siblings may be expected to complete homework immediately after school, a child who struggles with arousal and attention may require active engagement in high-energy activities before he can focus on this work. Consider ways to utilize routines—and the exceptions to them—to help children experience success on a regular basis.

In developing targeted routines, it is important to pay attention to key areas of vulnerability or difficulty, such as bedtime or mealtime. Many trauma-impacted children will struggle with basic physiological regulation (i.e., times of transition from one activity to another or from one state to another) and with times that have historically been associated with danger, fear, and/or deprivation. Although it may be particularly important to pay attention to building predictability in these moments, children may actively resist this predictability at first because it challenges their sense of felt control.

A common area of challenge for many children impacted by trauma, as it was for Elena, is bedtime. For example, Elena struggled to settle and often looked for additional connection and support at bedtime. Other children struggle with the transition itself, with increased anxiety, and with regressed needs. Because this is a time that children who have experienced trauma so often need support, we provide the following table as an expanded example of how to think about the use of routines in service of modulation and safety for targeted challenging areas.

Bedtime Routines

Teaching points		Bedtime is often a difficult time for children and adolescents, particularly for those who experienced abuse at a similar time or in the place they are now expected to sleep.
		It may be hard for children whose arousal is high during the day to calm their bodies in preparation for sleep.
		Bedtime routines help children decrease their arousal and learn to transition into sleep.
		Bedtime routines also offer a regular opportunity for connection and communication between caregivers and children.
Support caregivers in:		Developing a consistent bedtime routine, have child put on pajamas, brush teeth, have quiet time, etc.
		Problem-solving ways to keep bedtimes and their routines as consistent as possible. Pay attention to the location where the child is sleeping; work with caregivers to help child sleep in the same place each night. Pay attention to familial and individual obstacles.
		Identifying nighttime boundaries and coping with nighttime fears. For example, what will caregiver do if child awakes during the night? Work with caregivers to be consistent in follow-through.
		Minimizing child's engagement in highly arousing activities near bedtime. Decrease child's involvement in activities such as video games, overstimulating television shows, loud music, active play, etc.
General activities	Nurturing	Read a story, cuddle, or listen to soft music together.
	Bathing	Have child take a bath or shower about an hour before bed; this may help bring down arousal. Pay attention to issues of privacy, boundaries, and the possibility of these being a trigger.
	Safety check	Help children feel safe. Leave on a nightlight, hang a dream catcher, use transitional objects (stuffed animals, a small heart pillow under the child's pillow, etc.). Communicate clearly that the caregiver will keep the child safe during the night.
	Relaxation/quiet time	Allow child to read, listen to quiet music, etc.
	Movement activities	This point may seem counterintuitive, but children who experience high levels of arousal may need increased support to slow down. Often they need the caregiver to mirror and match their energy and then to begin to slow it down through coregulation—for example, rocking back and forth (or in a rocker) fast, to slower to slow; or bouncing a small child on the lap while gradually changing the pace from fast to slow. This point is covered in more detail in Chapter 11.

Bedtime routines: developmental considerations	Early childhood	Routines at this age should include the caregivers. Nurturing activities (e.g., reading a bedtime story) are a good way to build attunement and relax the child.
		Night is a time when generalized fears often emerge. Predictable nighttime routines are particularly important during this developmental stage.
	Middle childhood	Although children at this age will desire greater independence, bedtime is a natural place for nurturance, and traumatized children may show some developmental regression around bedtime.
		Developmental changes may shift the mechanics of bedtime: for example, may involve caregivers reading *with* their child instead of *to* them; may include independent activities (e.g., child brushes teeth, showers, gets in pajamas) as well as together time (e.g., caregiver enters room to say "good night").
	Adolescence	Balance is very important at this developmental stage. Some important areas to balance:
		▪ *Independence versus nurturance:* Adolescents need privacy. However, like younger children, they may also experience developmental regression around bedtime. Check in with your teen before bed—for instance, does he or she want a good-night hug? Allow some control, but don't assume that your older child no longer needs nurturance.
		▪ *Flexibility versus limits:* Although adolescents are independent, don't lose sight of the need for limits. Maintain expectations around bedtime (e.g., must be in room by 10:00 P.M.), but allow flexibility (e.g., can have quiet time—read, listen to music—and turn off lights when ready).

Additional Considerations

HOME ROUTINES

When working with families, it is important to acknowledge individual differences and the role of "comfortable chaos": Many of us have spent time (and continue to spend time) in environments in which a degree of chaos and spontaneity added to the richness of daily experience. The goal is not to replace spontaneity with rigid structure, but rather to buffer and surround experience with threads of continuity. It is important to provide psychoeducation for clients about the particular role of routine in the lives of children who have experienced danger in their young lives, the varying developmental need for predictability, and the ways that predictability can, over time, foster comfort with flexibility

It can be very helpful to educate caregivers about the role of routine through experiential activities. For instance, we have found that the session routine is as important in the caregiver work as it is in the child work. Caregivers learn to value routines when those routines provide them with a sense of safety. Caregivers are able to shift from their self-protective reactions (e.g., "Nothing will work") when they are able to build mastery within the context of their work with the therapist.

To the degree possible, it is important to involve children, as developmentally appropriate, in the creation of routines. Consider the child's particular needs, wants, opinions, and preferences, as well as the realities of the home or system. For instance: What elements will be most important to incorporate into bedtime routines? What level of independence and/or support will the child want or need in carrying out scheduled activities? How important is the particular routine to caregivers? Engage children and other members of the family system in developing daily/weekly routines that are realistic and helpful.

MILIEU ROUTINES

As in home settings, milieus offer a rich environment in which to provide predictability in experience. Many programs rely on rules, routines, and structure to organize daily experience, and this structure often supports children who have faltered in more relaxed or unstructured settings to experience success in daily activities and to build competency. It is not uncommon to hear of the child, for instance, who evidences extreme behaviors in the home setting but who thrives in the structured environment of school. Much of what has been discussed in regard to the building of routines in home settings similarly applies to milieu programs: identifying specific targets of focus (e.g., bedtimes, transitions), the role of modulation both in daily rhythm and in the incorporation of specific activities, and the incorporation of routine and predictability into key facets of daily experience.

With respect to building structure, we have observed two primary areas of vulnerability in milieu systems: (1) an overemphasis on structure and rules in the absence of understanding individual child needs; and (2) inadequate understanding of the impact of disruptions in routine on child functioning. Both areas are challenging: It can be difficult to be flexible around individual child needs when trying to address the needs and safety of many children at once, and is inevitable that there will be moments of disruption in a larger system. Despite these challenges (and with full empathy), we encourage those who work in systems nonetheless to focus on both of these areas.

In terms of the first area: Systematic routines are important because they provide continuity in daily experience. Most children will adjust and adapt, at least to some degree, to the requirements of the system. Some children, however, will struggle, to greater or lesser degrees, with some aspect of daily routine. When a child has consistent difficulty, for example, with a transition or some component of the schedule, consider ways to adapt that routine to the individual needs of the child to the degree possible, keeping in mind the ultimate goal of building child success.

In terms of the latter area: As structured as many programs are, many factors will introduce disruption (and occasionally chaos) into daily routine. Although it is not possible to account for all these disruptions, it is possible to anticipate that changes may stir reactions and difficulties. When planned variations occur, work to provide advance notice and to troubleshoot possible reactions. When unexpected changes occur, train staff to anticipate increased reactivity by children who may be sensitive to disruptions. Use caregiver affect management skills to manage staff's own responses to these reactions, and use attunement skills to support children in regaining their own equilibrium.

Children living in milieu settings are particularly vulnerable to common triggers such as felt rejection, abandonment, and loss due to separation from their primary caregivers. It is important to build routines around phone calls, visits, and family work, when applicable, in order to support modulation of associated arousal. For children who do not have caregiver involvement, it may be important to create individualized rituals when celebrations take place with other residents' family members. For example, have specific staff members assigned to a particular child, or offer the child an alternative to participating in the group celebration.

In milieu systems that are focused on teaching self-regulation skills, it may be important to create a routine approach to supporting modulation. Programs that we have worked with have modified their behavior management structure in order to incorporate this idea. For example, consider implementing a break system (to be distinguished from a time-out) in which children can take self-directed and/or staff-directed breaks when dysregulated. It is helpful to build a structure around the break process. For instance, a break might include an initial check-in, practice of a modulation strategy (or strategies), and a checkout; the content of the check-in and checkout may vary based on the needs of each program. Modulation strategies might include talking to staff, using a sensory tool, or taking a walk (if possible). See Chapter 11 for further examples of potential tools.

Celebrations, Traditions, and Rituals

Daily routines offer one type of predictability and coherence over time. Another important source of coherence is *ritual:* the repeated practice of traditions, celebrations, patterns of behavior, or experiences. Rituals are often passed among members of a family, culture, or community, and may repeat across generations.

Rituals offer a connecting thread, not just of the individual to him- or herself over time, but to other members of the family, community, or culture who share the same ritual. Rituals may be specific to a family (e.g., the singing of a particular song or eating of a particular food on special occasions) or to a larger community (e.g., attendance at midnight Mass on Christmas).

Shared rituals may provide a sense of belonging, of being part of a larger whole. Many groups and organizations, including schools, service organizations, clubs, religious/spiritual centers, and so forth, have developed varied rituals and traditions, from songs and chants to handshakes to traditional celebrations and activities.

The exploration, celebration, and creation of rituals with children and families, as well as with the larger communities in which children are often embedded, may provide a way to celebrate the threads of connection among and across the child and members of his or her surrounding system. Although much of this section focuses on daily routine, rather than larger rituals, traditions, and celebrations, we encourage providers to support families and systems in identifying and celebrating familial, cultural, and systemic traditions. This work often varies in relation to the context and the connection.

With *biological/kinship families,* the work may involve expression of curiosity about, and exploration of, the various traditions, norms, and celebrations in which the family currently (or historically) engages. In families in which celebrations are limited and/or have become associated with negative rather than positive experiences, providers can work with family members to create new traditions or celebrations.

In *foster and/or adoptive families,* children and caregivers often bring multiple, and sometimes disparate, traditions and celebrations to the system. Younger children may not have the capacity to hold the continuity of previous traditions; older children may be reluctant to engage in them due to a fear of disruption, a wish to engage fully in a new family, or a concern about caregivers' response. Consider the following example:

Leon, a 14-year-old African American boy, was placed at age 12 and adopted at age 13 by a Jewish couple. Early in his treatment, close to the winter holiday, Leon's new clinician asked him if he would be doing anything for Christmas, a holiday Leon had described celebrating as a young child. Leon shook his head quickly and said, "I don't celebrate any of that stuff now. My family does Hanukkah." On further exploration, Leon was able to state that he made a decision "to give all of that up" when he joined his current family, because he wanted to be "one of them."

This example illustrates both strengths and challenges: Leon's wish to integrate into his family and his willingness to do so speak to his desire and capacity for building relationship. A primary concern, however, is his felt understanding that, in order to do so, he needed to give up some aspect of self that may (or may not) have been important to him.

Work with family members to share and explore each other's traditions. New parents of a younger child may need to independently explore and incorporate aspects of his or her culture and tradition, whereas parents of an older child can work collaboratively with him or her to understand and share common and different experiences. Families may wish to create new "melded" or original traditions that combine aspects of all members' experiences and that are unique to the new family system, as well as to incorporate intact the traditions most important to each family member.

Milieu systems (e.g., schools, residential programs) often have their own unique culture and traditions. Making these explicit can contribute to community engagement and involvement. For instance, the monthly barbecue, the school song, the weekly election of a resident who exemplifies the program's strongest value, and the annual Halloween celebration are all ways to foster continuity and connection for both children and staff. As with families, milieu systems are often comprised of individuals with a diverse range of cultural experiences, including language, food, religion, race, gender, and the like. It is important for milieus to integrate opportunities to celebrate diverse cultures in addition to establishing a unique milieu culture. Pay attention to integrating celebrations from the many cultures represented by the individuals who are part of that system. Invite children to share their traditions—whether individual, familial, community, or cultural—with other members of the larger community. Build community-specific traditions and capture these concretely—say, in photos, on bulletin boards, or in weekly newsletters.

A word of caution about rituals: For many children and families who have experienced trauma, some rituals and traditions have become associated with negative experiences—for example, the Christmas when Dad became drunk and violent or the birthday when Mom did not show up for her visit. For children from nonmainstream cultures, dominant cultural rituals may enhance feelings of difference or loss. For many people currently struggling, times of celebration are experienced as particularly difficult. It is important to understand the meaning of specific holidays and other larger rituals for each individual and family.

Developmental Considerations

Routines will necessarily change over time as children shift across developmental stages, as felt safety in an environment grows or decreases, and as natural changes affect daily experience. For instance, a younger child may rely on a caregiver's external soothing at bedtime, whereas an older child or adolescent may have the capacity or preference to use more internal self-soothing strategies. Although this change is often organic, it is useful nonetheless to tune in to changes in routine and/or to the need for them.

In the following table we offer some developmental considerations in thinking about the role of routine and rhythm and the supports that may be required.

Developmental stage	Routine and rhythm considerations
Early childhood	This is perhaps the most crucial stage for building rituals and routines: 1. Younger children rely almost completely on caregivers for provision of structure. 2. Structure is a particularly salient need during this developmental stage. Young children love predictability: This is the age when children watch a video over and over until it breaks, notice when caregivers skip a word or a page in a favorite book—despite the fact that they can't yet read—and ask to hear the same stories over and over again. Most routines at this stage depend on caregiver involvement, and individual/self-structuring will likely be minimal. The goal here is not to foster premature/age-inappropriate independence, but to encourage growth of agency and exploration within a safe structure provided by caregivers. Having said that, there are certain independent routines that are age-appropriate. For instance, even very young children can develop self-care routines, such as brushing teeth or washing hands, with parental guidance. Age-appropriate chores may include picking up toys or helping parents place clothes in the laundry basket. These routines can build feelings of independence and industry, crucial over time to the development of agency. It is key, however, that there is family support for individual achievement, and most routines at this age are best accomplished with parental involvement and monitoring. Most young children have limited attention spans. When developing routines, keep this factor in mind. For instance, at-home activities, unless highly engaging, are likely going to need to shift regularly to keep the child's focus and attention; minimize expectations for lengthy independent play. Therapy sessions can be broken into 5-minute (rather than 20-minute) chunks.
Middle childhood	As children get older, there are increasing demands on their time: They enter school, join after-school activities, spend time with friends, etc. With the intensified daily schedule it is important for families to make an extra effort to schedule times to come together. Older children can begin to take a more active role in the creation of individual and familial routines and rituals. In addition, older children can be more autonomous in carrying out daily routines. However, caregivers should remain involved in the creation of expectations for routines, as well as in providing support for follow-through.
Adolescence	Family routines are increasingly challenging to adolescents. Teenagers normatively desire time outside of the home, greater flexibility, and more independence. They will take a larger role in creating autonomous routines outside of the home setting. Adolescents and their caregivers tend to travel in "nearby orbits," each with his or her own busy life. It is still important, however, for these orbits to overlap on occasion, and in routine, expected ways. Regular communication is both important and challenging in adolescence. Teach caregivers that adolescents will have things about which they do and don't want to talk. There can be expectations around communication even when family members don't see each other (e.g., leave notes). Work with caregivers to appropriately monitor adolescent activities.

🌐 Real-World Therapy

🌐 **Don't overdo.** The goal is not to rigidly structure every moment of a child's day, but rather to create a subtle sense of predictability. In fact, given the rigidity that many traumatized children bring to their interactions, comfort with flexibility is an important goal.

Rituals and routines can be thought of as the "bookends" that contain the daily living that happens in between.

● **Be realistic about expectations.** Know where a family or system is currently "at." Attempting to build overly expansive or inflexible routines will often create a setup for the child and caregivers to fail. Build slowly, and with the input of the child and the caregivers. As with any intervention, early success is essential.

● **Don't get discouraged.** Don't forget that the most common targets of routine are frequently those areas in which the child has developed what appear to be the most idiosyncratic behaviors—frequently in the service of anxiety management. Don't expect predictability to occur overnight; it is often in retrospect, after a lengthy period of "hanging in there," that the child's internalization of the routine becomes apparent.

● **Hang in there.** Predictability isn't always formalized in routines or rituals. The consistency that defies predictability is often as simple—and complicated—as sticking around, meaning what we say, and saying what we mean. With so many of the kids with whom we work, disruption of attachment becomes a regular occurrence as they are moved from placement to placement to placement. For this reason, it is quite adaptive of them to protect themselves from further loss by rejecting others first. Part of attachment work is sticking with these kids who present as oppositional, unlikable, or inconsistent, in order to prevent their further rejection. When you say you will show up—and you do—it is powerful. When you say you will remember to bring the glittery markers next week—and you do—it is powerful. Working and living with children who have experienced loss, over and over, is often about the long haul, about sticking it out for the journey. Don't underestimate the impact you have by just *hanging in*.

Part IV

Attachment

What Is Attachment?

■ One of the most basic human needs is connection to other human beings. We begin to connect from our earliest moments, and we continue to rely on relationships throughout our lives.

  ◆ The earliest relationship(s), built between the child and his or her primary caregiver(s), is referred to as the **"attachment system."** Why is this system so important? The attachment system **provides a model for all other relationships.** Out of this early connection, children form an understanding of *self* and *others*. For instance:

   ● A child who is loved, cared for, and listened to may believe that he or she is lovable and worthy and that others are generally trustworthy and will be available if needed.

   ● A child who is consistently rejected and ignored may believe that he or she is unimportant or unlovable and that others are uninterested, unavailable, and likely to reject any attempts to gain support.

   ● A child who is frequently hurt or excessively punished may believe that he or she is bad and that others are unsafe and potentially dangerous.

   ● A child whose parents are inconsistently available (e.g., due to substance use or mental health issues) may believe that adults are not able to handle things and are unpredictable in their responses. These children often feel overly responsible for the well-being of others, and may be controlling or clingy in their interactions.

  ◆ The attachment system provides the earliest training ground for **coping with and expressing emotions.**

   ● When children are born, they do not have the skills to deal with emotions on their own. They rely on parents to comfort them and help them manage distress. When children consistently receive nurturance from their parents, they learn that feelings are not permanent, that distress can be tolerated, and that it will eventually subside. When support is first provided externally, over time, children will internalize these same coping skills. Eventually, children are able to independently manage emotional experience.

- Children who receive inconsistent, neglectful, or rejecting caregiving have little support in managing the challenging experiences of early childhood. When they feel distress, they must rely on primitive and frequently ineffective or insufficient coping skills. As a result, two primary consequences emerge:
  - First, the child is unable to develop more advanced coping skills. While other children get better and better at dealing with emotions over time, these children continue to act and look like much younger children in the face of distress.
  - Second, children may become frightened by or guarded against emotional experience in general, as all feelings may be perceived as potentially threatening and overwhelming.

◆ The attachment system **provides a safe environment for healthy development.**

- Every developmental stage has key tasks that children work to accomplish. The attachment system provides the safety that gives children confidence in approaching these tasks. Success in relationships, school, identity, and, ultimately, independent functioning all stem in part from the support that the attachment system initially provides.
- When children do not have the safety net of a secure attachment system, the energy that other children are able to invest in accomplishments instead must be invested in self-protection and survival.

What Is the Caregiving System?

- Many children who have experienced chronic/complex trauma spend significant time in alternative systems of care (e.g., residential treatment centers, group homes, foster placements, specialized school placements). They may or may not have a consistent primary caregiver available to them.

- When a primary caregiver is available (e.g., biological, adoptive, or foster parents), treatment may focus on supporting parents in providing a safe environment that promotes children's healing process.

- For children who are in substitute care, professional staff enters into the role of the substitute caregiving system. Because this caregiving system is so crucial to child recovery, it is important to develop a system that is safe for both children and staff. Therefore, intervention will necessarily include a focus on staff-level understanding, behavior, and supports.

- For all children, it is important to also consider the range of adults with whom they will interact and who play a role in the children's surrounding system. These adults may include, for instance, the clinician, the child's teacher, after-school providers, or day care staff. Ideally, intervention will target multiple levels of the caregiving system.

Why Is It Important to Build Safety
(for Both the Child and the Caregiver)?

■ Children who have experienced trauma have a base expectation that the world and others are danger-ous. As a consequence, they are chronically in self-defense mode: They anticipate danger and react quickly when they think it is present. This response mode has helped them to survive in their young lives. However, this self-protective stance interferes with ongoing healthy development.

■ In order for children to move beyond a self-defense mode, they must be in an environment that provides some consistent degree of felt safety. Often, because the danger that these children have experienced is *relational danger,* they are highly tuned in to signs of danger in the people with whom they interact. This defensive stance makes it particularly important for all caregivers to develop skills to cope with this behavior

■ Maintaining safety with children who constantly anticipate danger is a significant challenge, and it can be draining for parents, staff members, teachers, clinicians, peers, and others who interact with these children. For this reason, it is important to pay attention to adult safety as well as child safety—and, ultimately, these two things will go hand in hand.

7

Caregiver Management of Affect

🔑 THE MAIN IDEA AND KEY SUBSKILLS

Support the child's caregiving adults—whether parents or professionals—in understanding, managing, and coping with their own emotional responses, so that they are better able to support the children in their care.

★ Psychoeducation about trauma and resilience
★ Normalization and validation of caregiver experience
★ Identification of both challenging and positive interactions and experiences with youth
★ Building self-monitoring skills
★ Enhancing self-care and supporting resources

★ Key Concepts

★ Why Build Caregiver Affect Management Skills?

■ A key role of caregivers within the attachment system is to help children learn skills in self-regulation.

■ Before a caregiver can help a child tolerate and modulate affect, however, the caregiver must also be able to tolerate, modulate, and cope with his or her own emotional responses.

■ One of the most salient components of a child's emotional climate is the affect of his or her caregivers. All children take cues from their caregivers' expressions and learn to interpret the world partly through these emotional reactions.

★ Trauma Behaviors That Challenge Caregiver Modulation

■ Children who have experienced trauma and attachment disruptions often struggle with intense emotions, difficulty with relationships, impacted systems of meaning, and behavioral dysregulation. The at-times significant needs of these children can be draining for caregivers. Child behaviors and interactional styles that challenge caregiver modulation may include:

- Triggered responses to caregivers
- Anger/opposition
- Demand for attention
- Patterns of approach and rejection
- Extreme emotional responses to stressors

■ The emotional impact on caregivers is complicated by the role of relational reenactments and child vigilance. Children who experience interpersonal trauma seek safety in various ways. One of their primary safety needs is the need for control in relationships. Children will often engage in behaviors (such as those listed above) that provoke intense reactions from their caregiver(s). Those reactions are often consistent with themes from a child's past such as punishment, shame, rejection, and/or abandonment. For instance, the child may act in a way that pulls for punishment or negative reaction from a caregiver, because this is the interactive style with which the child is familiar and has come to expect. This pattern is further complicated by the fact that children who have experienced trauma are often particularly vigilant toward the expressions of others and may interpret caregiver emotion in light of stark dichotomies of safety versus danger, approval versus disapproval, and acceptance versus rejection. This vigilance makes it especially important for caregivers to monitor and modulate their own feelings. However, this need for ongoing modulation and monitoring can be challenging for caregivers.

■ Many caregivers are coping with not just the identified traumatic experiences and responses of the children in their care, but with their own experiences of traumatic stress, some of which may be ongoing. This layering of affect (as an individual, as a caregiver–parent/provider) is particularly complicated for families or individual caregivers whose experience includes the legacy of historic trauma, systematic and structural injustice, and ongoing racism or discrimination. Any work supporting the emotional experience of caregivers must seek to integrate an understanding of the necessary role of self-protection, justified anger, and fear in the lives of many families.

■ It is also important to keep in mind that caregivers and families often face additional ongoing stressors that impact emotional experience and go beyond their child's specific identified trauma exposure, and which may or may not be identified as "traumatic" by the child or caregiver. Consider the role of experiences such as discrimination, economic challenges, familial mental health needs, housing instability, or mandated service systems involvement in their impact on the caregiver and family.

★ Common Caregiver Responses

It is nearly impossible to capture the full range of potential caregiver responses. Consider the following, however, as examples.

■ Challenges that arise in caregiving may lead to the following *emotional* and *cognitive* responses:

- ◆ **Reduced sense of efficacy** in the caregiving role, for example:
  - For parents: "Why is my child rejecting me?"
  - For teachers: "Why can't I get this child to listen?"
  - For providers: "Why can't I help this child calm down?"
- ◆ **Guilt and shame** about child experiences: "How could these things happen to my child?"
- ◆ **Anger and blame of the child:** "She's doing this on purpose! She's trying to manipulate me."
- ◆ **Anger and blame of the provider system:** "Why haven't people done more? Why is no one trying to help me/us?"

■ When faced with intense emotions such as these, it is not uncommon for caregivers, like children, to respond defensively in the service of coping. Common *behavioral and physiological reactions* include:

- ◆ **Shutting down or constricting** to defend against emotion—a reaction may lead to ignoring or minimizing the child and/or the child's needs.
- ◆ **Surges of arousal, involving intense physiological or emotional responses, that escalate quickly when confronted by difficult child behaviors.**
- ◆ **Overreacting** by trying to control or protect the child through overly punitive or authoritative response; this reaction may lead to stifling the child's expression and/or increasing triggered responses.
- ◆ **Being overly permissive** as a way to try to prevent the child's escalation. This reaction may lead to giving in or "caving" in the face of the child's affect.

Therapist Toolbox

What's the Stake?

■ For most of the families and systems we work with, the treatment "bid" emphasizes a *child* who has behaviors that are creating problems for those around him or her. Caregivers are referred to child-focused therapists, schools request child-focused consults, and milieu systems strategize around child-focused behavioral plans, all with the end goal of reducing or eliminating difficult child behaviors. As a result, providers may be anxious about placing an emphasis on or addressing the caregiver's emotional experience.

■ This reluctance may be particularly the case in systems that are not classically focused on mental health (e.g., schools, juvenile justice centers).

■ Our direct experience, in our own clinical practice and in consulting to hundreds of varying child-serving systems, is that despite this reluctance, a disproportionate (but not surprising) amount of our consultation time is spent in discussion of the emotions, reactions, and behaviors of the adults surrounding and caring for the child, rather than the child client. This focus only highlights for us how important it is to support adult emotional experience.

■ Acknowledgment of caregiver emotional experience is often felt as a relief, rather than a burden, so long as the acknowledgment is perceived as respectful, normalizing (rather than judgmental), and supportive.

■ Consider the following:

   ◆ Normalize adult emotional experience. This issue is covered in depth under Target #1 in the "Tools" subsection later in this chapter.

   ◆ Discuss, explore, and provide psychoeducation on why adult experience matters:

      ● Because adults matter. Even though the focus of a system or a referral may be on the youth, the experience of the adults is also important. Parents matter, teachers matter, milieu staff matter, and clinicians matter. Everyone in a system deserves to be supported.

      ● Because caregivers are more effective when they are regulated. An adult caregiver can have hundreds of tools in his or her toolbox, and every one of them will only be as effective as the person wielding it. A parent who sets a limit when enraged and screaming is less effective than one who does so calmly; an unsupported staff member will be less effective in trying to calm an out-of-control youth than a staff member with a support team.

      ● Because youth will respond to the emotional experience of the adults around them. It is not realistic—or even desirable—for adult caregivers to try to "get rid of" all feelings. A very important message for youth is that everyone has feelings and that feelings matter. Even intense affect, addressed and managed successfully, sends a powerful message to trauma-impacted children that feelings are okay. However, when adults are consistently stressed, distressed, angry, overwhelmed, depressed, or frightened, the emotions and behavior of the youth around them are likely to be impacted. A dysregulated caregiving system is likely to lead to a dysregulated child.

Behind the Scenes

Building the Foundation

■ It is an inherently vulnerable situation for caregivers when their own emotions are addressed. Caregivers often approach treatment assuming that the focus will be on the child, rather than on the caregiving system.

■ Providers themselves may be less comfortable or accustomed to tuning into their own emotional experience; reactions to youth and families; and experience of stress, vicarious trauma, and burnout; but awareness of and addressing internal experience is vital at all levels of the caregiving system, including the provider level.

■ In order to target caregiver affect management, it is important to have a common and respectful understanding of *why* this goal is important. Engage caregivers in the process by exploring and addressing the points above ("What's the Stake?").

■ It is vital that the provider maintain a nonjudgmental stance. Ideally, the provider is *teaming* with the caregiver (or caregiving system) in the same way that we want the caregiver to team with the child. In order for this connection to happen, there must be openness to, acceptance of, and tolerance for the caregivers' thoughts, feelings, ideas, and experience. As an example, if a caregiver states, "Sometimes I hate my child," it is vital that the provider be able to respond in a way that normalizes this experience and facilitates ongoing discussion.

■ At essence, the goal is normalization of caregiver experience and support of the caregiving system so that the system is able to support the child.

■ It is particularly important to normalize those affects that may be perceived as necessary and vital (for the safety of the child, for the safety of the caregiver, for other reasons). For instance, an African American mother expresses intense fear and distress to a clinician when talking about the behaviors of her 8-year-old son in school. She describes being afraid that he will be arrested or killed: "It's one thing now, at 8, but they're already looking at him like he's a criminal in training. What's going to happen to him when he gets bigger?" Trying to *change* the affect of the caregiver through unrealistic statements (e.g., "It's okay, he's a good kid, no one is looking at him like he's a criminal") is a clear misattunement that is likely to lead to increased intensity of distress and a break in the felt safety of the caregiver in treatment. Instead, it is crucial that providers seek to understand, acknowledge, and validate the protective value that many intense emotions continue to serve for caregivers and their children, and, when feasible, work to support caregivers in *managing the distress* associated with intense affects and experiences.

■ Caregiver affect management is a skill that serves as the foundation for all other skills in this framework. For instance, when modulated, a caregiver is better able to attune effectively to his or her child, respond consistently, support regulation skills, and foster competency.

Things to Assess

■ *For primary caregivers/parents:*

◆ Caregiver supports and resources. Who are the individuals, community resources, and systems to which the caregiver turns for emotional or logistical support? Does the caregiver have attachment resources in his or her own life? When and how does the caregiver access these resources, and what are the barriers?

◆ Caregiver stress management strategies. In what ways is the caregiver currently coping? What does the caretaker do to manage his or her life stress? Many caregivers may struggle to identify strategies for managing stress. It is common to hear statements like "I don't have time for myself"; "My husband and I haven't been out in years." Keep in mind that strategies in use may be less obvious, even to the caregiver. After much exploration one caregiver said, "I sit in my car by myself for 2 minutes when I get home from work and play a game on my phone." Caregivers may also be unwilling to identify strategies that seem unhealthy or undesirable, particularly if there is a perceived power differential with the provider. For instance, one caregiver may easily state, "I have a beer at night to relax," whereas another denies ever drinking. Normalizing even unhealthy strategies (e.g., "A lot of parents find ways to manage the hard times that they'd rather not talk about, like drinking, yelling, or finding ways to escape from the house. People don't always want to talk about these, but all of these make sense").

■ *For providers or caregiving systems:*

   ◆ What forums are there for staff/provider support? Whether in a residential program, school, mental health center, or other child-serving system, providers who interact directly with youth are vulnerable to experiencing, and reacting from, difficult emotions. All provider systems should evaluate what opportunities exist for (non-task-oriented) staff support and processing of experience.

   ◆ In what ways are staff members a team? Working with challenging youth can feel isolating and overwhelming. Provider systems should explore the ways that staff members have the opportunity to "tag team," work collaboratively, and feel like important and contributing members of a joint endeavor rather than individuals with sole responsibility for outcomes.

■ *For all:*

   ◆ What specific situations are positive for caregivers? Work with caregivers to identify child/adolescent behaviors, interactions, or other mutual experiences that elicit positive affect and pleasure for the caregiver. In what moments do caregivers feel best about their role?

   ◆ How aware are caregivers of their own reactions? Can the caregiver easily identify "clues" of frustration, sadness, helplessness, or other difficult emotion, or does the caregiver struggle to maintain or admit these types of reactions? The more difficulty a caregiver has with acknowledging his or her own challenging reactions, the more crucial parallel attunement by the provider will be (see Chapter 8).

   ◆ How much insight do caregivers have about the role of their own response? Be sure to target psychoeducation to caregiver blind spots.

■ How does the caregiver's or family's culture impact caregiver emotional display? It is important to understand what is considered normative within the family. For example, in one family intense speech and raised voices may indicate dysregulated emotion; in another, these same qualities are parts of a normative interaction style.

Helping Caregivers Identify Particular Challenges

■ When families or systems are experiencing distress, it becomes easy for them to develop a generalized perception of *hard:* in other words, it is not just that there are difficult moments, but instead *all* moments begin to feel difficult. However, for most caregivers the struggle is not with consistent and constant dysregulation or distress, but rather with specific situations that are challenging in some way.

■ Consider the following when exploring caregiver's trouble spots:

   ◆ Areas of insecurity for caregivers in parenting or other role fulfillment

   ◆ Child behaviors that have, in the past, been associated with crisis or significant events (e.g., hospitalization, assault, self-harm)

   ◆ Child behaviors or experiences that are perceived as potentially dangerous for the child/family due to societal stigma and interpretation

   ◆ The caregiver's own trauma history and triggers

- ◆ Areas of discrepancy between child and caregiver (e.g., cultural, generational, values)
- ◆ The role of external stressors (e.g., financial trouble, job stress)

■ Work with caregivers to monitor their responses in each of these situations, keeping in mind that "typical" responses may vary widely by stressor.

■ Build a plan that identifies specific coping strategies for identified challenge situations.

■ Consider the following example to illustrate this point.

> An adoptive mother of two young boys was generally relaxed, attuned, and supportive of her children's needs. When either boy was sad or worried about something, she was able to remain calm and provide comfort. However, she became very anxious when the boys' behavior would become more energetic. In the past, higher arousal had led to sexualized and aggressive behavior by the boys, behaviors that the mother found difficult to cope with, and which led to feelings of helplessness and self-blame. She worried that any energetic behaviors might lead to this same overaroused response. As a result, whenever the boys started to show high energy—even at normative levels for 6- and 8-year-old children—the mother would intervene and separate them.

In this example, although the mother's concerns are valid and real, her actions are communicating to her children that energetic play—an important component of healthy development in young children—is unsafe and unacceptable. In working with this parent, it will be important to (1) validate and help her understand her own emotional response and resulting behavior; (2) build her tolerance for normative, healthy levels of arousal and activity in her children; (3) build tools that will help her support her children in safe play; and (4) build a repertoire of coping strategies for those occasions when high energy might, in fact, lead to dysregulated behaviors.

What about the Provider?: Managing Your Own Affect

■ Because much of this section refers to *caregiver* affect management, it is easy to focus on the parent. However, it is equally important for therapists and other helping professionals to pay attention to their own emotional reactions and to build skills in monitoring and managing them.

■ Consider the following parallel process. A child who thinks that she is damaged and unlovable is convinced that she is unable to trust anyone. Placed in a new home, she feels afraid and anxious. Sure the new caregiver will reject her, she self-protects by keeping the caregiver at arm's length. In turn, the caregiver feels ineffective as a parent and rejected by the child. Feeling frustrated and helpless, the caregiver reacts by pulling away. Now what about the professionals working with this family? Faced with the increasing demands of the distressed system, the professionals also begin to feel frustrated and helpless, and to think that they are ineffective and incompetent. Over time, the professionals may feel themselves pulling away, ultimately terminating the therapy. With this "domino" sequence, the child's initial prediction of rejection has come true!

■ Throughout this section are techniques for teaching caregivers how to monitor their own experience, learn to recognize their vulnerabilities and typical coping patterns, and engage in self-care and other coping skills. It is strongly recommended that professionals practice these same techniques.

A Three-Way (or More) Parallel Process

	Child	Caregiver	Professional(s)
Cognitions	"I'm bad, unlovable, damaged." "I can't trust anyone."	"I'm an ineffective parent." "My child is rejecting me."	"I'm an ineffective clinician." "This family just needs to work harder."
Emotions	Shame, anger, fear, hopelessness	Frustration, sadness, helplessness, worry	Frustration, helplessness, indifference
Behaviors (coping strategy)	Avoidance, aggression, preemptive rejection	Overreacting, controlling, shutting down, being overly permissive	Disconnection, dismissing, ignoring, therapy termination
The cycle	"She's going to reject me anyway. I'd better not connect."	"He's just not interested in connecting with me."	"I don't think anyone could make a difference with this family."

Special Concerns

▪ Many caregivers—parents and providers alike—have their own trauma histories. Be aware that children's traumatic experiences and their resulting responses may act as triggers and reminders of caregivers' own historical experiences.

▪ Pay attention to **basic safety:** Are caregivers able to keep themselves and their children safe? Are any red flags present (e.g., significant caregiver depression, substance use, explosive or overly punitive reactions)?

▪ In the presence of red flags or other concerns, consider whether caregivers may need **additional supports** (e.g., their own individual therapy, increased supervision).

Understanding Vicarious Trauma

▪ For all individuals who care for someone who has experienced trauma—primary caregivers as well as professionals—there is a risk of **vicarious trauma** and, if unaddressed, **burnout.**

▪ *Vicarious* or *secondary trauma* has been defined as a process through which the caregiving individual's own internal experience becomes affected by engagement with the child's (or client's) traumatic material (McCann & Pearlman, 1990).

▪ Although the vicarious trauma response will differ across individuals, vicarious traumatization leads to a disruption of the same core issues that are impacted by direct exposure to trauma, including disrupted sense of safety, difficulties with trust, impaired self-esteem and self-efficacy, challenges with intimacy, and feelings of loss of control or helplessness (Pearlman & Saakvitne, 1995).

▪ For providers, understanding, recognizing, preventing, and addressing signs of vicarious trauma represent a primary systems-level intervention in targeting our own affect management. Excellent resources are available that discuss and address the providers' own responses (e.g., Pearlman & Saakvitne, 1995; Saakvitne et al., 2000; Stamm, 1999).

Considerations in Working with Primary Caregivers

■ Caregiver affect modulation should be assessed initially and taught either one-on-one or in parenting groups.

■ After basic skills are mastered, dyadic or family treatment may be helpful for practice and coaching in the use of these skills.

Considerations in Working within a Milieu

■ In any sort of a milieu system, consider the role of both individual supervision and group/team-level supports.

■ It is easy for interventions targeted toward staff affect management to feel inadvertently punitive (i.e., "You shouldn't feel that way"). As with primary caregivers, it is crucial that this process involve normalization of affect, staff supports, and skill building in specific coping strategies.

Primary Components of This Building Block

The primary components of this building block include the following:

■ Psychoeducation
   ◆ Depersonalization of child behaviors
   ◆ Education about the trauma response
   ◆ Validation of caregiver experience
■ Self-monitoring skills
■ Affect management skills
■ Building supports and resources

Teach to Caregivers

■ *Reminder:* Teach the caregiver the Key Concepts.

■ *Reminder:* Teach the caregiver the relevant Developmental Considerations.

■ The goal of affect modulation for caregivers is *not* to "fake" their emotions, to pretend that they have no emotional response or to deny internal experience. Rather the goal is to monitor affect; to maintain appropriate boundaries; to respond in a constructive rather than destructive way; and to communicate to their children that the adults around them can stay safe and calm and can handle difficult experience.

Teaching Point: Normalizing Caregiver Emotional Response

Target	Important points
Depersonalize: Provide education about the impact of trauma.	Teach caregivers basic information about trauma response in children and the impact of trauma on families. See caregiver handout "Introduction: Children and Trauma" (Appendix B).

Target	Important points
	Help caregivers understand the normative and adaptive nature of their children's responses.
	Help caregivers differentiate a child's *triggered response* versus opposition, rejection, etc. Identify: What is the *function* of the child's behavior? Consider: meeting emotional or physical needs *or* coping with perceived danger. Pair with education about triggers (see Chapter 2).
	If appropriate, teach caregivers about the parallel process, and the ways in which it manifests.
Integrate psychoeducation about normative developmental processes.	Intertwining with trauma-related responses are the normative developmental challenges of childhood. The particular temperament of the child, the developmental stage and needs, and the behavioral and relational expression of these can all challenge, feel overwhelming, and at times be misinterpreted by caregivers who are already experiencing significant stress. Part of the foundational psychoeducation and normalization process should include incorporating basic child development information.
Validate caregiver response.	Validate caregiver emotional reactions—as is true for children, all emotions are okay. The goal of affect management is to be aware of and effectively cope with emotional experience.

Tools: Teaching Caregivers Affect Management

■ *Target #1: Identifying difficult moments. Support caregivers in identifying factors that lead to greater adult reactivity, emotion, or distress.*

Identifying Difficult Moments

Target	Important points
The foundation: Normalize the experience of difficulty.	In order to effectively evaluate the experience of difficulty, a crucial starting point is to lay the foundation that *everyone* has difficult moments, difficult days, and some interactions or experiences that are harder than others.
	Although the caregiver's ultimate goal is likely, at least in part, to address difficult *child* behaviors, the ease with which caregivers are able to manage those behaviors will vary in relation to *their own* internal states. In other words, everyone—adult and child alike—is most effective when they are in control of their emotions, reasonably comfortable in their bodies, and have adequate access to internal or external supports.
	It is for these reasons that it is so important for all adults to be aware of "what makes a hard day."
Identify difficult situations or "push buttons."	Work with caregivers to identify challenging situations. Consider the following areas and helpful questions; providers should also consider these questions for themselves.
	Factors related to your child: ■ Are there child behaviors that are particularly hard for you to deal with or that "push your buttons"? ■ Are there child emotions that you find particularly difficult to cope with or respond to, or which lead to a strong emotional response in you? ■ What types of expressed feelings or behaviors have been the hardest to cope with or the highest risk in the past (e.g., led to family crisis, danger to self or other, or need for more intensive treatment)? Do these feelings or behaviors still occur? What are they like? ■ Are any of the child's feelings, behaviors, or experiences particularly hard for you to understand?

Target	Important points
	Factors affecting your world: ▪ What are some of the other stressful things happening in your life right now? ▪ Are there things that you find yourself worrying a lot about, like money, housing, or being able to take care of your family? ▪ How often do you feel like you "bring your job home"? ▪ What do you notice is different about your parenting/caregiving when you are tired versus when you are well rested? ▪ What other things affect your ability to stay centered (e.g., trouble at work, challenges in your own interpersonal relationships, external pressures)? **Factors stemming from your own experiences:** ▪ Are there situations that you know you find particularly hard because they remind you of hard times in your own life? ▪ In what kinds of situations do you feel the most and least effective? ▪ Thinking about many different experiences in your life, what have you learned about your own behavior or reactions when you are feeling confident versus anxious? Are there situations in which you often feel less confident? What types of situations are those? ▪ What do you think your most important values or beliefs are about how people should behave? Do any of your child's behaviors or actions ever challenge those values or beliefs? ▪ Do you feel like you routinely get enough sleep, enough rest, enough down time? What gets in the way of that?

▪ *Target #2: Working with caregivers to build a support system.* For both primary caregivers and professionals, it is important to have sources of support. Work to actively identify a range of resources.

Building Caregiver Support Systems

Target	Important points
Identify resources.	*Primary caregivers:* Work with parents to identify their support system. Consider the range of potential resources (e.g., significant others, peers, relatives, clergy, community supports, professional resources). Help parents identify the specific situations in which they are able to utilize particular supports (e.g., to whom can the caregiver go when worried and/or in need of reassurance, comfort, information). Pay particular attention to caregiver-identified trouble spots. *Providers:* It is important for providers to pay attention to both professional and personal sources of support. Within a system examine the presence or absence of professional supports such as supervision, peer support groups, and training. As for primary caregivers, providers should be able to identify which resources (professional and/or personal) are helpful for specific situations. *Systems:* A primary goal for administrators in provider systems should be the identification and/or development of support resources at all levels of staffing. These resources should focus on routine supports (e.g., supervision, provider team meetings) as well as crisis supports. For every staff member in the system, ask, "In what forum(s) does this individual routinely receive support for daily practices?"
Consider the role of caregiver-to-caregiver supports.	Caregiver-to-caregiver support is often particularly helpful. Trauma can be isolating for caregivers as well as children; it is not uncommon for caregivers to feel alone and overwhelmed in the challenge of parenting or caring for a trauma-impacted child. Support from other caregivers who have "been there" or are still there is often a valuable addition to the treatment.
Teach good boundaries.	When a support system is inadequate, caregivers may be more vulnerable to placing the child(ren) in the role of support system. However, not all caregiver emotions are appropriate to share with children. Help caregivers identify developmentally or situationally inappropriate experiences to share, as well as more appropriate alternative resources.

■ *Target #3: Building self-monitoring skills.* Help caregivers to identify their own typical responses in challenging situations. See handout **"Tuning In to Yourself"** (Appendix B).

Building Self-Monitoring Skills

Target	Important points	
The foundation: rationale for building self-awareness	Although an important goal is to identify and ideally get in front of the hard moments by becoming increasingly aware of them, the reality is that for most of us, the first "clue" that a situation is difficult may be the way we are reacting in the moment. By identifying and working to become aware of those reactions, adults can engage the strategies to manage them. Anchor in the end goal: to manage and support adult emotional experience, for the purpose of being better able to manage and support youth behavior and experience.	
Build self-monitoring skills: Teach caregivers to notice their own reactions, across domains.	Physiological	What is the caregiver experiencing in his or her *body*? Teach caregivers to pay attention to heart rate, breathing, muscle tension, numbness, etc. What warning signs does the caregiver's body provide of "losing control" or hitting a danger point?
	Cognitive	What does the caregiver *think* in the face of difficult situations? Consider automatic thoughts about self (e.g., "I can't do anything to help") as well as about the child (e.g., "She's doing this on purpose").
	Emotional	What does the caregiver *feel* in response to each identified difficult situation? Remember to check for common caregiver responses, as described above.
	Behavioral	What do the caregivers *do* in the face of strong emotion? Do they become punitive? Withdraw? Freeze? Work with caregivers to understand their own behavioral coping strategies.

Target #3 Tips

When trying to teach a new skill to anyone (child/caregiver), it is important to try to support him or her in experiencing a sense of competency and mastery with the skill. As with our child and adolescent clients, caregivers also need many opportunities for skill practice at times that are not associated as the most stressful.

For instance, this skill can be practiced with the use of displaced/nonthreatening situations/content. A parenting or other skill-building group might use a video clip and ask caregivers to monitor their responses in the areas identified in the preceding table. Over time, exploration can move to parental/relational situations with their own children, including positive "button" moments and challenging "button" moments.

The foundation of this skill can be applied by supporting caregiver curiosity about his or her typical responses when talking about difficult situations. Questions can be woven into routine conversation: for instance, when a parent states, "She's been completely impossible lately!" the provider might respond, "I'm sorry, that sounds so hard. I'm noticing you look really stressed out today. Is that how you're feeling?" If the caregiver is able to acknowledge his or her reaction, the provider might take some time to explore the nuances, rather than shifting directly or solely to the child's behavior.

Similarly, in supervision or other forum where providers are discussing youth, conversation about child/adolescent behaviors might incorporate reflection upon staff responses. For instance, a team leader might ask, "What are all of you noticing about how you react to Matthew? I've noticed he's pretty good at getting folks engaged in power struggles. Has anyone found that he kicks up feelings or reactions that aren't typical for you?"

Over time, caregivers can be given cues to support direct practice in this skill. For instance, if a caregiver states, "I just want to shut myself in a bathroom every time he starts screaming!," the clinician can prompt, "This week, I wonder if we can track that. I'm really interested in getting a sense of what's happening concretely when he starts to scream—what happens in your body, what you're thinking, and what you end up doing. Do you think you could try to jot down what you notice if that happens this week?" This type of active homework can engage caregivers directly in a skill set, but in a relatively contained and focused manner.

- *Target #4: Supporting caregiver modulation.*

- In Chapter 11 we discuss "Feelings Toolboxes" for children. It is often helpful for caregivers to create their own "toolboxes" 🔲 (e.g., a range of coping strategies and external resources) to support their own ability to maintain comfortable and effective arousal and emotional states. Many of the skills included below are described in greater detail in Chapter 11. Also, see caregiver worksheet **"Taking Care of Yourself"** (Appendix B).

- In building caregiver coping strategies, it is important to consider when and how a tool will be used; the most effective tools are those that are targeted to the need. Consider the following four categories of strategies to consider adding to the caregiver's toolbox.

  - *Advance preparation strategies:* These strategies include those tools that are useful when anticipating entering into a known stressful situation. The strategies, when practiced routinely, keep anticipatory anxiety down, support planning and preparation, help caregivers engage in strengths and proactively address anticipated needs.

  - *In-the-pocket strategies:* These strategies are useful for in-the-moment management of intense arousal, affect, or unexpected distress. The goal of these strategies is to help the caregiver get through the challenging moment without becoming overwhelmed by it.

  - *Recovery strategies:* These strategies involve purposeful attention to stress/distress relief after a difficult or challenging situation. Recovery strategies support "moving on," rather than allowing challenging situations to dictate emotion and experience long after the situation ends.

  - *Ongoing self-care:* Strategies used for ongoing self-care are designed to support a comfortable baseline level of arousal, to increase well-being, and to decrease stress, so that the adult caregiver is better equipped to manage difficult situations as they arise.

- Examples of these strategies follow.

Examples of Caregiver Modulation Strategies

Category	Possible strategies
Advance preparation	■ Engage in self-talk (e.g., "I know I can handle this"). ■ Have a plan: Troubleshoot each step of the anticipated situation. ■ Mental rehearsal: Visualize each step, mentally practice responding successfully to challenges, and imagine successful outcomes. ■ Remember the stake: Why is it worth it to hang in there for this challenging situation—that is, what are you trying to accomplish? ■ Identify supports: Who or what might be helpful in the moment? ■ Prepare physiologically: Get a good night's sleep, adequate food, and anticipate logistics to manage stress level. ■ Anticipatory relaxation strategies: for example, purposeful use of self-care strategies to avoid anticipatory high arousal.

Category	Possible strategies
In-the-pocket strategies	■ Deep breathing ■ Tense and release: muscle relaxation strategies ■ Personal mantra or self-talk (e.g., "I can do it"; "I'm strong"; I'm capable"). ■ Count to 10. Count to 20. ■ Walk away, if it's safe. Take a break from the stressful situation, then regroup. ■ Give yourself mental permission to make no major decisions—just get through the moment.
Recovery strategies	■ Call a friend. ■ Make a cup of tea or coffee. ■ Take 5 minutes to do something just for yourself. ■ Try to identify one thing that happened (in the day, in the situation) of which you were proud. ■ Do something active to release energy and reconnect to your body—exercise, do yoga, take a walk, turn on music and dance.
Ongoing self-care	■ Pay attention to the basics in your daily schedule, particularly sleeping, eating, and down time. If these areas aren't happening in healthy amounts, look at ways to support them by shifting the routine. ■ Identify a 10-minute block of time (at least) every day when you can engage in a pleasurable activity. ■ (Re)connect to family and friends. Pay attention to maintaining a support system. ■ Identify and engage in your community. Not every community source of support works for everyone—consider where your "fit" is comfortable. There might be a spiritual community, a work community, neighborhood groups, activist groups, hobby groups, adult education classes, library events, parenting groups, casual neighborhood get-togethers, etc. Identify your need for support (5 minutes a week? an hour a day?) and figure out ways to build a routine that allows for it.
Time-outs	In order to access affect management skills in the midst of intense emotion or conflict situations, caregivers may need to "take a break." Help caregivers differentiate safe versus unsafe situations and ways to separate from any unsafe situations. Help caregivers develop appropriate ways to communicate this need to their children (e.g., "I'm upset and need a few minutes to calm down. I'm going to go to my room, to take a little space, and when I come out, we'll talk about this").

Target #4 Tips

In-the-moment techniques are particularly important for preventing relational reenactments. Work with caregivers to pair specific techniques with their own identified cues of dysregulation. For instance, a caregiver who reports feeling shooting pain in her neck and back when upset about an interaction might practice muscle relaxation strategies; a caregiver who describes thinking "I hate him!" every time her son screams might try using a self-statement such as "This is just a hard moment" or visualizing a positive memory; and a caregiver whose cue is his or her own angry or threatening behavior might practice taking a time-out or a deep breath.

   In family based treatment or parent support work, it is recommended that caregiver modulation practice be built into each session. (Refer to Chapter 5 for ideas about how to structure this practice.) In individual or dyadic work it can be helpful for caregiver, therapist, and child to do this modulation practice together. The practice supports experiential learning for the caregiver and modeling for the child, and develops modulatory skills outside of stressful moments.

Developmental Considerations

Developmental stage	Caregiver affect modulation considerations
Early childhood	Young trauma-impacted children are almost completely reliant on adults to provide regulation. Therefore, it is particularly important for caregivers to have support in monitoring and modulating their own affect. In building support systems, consider what is realistic for caregivers of young children to access. At this stage, in-home supports, parent coaches and mentors, and parent–child groups may all be more easily accessed than outpatient parent supports.
	Developing distress tolerance in adult caregivers is crucial at this stage. Because early childhood dysregulation is so normative, the goal of eliminating child affect or difficult behavior is less realistic than the goal of surviving and managing it.
	Caregivers will need to be creative with self-care strategies at this stage. Consider supporting caregivers in identifying a range of "5-minute activities" they can engage in to support self-care.
	Positive dyadic experiences—moments of successful coregulation, sensory engagement, play, and rhythmic connection—will all provide important support to managing more distressing moments.
Middle childhood	Modeling of regulation skills begins to become important as children advance in their ability to observe others' experience. Work with caregivers to demonstrate affect regulation skills by naming what they are feeling (and how they are coping); for instance, "I'm feeling a little frustrated, so I'm going to take a deep breath," or "I'm worried about you."
	As children get older, it becomes easier for caregivers to take the time they need to self-regulate before addressing child behaviors and actions. Work with caregivers to find safe ways to delay response.
Adolescence	This developmental stage is often a particularly trying time for caregivers, as their adolescent children progress toward independence.
	Adolescents' repertoire for seeking independence may be limited to rebelling against caregivers, which can lead to heightened caregiver anxiety, frustration, or other strong emotions.
	Help caregivers to understand the following:
	Adolescents are increasingly able to develop an understanding of the impact of their behavior on others. It is not only appropriate, therefore, but important for caregivers to be selectively honest about their experience of adolescents' behavior and actions.
	Shame is a large issue for many trauma-impacted teens, so phrasing is important. Help caregivers balance honesty with empathy.

Applications
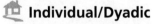 Individual/Dyadic

When working with children and families, normalizing, supporting, and addressing caregivers' emotional experience is often a primary and essential starting point. We address caregiver affect management from our first meeting by communicating (1) an understanding of trauma and trauma responses, (2) a belief that a child and family can be supported, and (3) a willingness to team with the caregiver in this process. When specifically targeting caregiver affect management, it is often important to meet with the caregiver(s) alone, so that there is adequate safety for the caregiver to explore and verbalize his or her experience. However, the clinician may integrate observations of dyadic or familial processes (e.g., "I noticed when we met together that it was upsetting for you when Jenny started to get really loud in the office. Is that something that happens other places? Is that the kind of situation that tends to be hard for you?").

Building affect management skills is an active process. A primary goal is to help caregivers cultivate their own curiosity and build active appraisal skills: By stepping outside of the difficult situation, caregivers are able to observe the moment rather than be overwhelmed by it. Work with caregivers to actively monitor difficult situations, their patterns of response, and the use (or lack thereof) of coping strategies. It is important that the clinician notice, name, and celebrate moments of success, even (and particularly) relative successes. As an example of the latter, consider the caregiver who identifies distress at having lost his or her temper. This caregiver has just experienced a moment of success by recognizing and seeking help with an area of vulnerability. When caregivers experience particular difficulties, explore these: What got in the way of using a coping strategy or remaining centered? Troubleshoot ways to cope with these situations in the future.

If there is more than one primary caregiver, it is important to pay attention to differential responses and to normalize these differences: It is exceedingly rare for two caregivers to have the exact same strengths and/or vulnerabilities. Pay attention to ways that each caregiver's response has the potential to support the other, and ways that these responses may undermine the other. Create a team: For instance, if one caregiver has a particular "push button," use the other caregiver for support; similarly, if one caregiver has a particular strength, tap into this in building parenting strategies.

🏠 Group

When appropriate for particular caregivers, support groups and educational workshops offer the significant advantage of being a natural forum for normalizing caregiver response. We provide an example of this from our own work:

> In the early period of developing this framework, we were conducting a training workshop for a group of adoptive parents that was receiving services using an adaptation of this curriculum. While focusing on "surviving the holidays" (the training took place in late November), we spent some time on normalizing the range of caregiver responses, from joy and excitement to anger, frustration, and helplessness. Despite inviting the attending caregivers to share their experiences, the room remained excruciatingly silent (from our perspective!) until finally one caregiver raised her hand. Invited to speak, she stated, "My name is _____, and I've adopted four kids. I love my kids, but I have to admit, sometimes I really just don't like them." In the aftermath of this statement, the room suddenly came to life: Parent after parent raised his or her hand and spoke of vulnerable moments in parenting and the emotions the parent was reluctant to share. Our normalization of difficult emotion and response was perhaps helpful, but not enough to provide permission; it was only after another parent was able to acknowledge these feelings that the remaining parents felt safe enough to speak.

Caregiver support groups have the potential to decrease some of the most common impacts of trauma: feelings of isolation, disconnection from others, secrecy, and shame. The skills provided in this section, along with those described in the remaining two attachment targets (attunement and effective response) may serve as a template for building group discussion and activities. A number of handouts provided in Appendix B may be useful.

🏠 Milieu

When working to build affect management within a milieu, the application takes place on a systems or provider level. Providers within systems that serve children and families exposed to trauma face many stressors that challenge our capacity to remain regulated. These include, among others, (1) the exposure to many different clients, all with different presentations, needs, and challenges, and the need to manage internal reaction to all of these and respond appropriately; (2) the frequent unpredictability that comes with working with youth in crisis; and (3) the helplessness that can come from working with systems over which the provider has no control. In systems serving higher-risk clients, such as residential programs or hospitals, affect management may be particularly challenging, given the very real threat to provider and other-client safety that may exist. Given these challenges, it is inevitable that providers—like primary caregivers—will experience a range of emotional responses and will have moments of reactivity.

It is important that interventions on a milieu or systemic level feel supportive rather than punitive (i.e., the goal is *not* to send staff the message, "You shouldn't feel the way you feel"). Work to build a programmatic culture that accepts that providers—like our clients— are people with built-in human emotions and danger–response systems. By building appropriate, boundaried forums for staff support, we reduce the likelihood that these emotions and responses will play out in our work with clients. Consider professional supports such as supervision, clinical or staffing meetings, and training. We often recommend adding a simple check-in process within the context of these meetings (e.g., "Where is your energy today?"; "What were the highs and lows of your week?"; "Did you struggle with any particularly hard emotions or have any particularly positive moments this week?") to support a culture of caring. Pay attention to forums that are *process* oriented as well as *task* oriented. This focus is particularly important in the aftermath of difficult and sometimes potentially traumatizing situations, such as the need for restraints or staff or client assaults. Building safe forums in which staff members can explore their own responses and actions—both positive and negative—is crucial to using these experiences as building blocks for future successes.

Beyond professional forums, it is important to pay attention to team building. Working in the field of trauma is too challenging to do alone, and it is important that members of a system feel supportive of, and supported by, their colleagues. In service of this effort, look for ways to explore and build an understanding of common goals and the role of all staff members in working toward these goals. Examine who supports each person on the team at every level. Build and support "fun" activities (e.g., staff retreats and celebrations), recognize and reinforce staff contributions, and normalize and encourage the importance of self-care.

⟳ Trauma Experience Integration: State-Based Skills Application

Distress Tolerance and Regulation

During early stages and in distressed states, the primary focus of caregiver affect management is to support the caregiver's own distress tolerance and "survival capacity" in (what are frequently) challenging moments. Emphasis during this stage is on engagement around and support of positive experiences, and development of internal and external resources to help the caregiver make it through the harder moments. A key strategy is to support the caregiver in identifying challenging situations and cues of caregiver dysregulation. As these are identified, the caregiver can be supported in developing proactive plans to access resources (when available) and to engage in distress tolerance when overwhelmed. Caregivers are also encouraged to practice regulation strategies in calm states, and to build practice of in-the-moment strategies as well as ongoing self-care into daily routine whenever feasible. In this phase it may also be helpful to engage caregivers in basic self-monitoring of their energy, affects, and cues in a way that is more strongly focused on their own experience than on understanding and managing responses to their children's experience.

Curiosity and Reflection

Caregivers who have gained some degree of safety in the therapeutic relationship, and/or are presenting in calm-enough states to reflect on their experience outside of the distressed moment, can often engage in the work of developing greater attuned understanding of their own patterns of regulation and dysregulation. Self-monitoring work can gradually be shifted to a range of caregiver experiences, including identified challenge situations or "push-button" moments. In addition to engaging and practicing the range of skills in the growing caregiver toolbox, clinical work can integrate an increasing awareness of ways that moments of dysregulation may be linked to historical or ongoing experiences of danger, and specifically support caregivers in working to identify internal and external resources and strategies that support safety.

Engaging Purposeful Action

As caregivers are increasingly able to build their awareness of challenges and resources related to affect management and to demonstrate the capacity to engage in the use of tools when needed, they begin to recognize areas of competence and to shift individual identity to a more strengths-based and adaptive view of self. In addition, as caregivers increasingly have the experience of *being* modulated despite distressed moments, they are better able to believe that they *can be modulated* in distressed moments, and therefore use their tools more purposefully both for themselves and for the children they are supporting. When this stage is reached, the goal of the work is to continue to support caregivers in applying their tools (understanding about trauma, trigger or push-button identification, observation/monitoring skills, and regulation strategies) *in the moment* in response to challenging child behavior. As reflective awareness builds, work with caregivers to gradually reduce the challenging moments through increased self-awareness and shifting of triggered or overwhelmed responses to children's behavior. In turn, these skills facilitate caregivers' increased ability to attune to their children. This is the topic of our next chapter.

Real-World Therapy

Have realistic expectations. Keep in mind that affect management is hard. Caregivers, particularly those who have an untreated trauma histories, may be starting in a very similar place as their children.

Build success. Success will likely be relative. Define realistic goals and encourage caretakers to take small steps toward reaching them. Offer praise along the way. Don't forget that caregivers need as much praise and encouragement as their children need.

Tap into empathy. When feeling frustrated with caregiver reactions, imagine living in a home with your client 24 hours a day, 7 days a week. Most caregivers have good intentions and are doing the best they can with the skills they possess.

Be aware of your own reactions to caregivers. Particularly for those caregivers who move slowly, a dual role as advocate for the child and support and educator of the caregiver may lead to frustration and blaming the parent. Pay attention to your own responses, as well as when it would be useful to bring additional clinicians onto the team.

Pay attention to cultural differences. These may influence your expectations of caregivers, your reactions to their behaviors, their reactions to you, and their feelings of vulnerability in doing this work. Be open to exploring and acknowledging differences as well as common ground.

8

Attunement

🔑 **THE MAIN IDEA AND KEY SUBSKILLS**

Support the child's caregiving system—whether parents or professionals—in learning to accurately and empathically understand and respond to children's actions, communications, needs, and feelings.

★ Parallel attunement: Respond empathically to the caregiving system.
★ Cultivate curiosity and help caregivers build an understanding of youth behaviors and communications.
★ Observe, validate, and put language to youth experience; use reflection to mirror child/adolescent communication.
★ Purposefully engage attunement skills to support youth regulation.
★ Look for opportunities to build fluidity and pleasure in dyadic engagement.

Key Concepts

What Is Attunement?

- Attunement may be defined as the capacity of caregivers and children to accurately read each other's cues and respond in a way that maintains rhythm, supports a coregulated state, and meets needs.

- Rhythm in relationship is built simultaneously on many levels and with many parts of our self: with language, emotion, behavior, and physiology. The ways we communicate are often nonverbal, and the needs—whether of the child or of the child's caregivers—may be expressed not in words but in action, in patterns of approach and avoidance, nuances of speech, and sudden emotional shifts. Attuned relational partners learn to go beyond language and to read and respond to these many layers of communication. Attunement is an important foundation of relationship, and in a caregiving system, is the facilitator of child and adolescent capacities and competencies. Accurate attunement allows caregivers to respond to the emotions and needs underlying children's behavior, rather than simply reacting to the most notable or distressing symptom.

- Attunement is a dynamic and ongoing process of learning about other. As needs change, behavioral expression changes, circumstances change, and effective responses change, and relationship partners must remain flexible and adapt in order to remain in—or regain—rhythm over time.

★ Trauma Behaviors That Challenge Attunement

- All children—not just those impacted by trauma—may communicate emotions and internal experience via behavior rather than words. One of the key challenges of attunement work is for caregivers—clinicians, parents, and/or staff members—to learn how to interpret the function behind children's behavior.

- Children who have experienced trauma may have more confusing, intense, and sudden feelings and reactions to internal and external experiences. Particularly when overwhelmed, they may lack the capacity to verbally communicate needs or to identify and cope with difficult emotions. As a result, these emotions, needs, and physiological (body) changes may be expressed in difficult behaviors.

- Often the behaviors that feel the most distressing to caregivers are simply "fronts" for unmet needs or unregulated affect, particularly those related to trauma.

- **Triggers,** or reminders of past traumatic experiences, may elicit intense emotion and/or numbing responses. Because triggers may not be obvious, it is particularly important to teach caregivers how to identify their children's triggering events and/or typical responses (see the upcoming "Teach to Caregivers" section for more detail).

📦 Therapist Toolbox
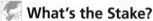 What's the Stake?

- The capacity to tune in to another's emotions, needs, thoughts, and perspective rests on the ability to be curious. In doing attunement work, we are asking parents and other caregivers to pause in their reactions to the youth in their care, step back, and wonder why the behaviors are happening. This is a big "ask" when a family or system is in great distress: The caregiver wants the behaviors to stop, and taking the time to get curious may feel secondary or unimportant.

- Cultivating curiosity will rest in large part on the provider's ability to be curious about, and attuned to, the family, and requires a reasonably regulated state. Consider the following two examples:

  > A mother expresses frustration to her young son's therapist about his escalating behaviors. She angrily states that she has tried everything she can think of and is considering sending him to live with his father. The therapist recalls that when she met with the mother in the waiting room, she noticed that the mother was talking loudly to her son, shouted at him when he asked to come into the room with them, and walked away without saying goodbye. The therapist states, "It looks like he might be reacting to some of your emotions—you said you've been pretty depressed lately. I wonder if he's just trying to get your attention." The mother rejects the therapist's statements, saying, "He gets plenty of attention—he's just acting like a brat. You think you can do better, he's all yours," and then walks out of the room.

- The therapist feels frustrated and unheard, and concludes that the mother is unable to attune to her child. But let us consider an alternative way she might have approached the situation.

> When the mother expresses her distress, the therapist states calmly, "I'm so sorry to hear that things have been so difficult at home. I could see in the waiting room how frustrated you were feeling. Did the two of you have a hard morning?" The mother reports that her son had several tantrums that morning and threw one of her small decorative statues, breaking it. The therapist sympathizes, saying, "What a tough day you've had. No wonder you're feeling tapped out. I know you're usually able to be pretty calm with him, but it sounds like he's really pushing all your buttons today. I can imagine anyone would be at their wits' end after a morning like that." The mother visibly relaxes and says, "Yeah, some days are crazy, right?" The therapist agrees, but notes, "The thing is, they're not all quite this crazy, are they? So I wonder what might be going on that's getting him so revved up."

- In the first example, the parent is unable to engage in curiosity about her child, because she feels completely unheard herself. In the second, when the caregiver is seen, mirrored, validated, and supported, she is in turn able to self-regulate (or coregulate, with the support of the provider), and become open to being curious about her child.

- At all levels of the caregiving system, attunement to other requires a regulated state. As providers, we must be regulated and aware of our internal spaces in order to attune to the youth and families we work with; primary caregivers require the same. Our attunement capacities will rise and fall according to our emotional and physiological states, and the more we integrate our affect management skills in supporting this goal, the better we will be able to engage ourselves and the caregivers with whom we are working.

Behind the Scenes

- We have had the privilege of working with many caregivers who have taught us valuable lessons about attunement. As we discussed in the previous chapter, trauma challenges caregivers in many ways. There have been many caregivers who have struggled to attune to the impact of traumatic experiences on their children. Although this can be frustrating for providers, we often challenge clinicians to read the message behind (or underneath) caregiver behavior.

Factors to Assess: Caregiver

- How consistent is the caregiver's response to the child? For instance, does the caregiver routinely have difficulty reading child cues, or is the problem situation-specific? Target intervention to the needs of the dyad.

- Can the caregiver tune into cues of positive affect as well as problem situations?

- Pay attention to caregiver boundaries. Some caregivers are overly involved with their child, whereas others are dismissive or withdrawn. Work to build developmentally appropriate involvement.

- How does the caregiver conceptualize his or her child's symptoms? Consider the following example.

> An adoptive mother of 13 children met with the evaluator of her 9-year-old son. When asked whether her son had difficulties with attention or impulsivity, she stated that he did not. When the evaluator asked more specific questions about the child's daily functioning, the mother described him as "constantly moving"; during a typical family dinner, for instance, she stated that her son might be up and down from the table over 20 times. When asked about this discrepancy, she appeared surprised, noting that she did not consider his behavior problematic.

In this example the family views a behavior as normative and likely would not identify it as a treatment target. However, in other contexts, this same behavior might lead to significant difficulty and, in fact, be a primary reason for referral. This child, for instance, was failing his current grade due to ongoing difficulties with sustaining attention. This case highlights one of the common balancing acts in treatment: reinforcing a caregiver's ability to accept his or her child's behaviors and typical responses, while building the caregiver's attunement to the impact of the behavior on the child's functioning in other contexts.

■ What level of insight does the caregiver have into the reasons behind the child's difficult behaviors? Does the caregiver understand the contribution of trauma? There are many reasons caregivers may have difficulty acknowledging the role of trauma in their child's presentation. For instance, we have worked with many caregivers who have played a direct and/or indirect role in their child's traumatic experiences. This involvement creates overwhelming and sometimes intolerable feelings of shame and guilt. It is simply too painful to acknowledge and often leads to avoidant coping on the part of the caregiver. Acknowledgment and support for the range of emotions caregivers experience will be crucial, along with psychoeducation.

■ What roles do race, culture, and intergenerational experience play in the caregiver's understanding of the meaning and impact of the child's individual trauma experience? In some cultures, for instance, a child who has been sexually abused may be viewed as permanently damaged and possibly ostracized by community members. For another family, the child's experiences of trauma may be embedded in and mirror not just the parent's but the larger community's exposure to and experience of historical or individual trauma. It is important to work with the child and caregiving system to understand the particular meaning and interpretation of behaviors and experiences.

Factors to Assess: Child

■ Although the primary goal of attunement work is helping caregivers to accurately read their children's cues, a secondary goal is to help children accurately read their caregivers' responses.

■ Trauma-exposed children may be *overly tuned in* to their caregivers, feeling an age-inappropriate responsibility to take care of the adults around them; they may be *misattuned,* reading signs of anger, rejection, or abandonment where there are none; or they may have learned to withdraw from interaction (i.e., to *nonattune*) as a survival skill.

■ Although children's ability to accurately identify emotion is covered in greater detail in the "Regulation" section, it is important to assess each child's attunement style with his or her caregiver in order to help the caregiver adjust his or her response to that of the child.

Family Norms

■ "Attuned" behavior looks different across families, and level of attunement may not always be measurable by surface behavior. Consider these two examples.

> *Example 1:* A single father appears constricted and disconnected in response to his 10-year-old son's affect. Observation and report indicate that he is rarely emotionally nurturing toward his child. However, he frequently spends time teaching his son life skills and other tasks, such as fishing and farming. Over time, the clinician learns that this father's early caregiving environment lacked warmth and affection. Determined to respond to his own child's needs, the father has made a point of spending time with his son. The son describes his father as responsive and caring, citing as evidence a recent day in which his father took the time to teach him how to take an engine apart.

> *Example 2:* A mother with a 5-year-old daughter appears highly responsive to her daughter's needs. She checks in frequently with her child, often naming an affect before the child expresses it. Over time, the clinician notices that the child rarely responds to the mother's statements and often appears to withdraw as the mother becomes more responsive.

In both cases, the surface behavior is in contrast with the true level of attunement. In the first, the apparently disconnected father is well aware of his son's needs and is providing affection through dyadic tasks—a forum that is comfortable for both him and his son. In the second case, the apparently responsive mother is overly intrusive, often misreading her child's affect and missing the child's cues for distance. The key question in attunement is often the extent to which the caregiver is able to *accurately identify the child's need* and then respond in a manner that adequately meets that need.

■ Cultural background, across dimensions, is one of the factors that influences family norms about caregiver–child interactions. Consider, for instance, the influence of the caregiver's own family of origin on ways of connecting, including beliefs about affection, respect, physical contact, play, and so forth. It is important for providers to elicit information about clients' cultural norms, rather than making inadvertent assumptions.

Provider Attunement

■ *Provider attunement to caregiver:* Engagement of the caregiver is one of the most critical steps in the treatment process. The caregiver has to build a connection with the provider and trust, on some level, that his or her child is in good hands. Establishing this attunement can be extremely complicated in work with families that have had multiple providers, system involvement, and long-term struggles with child behaviors. This may also be particularly complicated in situations in which the apparent life experience of the provider is, or is perceived to be, clearly discrepant from the life experience of the child and family system. In the previous chapter we discussed many strategies for normalizing caregiver affect. Here we encourage the therapist to attune to caregiver affect as it emerges throughout the treatment process.

■ A challenge of working with children is often the multiple members of the system with whom the provider is working. As a result of taking on the role of child advocate, we may fall into the trap of demonizing the caregivers. Attunement toward the caregivers is as important as attunement toward the children. More often than not, we are working with parents or other caregivers who are doing their best in often challenging situations. As with children, when a caregiver is unable or unwilling to engage in treatment, learn or practice a new skill, or respond appropriately to his or her child, use your attunement skills to try to understand the caregiver's experience and perspective.

■ It is common for caregivers to send messages to the provider through their words and actions. For example, it is common for providers to identify difficulty working with a caregiver because the caregiver says things like "This won't work"; "I already tried that"; "I really don't see the point of this." These statements tend to push provider buttons, but if we take a step back and think about the underlying experiences of the caregiver, we can clearly see themes related to feelings of hopelessness or helplessness in the face of challenging circumstances. It is important for providers to learn to identify and validate underlying emotions in caregivers. Doing so often supports caregiver engagement.

■ *Provider attunement to child:* Along with helping caregivers attune to their children, providers should practice these same skills. Children and families who have experienced trauma may present with an array of challenging behaviors. As a provider, it is easy to target and respond to the behavior rather than to the underlying affect. Children may reenact key relational dynamics with their providers, may play out distress through behavior, and may test the provider in the same way they do their caregivers. Consider the following examples.

> *Example 1:* A clinician is in session with a 5-year-old boy who has a history of complex trauma. After completing a feelings check-in, the boy appears to become increasingly dysregulated, playing with a toy truck and banging it into walls. The therapist, worried about the noise and about safety, tells him to stop banging the truck. In response, the boy begins banging the truck harder, and the therapist warns him that if he does not stop, she will have to terminate the session.

In this example, the clinician was appropriately worried about the child's safety, but got caught in the trap of limit setting and the ensuing power struggle, rather than attempting to respond to the boy's underlying message, "I'm feeling distressed." Although safety is obviously a primary concern, the clinician's anxiety about the child's behavior prevented her from accurately attuning to the dysregulated affect driving his behavior.

> *Example 2:* A 15-year-old girl in residential treatment is in her room shortly after a phone call with her mother. A passing staff member notices that she is sitting on her bed, kicking her dresser and swearing loudly. The staff member provides a warning that sanctions will occur for swearing and dangerous behavior unless she stops. A minute later, staff hear a loud crash and enter the room to find the girl kicking with enough force that her lamp has fallen off the top of the dresser; she curses at the staff members and tells them to leave her alone. The situation escalates, leading to a physical hold.

In this example, the first staff member appropriately tries to maintain programmatic structure and safety by setting a limit. However, the staff member misses the way that the behavior reflects emotional dysregulation in response to a trigger. Observation of the girl's affect and energy, validation of her experience, and support and cuing in modulation skills may have prevented escalation.

■ As is the case with caregivers, affect management is a key first step for professionals in building our own attunement skills. Keep in mind the skills from the previous section, including self-monitoring. Know your own "push buttons" and the behaviors likely to interfere with your ability to respond versus react. Be conscious of self-care strategies and other in-the-pocket coping skills. When regulated and able to respond, the provider may act as an important model of attunement for the caregiver.

■ In this section highlighted skills include becoming a "feelings detective" and the use of reflective listening. These skills can be applied to the therapeutic relationship as well as to the dyad. Nonverbal attunement exercises, including the examples that follow, may also help to build clinician–child attunement and can often serve as the basis for coregulation.

■ Therapy with dysregulated children is often a dance; these children have varying degrees of ability to tolerate relationship, engagement, play, or discussion. Remember to pay attention to behavioral and physical cues that the client is distressed, excited, sad, or angry, and modify the session accordingly. The majority of our clients' communication is nonverbal. It is important to remember to actively observe all levels of communication and the ways this communication shifts and changes over time, and not just during moments of obvious distress and/or joy. It is one of our primary challenges to "hear the message" and respond accordingly. Consider the following example.

> Example: A 17-year-old girl with a long history of interpersonal trauma presented for her session with her therapist. She was experiencing an increase in trauma-based coping behaviors (sexual activity, substance use) in response to a trauma trigger. The therapist conducted the session and then realized at the very end that the client had sent her a nonverbal message during the greeting in the waiting area when she reached out and touched the therapist's shoulder while saying hello. This client rarely initiated touch with caregivers because it was a significant trigger. She had never initiated touch with the therapist. The therapist shared her observation with the client and inquired about the need behind it. The client was able to acknowledge her need for comfort. The therapist provided comfort and then brought the client's mother in to physically comfort her daughter—a very rare occurrence in this family.

In this example the client was not able to verbally communicate her need for comfort. She may have not even been fully aware of this need, but she was able to communicate it through this small but powerful nonverbal gesture.

■ Attunement is often about more than emotion. Sensitivity to our clients includes an awareness of creating an environment that welcomes and tunes in to diversity. Children and families who have experienced trauma often feel "different." Although it would be impossible to change the therapy room for each new client, clinicians can attempt to create an environment that invites the client to explore, create, and contribute, and that reflects the experience of the child or family on some level. Consider dolls from various cultures, male and female puppets, a tree house in addition to a dollhouse, books that include nontraditional families, forms that pay attention to the nuances of gender identity and family structure, or visuals that are reflective of the client population.

Teach to Caregivers

■ *Reminder:* Teach caregivers the Key Concepts.

■ *Reminder:* Teach caregivers the relevant Developmental Considerations.

- Keep in mind: Attunement happens on an ongoing basis. It is not just about monitoring and responding to intensive experiences, but also about day-to-day interactions. Teach caregivers to respond to children's cues across situations, whether in play, conversation, or general interaction.

Read the Message—Understanding the Function of Trauma Behavior

- In the earlier chapters of the book we referenced a three-part model for understanding child behavior. We have found it to be a helpful frame to teach to caregivers about the etiology of many behaviors that we encounter. This model presumes that many dysregulated child and adolescent behaviors can be understood through a three-step sequence: (1) the child's vigilance to danger; (2) the child's behavioral responses to perceived danger, designed to seek safety and meet needs; and (3) the child's difficulty recovering from the danger response.

Part I. The Assumption of Danger

CHILD VIGILANCE AND ATTUNEMENT

- A primary foundation for building attunement is to help caregivers understand and learn to recognize the child's danger response. Dysregulation brought on by a triggered response is often a primary source of caregiver distress.

- Children who experience trauma are often hypervigilant. They expect bad things to happen in relationships and in their world. Child vigilance of caregiver expressions may lead to moments of misattunement between child and caregiver. Awareness of the role of child vigilance may help caregivers recognize and respond to these moments.

- For expanded information and teaching points, see caregiver education handout **"Understanding Triggers"** and caregiver worksheets **"Identifying Your Child's Triggers"** and **"What Does Your Child Look Like When Triggered?"** in Appendix B.

Child Vigilance and Attunement

Child vigilance to caregiver expression may result in:
  - Misinterpretation of parental cues (e.g., overreading anger).
  - Minimizing or denying own needs due to prioritization of caregiver needs (e.g., parenting the parent).
  - Feeling overwhelmed by or afraid of signs of caregiver affect.

Help caregivers respond by:
  - **Taking the time to understand the child's perspective.** If the child reacts strongly to minor statements, try to understand what brought on the overreaction. What does the child think you're feeling? Saying? Reflect what you see, and elicit the child's thoughts or feelings (e.g., "It looks like you just got really worried when I said that. Can you help me understand why?").
  - **Being respectful of what the child is feeling.** Don't argue that the child is wrong—what he or she feels is just that (e.g., "It makes sense that you would feel really worried if you thought I was angry").
  - **Correcting misperceptions.** Once the caregiver understands the child's reaction, correct misinterpretations (e.g., "I'm so sorry that you thought I was angry. What I was trying to say was, I'm worried about what would happen if . . . ").

UNDERSTANDING TRIGGERS

Understanding Triggers

What are triggers?	A **trigger,** as commonly defined within the traumatic stress field, may be thought of as any cue that is interpreted by an individual as a sign of imminent danger; in the face of this cue, our brains assume that we are in danger *right now* and initiate a series of rapid responses designed to help us survive the danger. These cues, or triggers, become associated with danger because of historical or ongoing danger experiences, and the more frequently the cue has been associated with historical or current danger, and/or the more intense the danger, the stronger the likelihood that the trigger will lead to a survival response in the present. Triggers can be *external*—such as a facial expression that reminds a child of a past abuser, or a smell that reminds a child of a lost parent; *internal*—such as feeling hungry, frightened, or highly aroused; or a *combination*—such as an interaction that leads to a child's feeling vulnerable.
Common triggers for children who have experienced trauma	Unpredictability or sudden change Transition Loss of control Feeling vulnerable Feeling rejected Confrontation Loneliness Sensory overload (too much stimulation from the environment) Intimacy (safety, love, security, family) Peace/calm/quiet
Intersection between attachment and triggers: What caregivers should know	In the face of strong emotion, children who have previously experienced danger, rejection, or neglect may: ■ Avoid or withdraw from caregivers. ■ Become overly clingy and appear unable to take in support. ■ Freeze. ■ Appear "manipulative" or attempt to control caregivers. ■ Engage in conflicting approach and avoidance behaviors. When under stress (e.g., after being triggered), one of the biological mandates of human beings is to seek security from the primary attachment figure (i.e., the caregiver). As described above, however, the alternative strategies developed by traumatized children may prevent them from proactively seeking and taking in support. Therefore, it is particularly important for caregivers to be attuned to signs that their children are feeling overwhelmed or distressed.

Part II. Behavior Addresses a Need

Behavior Addresses a Need

What are the primary functions of trauma-related behaviors?	**Avoiding danger.** In the face of a cue of potential danger (a trigger), our brains will initiate a rapid series of biological, physiological, and behavioral changes designed to help us survive. For these changes to be initiated, there does not need to be actual danger; just the perception or interpretation of danger will lead to the same response set. For youth who have experienced frequent or intense early danger, a high vigilance toward possible danger, combined with a wide array of cues perceived as signaling danger, may lead to frequent self-protective responses.

Getting needs met. Many youth with whom we work have had repeated experiences of physical, emotional, and/or relational needs going unmet. In the face of cues such as *rejection or abandonment, deprivation, loss, hunger, denial,* and others, children and adolescents may engage in behaviors designed to help them get needs met.

What are the primary danger avoidance strategies?

Fight: A high-arousal response that may look like aggression (verbal or physical, toward people or objects), but may also look like hyper, silly, or behaviorally disorganized responses.

Flight: A drive to escape a dysregulating, frightening situation. Escape may be physical, such as running out of a room or withdrawing to another location; or it may be relational, such as ending a friendship.

Freeze: A stilling response that is also marked by high arousal. When danger is perceived that a person can neither fight nor escape, he or she may freeze and become hyperalert toward the identified source of the danger. The freeze response is a state of highly alert readiness.

Submit or comply: Submission and compliance in the face of danger that is perceived to be inescapable is a survival strategy. Children may deny their own needs, give in to others for the sake of relationship, present with a false "cheerfulness" ("Everything is fine"; "I'm happy") that does not match their presentation; or appear disconnected or spacy.

What are the primary need fulfillment behaviors?

Needs may be primarily grouped into two categories: physiological needs and emotional and relational needs. Examples of associated behaviors are listed here. However it is important to note that needs can often substitute for each other: for example, a child may attempt to meet a relational need with something concrete, or a physiological need through relationship.

Physiological needs: Strategies involving the use of concrete objects to meet needs—for instance, hoarding food or other objects, stealing, and intense attachment to a specific object.

Emotional and relational needs: Strategies used to manage relationship and internal experience. These may include, for instance, whining, engaging in negative action to gain attention, attempts to be perfect, lying, and sexualized behaviors are all common examples of this category of behavior. Children who frequently engage in need-fulfilling strategies in this category are often described by others as "needy" and/or "manipulative."

Part III. Difficulty Returning to Baseline

Difficulty Returning to Baseline

Why do the behaviors and emotions get so intense and last so long?

When someone experiences an intense emotion or physiological response, the ability to recover from that response is affected by the individual's *internal* and *external* resources. The more resources we have, the more easily we can recover; the fewer we have, the harder it is to return to a comfortable state. Children and adolescents who have experienced chronic developmental trauma may have a number of impacted capacities that make recovery difficult.

What are some important resources for managing overwhelming responses with which trauma survivors may struggle?

- Frustration tolerance
- Availability of social support
- Trust
- Problem-solving ability
- Impulse control
- Self-soothing ability
- Cognitive organization

What alternative strategies might trauma survivors use?	In the face of overwhelming affect and physiological distress, and in the absence of adequate resources, children, adolescents, and adults may turn to alternative methods for managing their experience. These *coping strategies* may themselves present as "problem behaviors" that caregivers are seeking to address. Examples include:

- Substance use
- Self-injury
- High-risk behaviors
- Disordered eating (over/undercontrolled)
- Primitive self-stimulating/self-soothing behavior (rocking, head-banging, biting)
- Sexualized behaviors

Understanding developmental state	When children experience trauma, the developmental stage at which they are functioning may differ from chronological age. This may be true across domains of development, and/or may be particularly true when the child is in a distressed state. For instance, a 15-year-old experiencing strong feelings of shame and perceived rejection, and feeling sad and overwhelmed, may suddenly seem more like a 7-year-old with regressed behaviors and increased neediness.
	An important teaching point and area of exploration with caregivers is therefore the concept of "stage, not age": asking caregivers to be curious about the developmental stage that the child appears to be operating at *in a given moment* and *in a given state,* and working to meet the child where he or she is at.

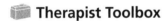

Therapist Toolbox

Skill #1: Building a Repertoire for Understanding Children's Communication: Be an Observer

- Attunement is a skill requiring parents and caregivers to become "feelings detectives." A primary goal is for all caregivers to approach behaviors and interactions from a position of curiosity: that is, when thinking about how to respond to a behavior, start with asking, "I wonder why that behavior is happening?"

- Once caregivers learn to "read" their child's cues and patterns, they can better respond to the emotion underlying the overt behavior, rather than to the behavior itself. Caregivers can then use **reflective listening skills** (see "Verbal Skills for Mirroring," below) to mirror back to the child what they are seeing in an age-appropriate way.

- It is important to give caregivers permission to start with just observing their child. Often they don't have to *do* anything. We find it useful when introducing this skill to focus on the observation aspect and to be clear with caregivers that they are not being asked to form a response to what they see just yet—unless there is imminent risk or a safety concern.

- Caregivers should learn their child's individual communication strategies. What does the child look like when he or she is angry? Sad? Excited? Worried? Joyful? What are the child's cues? For each emotion, help parents track the communication channels noted in the following table. (See caregiver education handout **"Learning Your Child's Language"** and the worksheet **"Learning Your Child's Emotional Language"** in Appendix B.

How Children Communicate

Facial expression	Includes both intense expressions and lack of expressiveness
Tone of voice	Higher-pitched, louder, softer
Extent of speech	Very verbose or very quiet; rate of speech
Quality of speech	Organization, maturity (e.g., regression)
Posturing/muscular expression	What does the child's body look like? Is the child curled up, fists clenched, muscles tense or loose, posture closed or open?
Approach versus avoidance	Does child get withdrawn, overly clingy, or both?
Affect modulation capacity	Does child have a harder time being soothed and/or self-soothing? Does child start to need more external comforting? How receptive is the child to soothing—does this change in the face of stress?
Mood	Does child's mood change overtly? For instance, is child normally even-tempered, but becomes more labile in the face of intense emotion? If so, that lability can serve as a warning sign to parents.
Behavior/coping strategies	How does child attempt to manage own mood or affect? Sucking thumb? Withdrawing to bedroom? Seeking more attention/connection from caregiver? Picking a fight with a sibling?

WAYS TO CULTIVATE CURIOSITY

Learning to be curious about a child, whether as a primary caregiver (parent, grandparent), caregiving system (teacher, milieu staff), or other provider is a skill that is built over time. The pace of the work is important to pay attention to, as some caregivers will have a more challenging time than others in developing curiosity to replace reacting in the moment.

When asking a caregiver to be curious about a child, keep in mind that the most challenging context in which to learn a new skill is one that is distressing. Because of this, it can be helpful to ask caregivers to focus first on positive affect (e.g., "I know there are a lot of hard times, but what are the moments that you feel really connected to your daughter? See if you can tune in to when those happen this week") and then gradually move into distressing behavior. Because strong affect will derail curiosity, caregiver affect management skills should be integrated into this work. It is important to emphasize to the caregiver that the first step in learning how to manage a behavior is to observe the behavior (unless there is imminent risk).

The skill of being curious can be cultivated by using displacement (i.e., presenting a fictional person/character with the skill) as well as directly.

- **Engage curiosity via displacement.** It is often helpful to teach the skill in relation to someone other than the caregiver. For example, use yourself to model cues (facial expressions, movement, energy changes, body posture) and ask the caregiver to fill out a "detective" sheet about you. Show the caregiver a video and ask him or her to fill out the sheet for a specific character or to engage in a charades activity.

- **Engage curiosity directly** about identified emotions or behaviors. This can be done proactively, often through conversation but also through completion of written worksheets or other documents, particularly in treatment systems. It can also be done in the moment, when discussing a difficult interaction or situation. Work with caregivers to identify:

◆ In-the-moment clues: What does/did the child look like when . . .

◆ Lead-in clues: What was happening just beforehand?

◆ Triggers: What are some of the things that seem to lead to the behavior/reaction?

◆ Need: What does the child seem to be attempting to accomplish with his or her behavior?

◆ Effective responses: What helps/makes things worse?

◆ Adult reactions: What is the adult caregiver's reaction/response in the moment?

Skill #2: Skills for Mirroring Child Experience

■ An awareness of the importance of *mirroring* helps caregivers actively *hear, validate,* and *communicate support* to their children. Mirroring someone's experience can be done verbally, as with reflective listening, or nonverbally, as with matching a child's energy or posture. Reflective listening skills have their roots in Rogerian client-centered therapy (e.g., Rogers, 1951) and can be used to build caregivers' capacity to actively and empathically respond to their children's communications (whether verbally or nonverbally).

■ Teach caregivers the range of mirroring skills; have caregivers practice in session with you and/or child. In addition, providers should be conscious of using these skills actively in their work with children and caregivers.

Setting the Foundation: How to Be an Active Listener and Observer

Step	Description
1. Accept and respect all of a child's feelings.	There should never be a hidden agenda to "change" the child's feelings (e.g., *not* "You shouldn't be angry").
2. Show child that you are listening and observing.	Work to be present with the child. Engage actively in relationship or interaction. Apply active listening skills: Use eye contact, nod your head, respond verbally, etc.
3. Don't rush to *do* too soon. Offer advice/suggestions/reassurance/ alternative perceptions *only* after helping child to express how he or she feels.	Particularly when we perceive there to be a "problem," the urge is to "fix it." It can be important, though, to mirror and tune in to experience (i.e., actively observe) before rushing to action. Don't jump to problem solving until you've taken the time to hear what the child has to say or demonstrated that you see what a child is showing you with his or her actions and behavior.

Verbal Mirroring Skills

Skill	Description
Reflect	*Definition:* Empathic observation or witnessing of someone's experience. *How to:* Reflection involves putting language to someone's experience by observing and naming what is seen. Observation can be surface level ("Boy, is your body wiggly") but can also go beneath the behavior to what is driving it ("It looks like you're feeling really upset right now").

Skill	Description
	Examples: ■ "I notice your energy just got really high!" ■ "Your face looks so sad right now." ■ "Boy, something is off in our interaction—you seem really frustrated with what I'm doing right now."
	Caution: It is important that reflective observations leave room for error: An observation is an interpretation, rather than a fact, and children should always be allowed to reject our statements. Observations should be made either empathically or factually; if there is judgment, there is no empathic mirror for the child.
Validate	*Definition:* Acknowledging an individual's "truth" or reality.
	How to: When we validate, we are communicating that a person's response matters and makes sense based on his or her perception. Validating is different from agreeing with the perception or approving of the resulting behavior. We validate by naming/observing an understandable link between a child's emotion or reaction and its context.
	Examples: ■ "It makes sense that your energy is really high right now. I know you just visited your mom and it's been a long time since you've seen her." ■ "I can imagine that you felt really angry about the way your teacher talked to you, and that's why you shouted at her." ■ "People sometimes do things that they wouldn't normally do when they're really upset, like when you broke your mother's vase."
	Caution: Because the link made between the child's behavior and its cause is often based on the adult's observation, rather than the child's, the child may reject it ("That's not why I'm mad!"). Validation may be a harder skill for adult caregivers to develop because it can feel as if we are giving permission for a negative behavior or reaction.
Normalize	*Definition:* When we normalize something the child has done or expressed, we affirm that the child is not the only one who has ever had a particular reaction, emotion, or behavior. We include the child or adolescent in a community of others who sometimes get angry, feel frightened, get overwhelmed, hate everyone, don't know how to make friends, etc.
	How to: We normalize by making a statement that links the child's behaviors or emotions to those of other people. This can be a direct linkage ("I know it's really hard to make friends sometimes; I worry about going to new places, too") or an indirect/broad one ("Lots of kids might worry about going somewhere new").
	Examples: ■ "I would imagine anyone might feel frustrated by that." ■ "I've known so many kids who get anxious when they have to go to court." ■ "A lot of our students are confused by the rules when they start in our program."
	Caution: Although the intent of a normalizing statement is to support children in feeling less alone, they may feel as if the statement "steals" their unique reactions, feelings, and experiences. It is not uncommon for a child to respond, for instance, with "No one else knows what I feel like!" It is important to provide permission for this kind of response: "You're right, no one does know what it feels like to be you. I've known a lot of kids who have had hard feelings, but all of them are different in their own ways."

As with building curiosity, this skill is developed over time, and the teaching of it may move from a displaced approach to a direct one.

Skill #3: Using Attunement Skills to Coregulate Child Experience

Mirroring of experience takes place on many levels that go beyond language. We mirror those around us with our whole self. This may include energy, pace, and tone of speech or movement and posture. If a child is talking to a caregiver excitedly about something that happened at school and the caregiver responds quietly, slowly, and unenthusiastically, then the child will not experience the caregiver as attuned. In addition, caregiver attunement supports many of the regulation skills that we highlight in following chapters, including the child's ability to learn to increase/decrease arousal. When the caregiver uses his or her own attuned responses to actively influence a child's experience, the outcome can be thought of as *coregulation*. For instance, a caregiver might intentionally move from direct mirroring of the child's experience toward a purposeful shift in his or her own arousal (e.g., caregiver meets child's excitement with his or her excitement and then slowly decreases the rate and rhythm of speech to ease down the child's arousal).

When the provider is mirroring and coregulating the child's experience, and/or teaching caregivers to do the same, it is helpful to engage actively in this process through games and shared/collaborative activities. Examples of dyadic attunement exercises are supplied here.

DYADIC ATTUNEMENT EXERCISES

▦ The following exercises can be used in both dyadic and individual therapy. In dyadic therapy the caregiver and child should do the exercises together, with the clinician as observer/facilitator.

▪ It is particularly important to include these activities in the context of the material covered in "Teach to Caregivers," as well as the skills covered previously.

Dyadic Attunement Exercise Examples

Activity	Variations	Description
Feelings charades	Basic	Caregiver (or clinician) acts out a feeling state; child must guess. Child then takes turn acting, while caregiver guesses.
	Reverse	Caregiver acts out what child looks like during a particular feeling state; child must guess. Roles are then switched, and child acts out what caregiver looks like.
	Triggering situation (variation 1)	Caregiver and child pick a feeling; caregiver or child acts out a situation that might elicit that feeling, and partner guesses the situation.
	Triggering situation (variation 2)	Caregiver acts out a difficult situation; child must identify potential emotional responses. Roles are then reversed.
	Identify the person	Caregiver and child pick an emotion together. The actor portrays a known individual (e.g., someone in the family) in that emotional state; partner must guess the individual.
	There is an infinite number of variations on this game; target the game to the family's needs.	
Follow-the-leader games	Music	Use drums or other musical instrument. One partner creates a rhythm; the other must follow and/or build on the original rhythm.
	Dance/movement	One partner creates a physical movement; the other must follow or build on the original movement.
	Mirroring	Two partners face each other. One partner engages in slow movements; the other must follow. Goal is to be attuned to the point that an observer cannot discriminate the leader from the follower.
	Follow the leader	For younger children, pick a fun movement (e.g., walking across the room like a duck); all in the room must copy the movement.
	Classic follow-the-leader games	Consider games such as Simon Says, Red Light/Green Light, etc., to build attunement.

Activity	Variations	Description
Parallel "self" books		Work with caregivers and children to create a joint "All about Us" book. The book should contain parallel entries by caregiver and child. For example, pick an event that happened over the past week and have each describe his or her feelings, favorite part, least favorite part, etc.
Play		Work with caregivers to play *with* their children. Any type of play will work: board games, imaginary play, expressive arts, etc. Teach caregivers to follow their child's lead and not to instruct or direct. Teach caregivers to use reflective listening skills.
Comfort		Work with caregivers to create opportunities to provide shared experiences of comfort. This may be as simple as sitting together on the couch, reading a book together, a moment when a child sits in the caregiver's lap, etc.

Skill #4: Putting It All Together: What to Do When a Child Is Triggered

■ All caregiver skills in this framework provide a foundation and a support for the child/adolescent skills discussed in Parts V (regulation) and VI (Competency) of this book.

■ As mentioned previously, sensitive caregiver attunement is a primary tool for supporting child regulation skills, particularly when a child is triggered.

■ As you work with children on regulation skills, teach caregivers the following sequence for supporting child modulation. Note how the steps parallel child identification and modulation work.

Steps toward Supporting Child Modulation

Step	Description
1. Be attuned: Keep on your detective hat.	Be aware of shifts in the child's feelings. If you are not sure what the child is feeling, notice the energy: Is it high or low? Withdrawn or active? Look for the cues that were identified during "feelings detective" work (Skill #1), particularly those indicating that the child has been triggered. The goal over time is to get in front of the big reactions by anticipating and recognizing them as they start to occur.
2. Keep yourself centered.	Check in with yourself. Use your own affect management skills. Even if nothing else feels in control, you can try to stay in control of your own emotions and actions.
3. Reflect, simply, what you are seeing.	Name what you see, but keep it simple. Keep in mind which part of the child's brain is in charge. The purpose of reflection when a child is very dysregulated is to begin the coregulation process and/or cue him or her to use modulation skills (e.g., "I can see that your energy just got really high. Let's see if we can bring it down a little bit so we can talk").
4. Cue child in use of skills.	Be aware of the range of modulation skills on which the child is working in treatment. Offer simple suggestions of a tool the child might use, either with you or independently (e.g., breathing deeply, sitting quietly, moving to the calming-down space, using a stress ball). Early in treatment it is suggested that you engage the child in learning these skills in order to practice regulation strategies and effectively model them for the child. Pay attention to opportunities for giving the child control; for example, allow the child to actively decide among alternatives (one tool or another, alone or with supports) as a way to decrease his or her felt danger.
5. Support, and engage with the child in use of skills.	One of the primary goals here is to help the child tune in to his or her own physiological experience. consider the following wording as a template for helping the child acquire this skill: "Right now, you are having big feelings. Everything feels hard. I am wondering if there is something that we can do together to make things feel a little better? See if you can notice your breath and now notice your breath slowing down, slowing down, slowing down."

Step	Description
6. Reinforce the use of modulation skills.	Be sure to tune in to the child's attempts to modulate (e.g., "I'm really proud of you for trying to calm down your energy"). Remember that success is relative; just noticing that an emotion is dysregulated may be a success for some children.
7. Invite expression.	Once the child is calmed, invite expression/communication. Put the rest of those reflective listening skills to work!

ᛘᛘᛘ Developmental Considerations

Developmental stage	Attunement considerations
General considerations	Teach caregivers what is normative versus atypical at a given age. As an example, it is normative for 2-year-olds to assert their independence by saying "no"; this is part of appropriate and healthy development and *not* about being "oppositional," as it might be for an older child.
	One of the challenges in caregivers' understanding of normative behavior is the impact of ongoing cultural changes in the experience of children at a given age. A 15-year-old in 2018 will have a very different experience than a 15-year-old did in 1975. Acknowledge these differences, and when feasible, invite a dialogue. Allow caregivers and children to teach each other about their lives.
	Regardless of age, using language to communicate their needs is often difficult for trauma-impacted children. With less practice in safe forms of expression and lower frustration tolerance, these children often have no choice but to communicate their needs through their behavior.
	Children in substitute caregiving systems may have a different cultural background than that of their caregiver(s). Given the influence of culture on social interaction and emotional expression, attunement may be a particular challenge (both for the caregiver and the child). Again, acknowledge differences and invite a dialogue.
Early childhood	Young children are increasingly able to use language for communication. However, although they become efficient at communicating wants and needs through words (e.g., "I want apple juice," "I want that toy"), feelings continue to be primarily communicated through behaviors and physical states (e.g., temper tantrums as a sign that child is frustrated; upset stomachs as sign child is anxious or worried; shutting down/withdrawing as sign of need for reassurance).
	As children become more sophisticated in language use, adults may overestimate their reasoning ability as well as their capacity to use language to communicate internal state. Therefore, it is particularly important for caregivers to understand where their child is "at" developmentally and to learn to interpret behavioral cues.
	Part of how attunement helps young children is to provide a foundation for the building of affect identification, expression, and regulation skills. By using verbal labels to identify children's states, caregivers are supplying the building blocks of emotional knowledge.
	Attuning to children's emotions and helping them to attune to the experience of others also act as a foundation for the building of empathy and interpersonal interaction skills.
Middle childhood	Children at this age are increasingly tuned in to caregiver expression and feeling states. This can be positive for building empathy and perspective taking, but has multiple pitfalls for overly vigilant, trauma-impacted children.
	The elementary school years are the peak age for somatic expression of symptoms (headaches, stomachaches, etc.). Caregivers should pay attention to signs that the child's body may be holding/communicating affect for him or her.

Developmental stage	Attunement considerations
Adolescence	The key word for attunement in adolescence is *balance:* between connection and independence, privacy and disclosure, and so on. Although caregivers often want to know *more* about their children during this higher-risk period, it is normative for adolescents to want to communicate *less.* Some of the negative behaviors, emotions, and interactions that emerge at this point may, in fact, be reconceptualized as the teen's striving for independence and separation.
	Adolescents often have ambivalent feelings about their need for nurturance versus their desire for independence. Because of this ambivalence, it is important for caregivers to provide opportunities for connection while respecting adolescents' negotiation of closeness and distance.
	An important part of attunement at this age is respecting privacy. Negotiate this area actively: Where can the adolescent maintain privacy, and where does the caregiver draw the line in terms of "need-to-know" information?

Applications
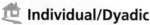 Individual/Dyadic

Work with caregivers in individual caregiver education sessions or, if necessary, by phone. Consider using ARC caregiver handouts and worksheets (Appendix B), if appropriate. Intervention in this section involves psychoeducation as well as active exploration, practice, and homework. For instance, than simply teaching caregivers about the ways a child may communicate, ask caregivers to track signs of anger or distress in their child over the course of a week, or complete a detailed detective worksheet ("Being a Detective: Understanding a Child's Patterns") in session about a particular child emotion or experience and the ways in which it manifests. Educating caregivers about triggers and exploring ways in which the child demonstrates triggered responses are crucial aspects of this intervention target.

Once caregivers have a basic understanding of the concepts, it is important to apply attunement skills "in the moment." For instance, consider the following example. About her adolescent daughter, a mother states: "She was driving me crazy this morning—she was all over the place, bouncing off the walls. She wouldn't listen to anything I said, and then got all snarly when I tried to send her to her room." Rather than focusing on the behavior of the child, the therapist might consider working with the mother to go *beneath* the behavior to the likely emotion driving it, the precipitating factors, and/or the function of the current behaviors. It is important, when doing this, to also validate and normalize the caregiver's frustration with the behavior itself, and to explore the caregiver's own use of affect management skills.

Experiential practice of self-monitoring and self-regulation for the caregiver can be a valuable tool. Often the caregivers themselves have had little exposure to the self-care strategies discussed in the previous section. Consider building ongoing practice of dyadic attunement activities and modulation support steps into session routines in order to increase comfort with use of the various skills.

Group

Caregiver groups can be an invaluable way to teach key skills and provide information, while simultaneously providing caregivers with support from others who have had similar experiences. Use the "Teach to Caregivers" section as a guide for curriculum content. Active teaching is better than passive: Invite caregivers to share ideas of ways in which their children communicate, evidence they have seen of triggered responses, and the like. Hearing from other caregivers often helps normalize behaviors caregivers have observed in their own children. As with individual caregiver education sessions, keep in mind the value of application and practice.

Milieu

In a milieu system, staff at all levels and particularly direct-care staff are in the role of substitute caregivers. Education and training in trauma response and triggers for all milieu staff are crucial. It is important to make this training "real": Rather than speaking in the abstract, apply the concepts to the residents/students/clients served by the system. For instance, pick a particular child and ask staff to consider (1) ways in which that child demonstrates the fight, flight, or freeze response; (2) observations about situations that trigger the child; and (3) strategies that appear to help (i.e., those strategies that increase child felt safety) versus make things worse (typically, strategies that increase felt helplessness or perceived danger). Compare different children: How does Resident A, who has many externalizing behaviors, show a triggered response, and how is that different from Resident B, who is generally quiet and constricted?

Help staff to understand the range of ways in which children show their feelings. Integrate these concepts into routine clinical discussions, staff meetings, or other forums in which youth behavior and functioning are discussed. Ultimately, the goal is for staff to develop a repertoire for understanding the "communication strategies" of every resident/client, and to learn to read these messages and respond in a way that supports longer-term goals, rather than reacting to immediate behaviors. Consider building in systematic tools for supporting modulation within the milieu itself in order to increase implementation by both counselors and clients. For example, when possible, create a safe space for use of modulation strategies. Have modulation-related activities readily available to staff and clients. Examples of such activities are discussed in greater detail in Chapter 11.

The Value of Misattunement and Mess-Ups

Be sure to pair caregiver affect management skills with efforts to build attunement for all levels of intervention, and to normalize the frequent "misattunements" that occur. It is impossible for a caregiver to remain attuned at all times, and in fact, the missteps can strengthen an attachment bond, if handled well. Support caregivers in backtracking, reviewing difficult interactions, and considering alternative responses. Whether this is done as a supervisor in a residential system with milieu staff, or as a clinician in your own supervision, or with an individual parent, it is crucial to pay attention to safety: Caregivers must feel safe enough to acknowledge the "mess-ups" and the missed moments. Use these moments constructively:

They are all part of a learning process. When necessary, support caregivers in taking steps toward reparation or resolution. These moments are often as important as the moments that are attuned: It is rare for a child to hear an adult express regret at the way a situation or interaction was handled, so such an experience can be infinitely valuable for both caregiver and child in building real-world relationships.

◌ Trauma Experience Integration: State-Based Skills Application

Distress Tolerance and Regulation

During early stages of treatment or when caregivers are experiencing more intense stress, attunement work will necessarily focus on attunement to caregiver experience, rather than emphasizing the caregiver's attunement to the child. As such, parallel attunement is an important subskill of this phase because it provides the foundational support for caregiver regulation that will, over time, allow the caregiver to attune to the child. Caregivers in overwhelmed states can and should be supported in acquiring a basic understanding that child behaviors are communications ("It makes sense that . . ."), and ongoing education about trauma, attachment, and child development may help to normalize the child and family's experience.

Curiosity and Reflection

In moments when the caregiver is able to engage in curious observation and "feelings detective" work, attunement work can focus on a wider range of goals, including identification of child triggers ("When I raise my voice, I notice that Ethan gets hyper and has more difficulty listening to what I'm asking him to do"); recognition of patterns ("Every morning after tooth brushing, Ethan goes into his room and gets very quiet for about 5 minute—I'm not sure why this is, but I am sure that it happens every day"); and building awareness of the function of behaviors ("I'm wondering if the reason that Ethan gets so hyper is because when his dad used to yell at me when we were together, Ethan would run to his room and pretend to wrestle his stuffed animals").

Engaging Purposeful Action

Over time, as caregivers build mastery of attunement skills they will begin to apply those skills in the moment by mirroring child experience and using active attunement skills to meet needs, coregulate moments of dysregulation, and enhance overall felt safety of the child and family. For instance, caregivers can take part in actively and collaboratively engaging their child in gaining a shared understanding of the function of trauma-related behavior, triggers, and patterns across a range of experiences and affective states. This new understanding, in turn, supports child identification skills (covered in Chapter 10). Caregiver attunement will also increase and support child regulation strategies in the moment of child dysregulation. When consistency with regulation support grows, so too does the child's modulation toolbox (see Chapter 11).

In addition to supporting child regulation, caregivers can use mirroring skills to reflect on areas of child identity, including positive and unique attributes, to begin to expand the child's sense of identity so that he or she can begin to build a life narrative that includes, but is not exclusively about, traumatic experience. Ultimately, trauma processing can be supported by the attuned system.

Real-World Therapy

Match the work to the caregiver. As with other principles in the "Attachment" section, keep in mind that attunement may be more difficult for caregivers with unresolved trauma. In particular, these caregivers may, like their children, vigilantly attend to others' expressions and/or feel shame or guilt about their children's emotions. It is important to match the caregiver affect tolerance work with the attunement work.

Have realistic expectations. Define success in terms of where the dyad started and build success step by step.

Pay attention to vicarious trauma. Tuning in to strong emotions can kick up difficult emotions in both the clinician and the caregiver. Pay attention to your own self-care needs.

9

Effective Response

 THE MAIN IDEA AND KEY SUBSKILLS

Support the caregiving system, whether familial or programmatic, in building predictable, safe, and appropriate responses to children's behaviors in a manner that acknowledges and is sensitive to the role of past experiences in current behaviors.

★ Proactive identification of target behaviors
★ Use of attunement skills to identify and understand patterns of child behavior
★ Implement "go-to" strategies (meet needs, support regulation) to reduce and address identified behaviors.
★ Identify, experiment with, and enhance other behavioral response strategies (problem solving, positive reinforcement, limit setting) that increase youth and environmental safety.

★ Key Concepts

★ Why Do We Need to Think about Trauma in our Response to Behavior?

- An important part of building a safe environment is building safe and effective caregiver responses to child and adolescent behaviors.

- For children who have experienced trauma at the hands of their primary caregivers, limits may have been associated historically with powerlessness and intense vulnerability. Previous caregivers may have been perceived as out of control, punitive, and frightening.

- Even for children who were not harmed by primary caregivers, trauma itself is often perceived as an unpredictable punishment from the environment.

- Following these early exposures, children's behaviors often become dysregulated and impulsive, and are frequently the reason for referral to mental health or other services. Behaviors may be viewed as oppositional, manipulative, impulsive, overwhelming, and difficult to control, and as a result caregivers may enter a cycle of reactive and often ineffective responses that further escalate, rather than decrease, the behaviors.

141

- A caregiving environment that provides safe, predictable responses to behavior provides children with reassurance that there are meaningful rules and consequences, both positive and negative, for behavior; that there are lines and boundaries defining appropriate behavior; that there are caregivers who are able to keep children safe; and that there are expectations for which children are believed to be capable of fulfilling. When caregiver responses are embedded in an attuned understanding of *why* behaviors are occurring, the need for the behaviors decreases over time. Eventually, children begin to relax some of their vigilance and control, and to invest their energy into tasks of normative development.

 ## It Takes Two: Child and Adolescent Factors That Interfere with Effective Caregiver Responses

- All rules (in families, in systems) presume—on some level—a shared belief system about the world. For instance, a rule such as "Don't steal" presumes that someone's needs can be met in a more prosocial way; a rule such as "no fighting" presumes that there is a better way to keep yourself safe. For youth who have grown up in unjust, unsafe circumstances, there is often a very different sense of social justice guiding their actions.

- Even when children and adolescents agree, in calm states, with rules and behavioral guidelines, when they are in a state of heightened arousal (i.e., when the danger response goes off), they will have greater difficulty responding to adult cues and limits. Keep in mind that the survival drive will always trump the child's ability to cooperate.

- In the face of unpredictability and chaos, such as that associated with trauma, one of the adaptations children often make is to attempt to control their environment and others around them. This controlling behavior is the child's best effort to achieve safety in what is perceived as an unpredictable and dangerous world.

- Although clear, consistent limits and boundaries help children feel safe and are crucial for healthy development, children impacted by trauma may be reactive to and triggered by both limit setting and praise, as these responses are initially perceived as a threat to their own control.

 ## Therapist Toolbox
 ### What's the Stake?

- Challenges with behavior are often the primary reason for referral, and it is typically not difficult to get caregivers or other caregiving providers to sign on to the idea that youth behaviors should be a point of focus for any intervention. What may be more challenging for caregivers, however, is the idea that they, the caregivers, may need to shift their responses or actions in order to manage children's behavior more effectively.

- Because difficult behaviors are so often a point of distress (for a family, for a caregiving system), talking about behavior and adult response patterns is a natural point of entry. However, the choices we make as adults—whether in parenting or in responding to a child's behaviors professionally—often feel very personal and very loaded. Most adults have strong beliefs about what children should or should not do; about the best way to handle behavior; about the values children should be taught throughout their growing-up years; and about the messages adult actions send to children about those behaviors. These beliefs may be drawn from the ways we adults were raised ourselves; from our personal value system; from our cultural background and influences; and from the communications we receive from others in our families, communities, or surrounding environments. Addressing adult responses can easily feel like criticism: a judgment not just of the individual parent or caregiver, but of his or her beliefs, background, and culture.

■ Particularly for primary caregivers, there is little that feels like a more personal reflection on ability as a parent than a child's behaviors, and attempts to manage those behaviors—particularly when they are challenging—may easily become intense, reactive, and rigid. Because of these factors, any discussion of behavior management strategies that focuses on what the parent/caregiver is/is not/should be doing, in the absence of an attuned understanding of the caregiver's experience or goals, is likely to fail.

■ In working to build effective behavior response strategies, there are several points of entry that we have found to be essential:

1. **Engage the caregiver in discussing his or her values or beliefs.** Who does this person want to be (as a parent, as a child care provider, in relationship as a youth worker, etc.)? How does the caregiver view his or her role? What values does the caregiver want to bring to relationship with the child, and what values is he or she hoping the child will internalize over time? In what ways do the child's current behaviors challenge those values?

2. **Explore history of caretaker's caregivers.** Most caretakers will bring their own experiences to the table: in being parented themselves and in learning to manage their own behaviors. It is not uncommon to hear statements such as "Well, my mother did it and it worked for me!" or "I learned to control myself and I came from the same background." Challenging the strategies of someone who feels that those strategies were successful in shaping his or her own life can feel like a direct criticism of the individual (or of important others in the individual's life). Get curious about identifying where the person's strategies originated, what aspects of those strategies worked (e.g., was it being hit that was effective, or was it knowing that there were consequences for behavior?), and what values and beliefs the individual has brought forward from those experiences.

3. **Be curious about the ways the child's behavior may be impacting the child, caregiver, or family's experience.** For many parents, one of the primary reasons they want to stop a child's behavior is because of the fear or worry they have about the impact of the child's behavior on the child's safety or on the family's safety. Parents may be realistically afraid of the way their child will be treated in school, by community members, by law enforcement, or by other relatives, and the sense of urgency they feel is linked to these anticipated consequences more than to the child's actions themselves. Understanding these fears is often crucial to engaging caregivers in experimenting with and building effective responses to child behavior.

4. **Be attuned to the caregiver's affect.** There are few things more destined to lead to failure in attempts to address behavior response strategies than ignoring the experience of the adult engaging in those strategies. To use any response strategy effectively, the adult must have some degree of awareness of his or her internal state and the ability to manage it. The starting point for helping caregivers to acquire this ability is often

to acknowledge, explore, and support their affects in the face of youth behaviors. The truth is, many of the behaviors of trauma-impacted children and youth that lead to services are distressing and overwhelming for adults caring for them, and it makes sense that caregivers go to extreme measures at times to manage those behaviors. Witnessing, affirming, understanding, and acknowledging adults' experiences lay an important foundation for any skill-building.

5. **Acknowledge differences.** As providers, we may differ in many ways from the families, colleagues, or systems with whom we work. We may or may not have children, we may come from different parenting backgrounds, have different cultural or religious influences, and have experienced different types of stress or resource in our lives. In broader society, negative behaviors may be viewed through a different lens for some youth than others, and there are often more significant consequences for youth of color, youth from impoverished backgrounds, youth whose behavior does not follow gender norms, and many other social groups for whom society continues to carry prejudicial and extreme responses. These real-world consequences may make caregivers' own responses more extreme, more emotionally loaded, and more fear-based than in other circumstances. In our work with caregivers, we have found that it is crucial to acknowledge differences in experience, to be open to learning and understanding about the world of the adult and child, and to work together at all levels to support caregiving choices that ultimately support safety of the child.

Behind the Scenes

■ The goals of building trauma-informed behavior responses in caregivers are twofold: (1) incorporating the caregiving system's understanding of the role of trauma in shaping child behavior into the caregiver's responses to those behaviors (i.e., incorporating attunement skills into child management strategies) and (2) building a capacity to respond to behaviors in a way that is consistent, appropriate, and sensitive to trauma influences on the child's responses.

■ When addressing the area of behavioral response in the home environment, the target of intervention is generally the primary caregiver(s), along with appropriate collateral or substitute caregiving systems (e.g., school settings, foster care), and ideally with the collaboration of the child. In a system, the target is typically the pattern of responses within the system as a whole, across and among staff members.

■ Norms about what is considered "appropriate" caregiving vary widely across cultures. Behaviors that might be considered abusive in one context are considered acceptable and responsible parenting in another. Research shows, in fact, that effective parenting strategies differ across culture and context. It is important to understand the belief system of your client as well as contextual variables prior to developing treatment targets. Consider the following example.

> Keon was a 12-year-old African American boy being raised by a single father in an urban inner-city area. Keon came to session one day and angrily reported that his father had given him a "whupping" the night before. When the clinician spoke with the father, he acknowledged disciplining his son with a belt after his son brought home a negative report from school that led to a week of detention.

In this example, the clinician is faced with a dilemma. Striking the child with a belt may be considered an incident requiring a mandated report. However, in this family's culture, the father's discipline of his son is considered appropriate, and in fact responsible, parenting. In conversation, the father discusses the discipline he received as a child, his own mistakes during his teen years, and his determination that his son will succeed. In this, as in many situations, clinicians are faced with the challenge of balancing validation of the caregiver's values, belief systems, and cultural norms with accommodation to societal laws.

■ Our own experience with parenting (as child and as caregiver) may influence our beliefs about what constitutes "good parenting." Pay attention to your own biases.

■ When assessing parenting behaviors, it is important to understand not just the action but the intent behind the action. Consider this example.

> A grandfather with significant health issues is caring for his two young grandchildren who have recently emigrated from Cuba; the children's parents remain behind. The family lives in a housing project in a dangerous neighborhood, and the grandfather reports significant drug activity and other violence in the building and surrounding area. During an evaluation, the children report that their grandfather frequently sits at the door to the apartment with a belt in his lap and hits them if they try to go out the door. The grandfather reports significant fears for the safety of his grandchildren, and concern that, due to his own physical disability, he would be unable to go after them if they left without permission.

In this example the grandfather's *intent* is to keep his grandchildren safe from the significant violence in their environment. His *action* is one that has raised significant concerns by treaters and child welfare. In working with this family, it is essential to understand and validate the intent behind his actions.

Intergenerational Layers

■ Many children who experience chronic, complex trauma have parents or other primary caregivers who themselves have experienced, to some degree, stress within their own families of origin and a lack of appropriate parenting.

■ In the absence of a model of appropriate and attuned parenting, stressed caregivers and caregiving systems will make attempts to care for their children, and to manage behavior, in as effective a manner as they are able.

■ It is our experience that the majority of parents are doing the best they can, based on the resources, supports, and experiences available to them. Given this starting point, it is crucial that the intervener work to develop an empathic attunement to the caregiver. Although as professionals we must balance this support with our obligation to protect, a crucial foundation of the work described in this chapter is attunement to the caregiver and the understanding that, as with children, *the behaviors of the caregiver make sense.* We are at our most effective in working with caregivers when we first attempt to step into their shoes.

■ Along with attunement, it is crucial to maintain an awareness of the importance of caregivers experiencing success as they learn and practice new skills. Behavior management strategies are hard work, when first attempted; build skills slowly and in manageable steps.

■ When caregivers struggle to consistently implement behavior management strategies, it may be a result of strong emotional responses to child behaviors. When caregiver affect is driving behavioral response—which happens for all caregivers some percentage of the time, even in the best of circumstances—it is common for caregivers to impulsively select ineffective strategies. Examples of these ineffective approaches may include the "Just stop it" approach, the "Talk until your blue in the face" approach, the "You need to . . ." approach, and the "Forget it—I'm done!" approach. These strategies are often *reactions,* rather than *proactive attempts to address behavior,* and are typically ineffective in the long run and may actually increase, rather than decrease, the child's provoking behavior.

■ Keep in mind that it will be important to employ these same skills in building safety and predictability in the therapeutic relationship and the therapeutic space. Although limits and rules will necessarily differ from those in the home setting, clear expectations and boundaries in the therapeutic space are essential.

■ A number of strategies can be used to support caregivers in building increasingly effective behavioral responses. Consider the following broad approaches to support this skill set; specific steps and techniques appear in the next section.

Parallel attunement and curiosity	Get curious about the caregiver: How did the caregiver learn to respond to behaviors? What is the caregiver attempting to do in his or her responses? Take the time to learn about the caregiver's values and goals in caring for the child.
	Work to understand the caregiver's own experience. In examining patterns of behavior, the *caregiver* experience is as important as the child's experience.
Psychoeducation	Describe why it is often harder to change behavior in children who experience trauma because of the entrenched nature of survival-based behavior.
	Discuss common caregiver responses and emotions that interfere with consistent limit setting.
	Explain how no two children respond the same way to any single strategy and about how any single strategy is not likely to work for every behavior.
Behavioral skills training	Teach appropriate use of behavioral strategies, including praise and reinforcement, appropriate limit setting, and effective problem solving, as described in the upcoming sections.
Practice	Help caregivers to role-play skills in session; target both typical day-to-day scenarios as well as potential trouble spots.
Caregiver coaching	It can be particularly useful to hold dyadic sessions with the child in order to support the caregiver's application of these skills.
Modeling	For caregivers who have difficulty with application, clinicians can model the skills in dyadic sessions.
Homework	Don't just talk about the skills; have caregivers actively practice and track the outcome of at least one skill (specified in advance) each week.

■ The following broad considerations can be useful in increasing the likelihood of treatment success.

Collaborate in target selection	Caregivers need to be engaged in selection of targets. Collaboration is essential for behavioral skills training to be successful. Caregivers will often want to target the most distressing, entrenched behaviors first. However, doing so may be frustrating and demoralizing. Work with caregivers to break down difficult targets into smaller steps. Balance caregiver identification of the most pressing "wants" with your own assessment of the family's needs.
Start small and build	For caregivers to be successful, targeted skills should be realistic. Never target more than one or two behaviors at a time. Start by teaching reinforcement rather than limit setting. Target behaviors in which the child already engages, to some degree. With limit setting, don't start with the most difficult behaviors.
Use successive approximations	When targeting difficult behaviors, follow the rule of successive approximation: Success builds in small steps, not large leaps. *Example:* A child consistently punches a sibling when angry. The goal is to reduce *dangerous* expressions of anger, and *then* to build healthier coping strategies, including use of modulation tools and healthier expression. *Step 1:* Reinforce any expression of anger that does not involve physical harm to self or other (e.g., punching a pillow or slamming a door is considered a success in this first step). *Step 2:* Reinforce use of modulation skills, such as those built during self-regulation work (e.g., the child's "Feelings Toolbox"). *Step 3:* Reinforce the use of verbal expression—or the child's ability to communicate safely to others—to convey that he or she is feeling angry. Keep in mind that this is the most difficult step.
Predict pitfalls	Collaborate with caregivers to predict trouble spots. Potential trouble spots may be a result of: ▪ Child triggers (e.g., transitions, anniversaries, locations). ▪ Caregiver "push buttons" (e.g., whining, nagging, lying); in a system, consider individual push buttons as well as systemically vulnerable areas. ▪ Atypical routines (e.g., vacation days). ▪ The presence of multiple caregivers. ▪ The presence of additional stressors, including positive ones (e.g., birthday parties, playdates).
Experiment	Encourage caregivers to try new techniques. Predict in advance that some may not be successful. (However, remind caregivers that nothing will be successful if not applied consistently, over a realistic time frame.)
Assign homework	Remind caregivers that learning new skills takes practice. Select specific targets and have caregivers practice and track the new skills each day. Check on the application of skills, successes, and trouble spots each week. When possible, it may be helpful to be available to caregivers for "on-the-spot" telephone consultation at the start of applying a new skill.
Provide reinforcement	Work with caregivers to identify and use both verbal and concrete forms of reinforcement with their children on a consistent basis. Help them praise child effort as well as success. Be sure to reinforce caregivers for success.
Track progress	With difficult behaviors, it is often helpful for clinicians to track weekly change (e.g., using charts or tables). Small change is often easier to identify over time with the help of concrete markers.

📋 Teach to Caregivers

- *Reminder:* Teach the caregiver the Key Concepts.
- *Reminder:* Teach the caregiver the relevant Developmental Considerations.

Skill #1: Be Proactive

Behavioral response strategies are often reactive: A child engages in a challenging behavior, and the caregiver reacts to address it. When the caregiver's response is ineffective or the behavior is intense, both the reactive caregiver response and the youth behavior can escalate over time, leaving both parties feeling highly aroused, frustrated, and overwhelmed.

Teach caregivers the following:

- Frustration with a child's or adolescent's behaviors can lead us to be reactive: to respond with escalating consequences (or increasing disconnection) every time the behavior occurs. That response can actually increase the difficult behavior and leave us feeling frustrated and helpless.
- The first step of an effective behavior plan is to concretely identify the behaviors we want to address. By taking the time to identify and define a behavior, we can begin to get in front of it.
- Start by identifying a limited number of behaviors to address (no more than two or three at a time). Define and describe these behaviors concretely: What is the specific behavior of concern, and what would you like to see happen instead?
- Be sure to identify behaviors you want to increase, as well as those you want to decrease.

Skill #2: Every Behavior Has a Function: Identify What is Driving Child Behavior

- In Chapter 2, we provide a three-part model for understanding the development of trauma-based behavior, and we review that model in Chapter 8. When working to address challenging youth behaviors, a crucial first step is to identify patterns and understand why a behavior is occurring. A foundation for doing that is to understand that trauma-based behaviors develop for very specific reasons. Without reviewing all teaching points in depth here, it is important to address the following key points:

From Where Do Trauma-Based Behaviors Come?

Remember the child's lens of the world	Youth who have experienced trauma approach the world expecting that bad things will happen. Vigilance is high, arousal is high, and behavioral responses to perceived threats are often reactive and intense. It is important to keep in mind that what triggers a child can be as subtle as the way someone looks at him or her, or a feeling of rejection or deprivation.
Behavior always serves some purpose. There are two primary functions of (trauma-related) behaviors. (Note that these behaviors are described in depth in Chapter 8.)	*Function 1:* Seeking safety or avoiding danger (fight, flight, freeze, submit or comply). Typically a high-arousal behavioral response that helps the child protect him- or herself. *Function 2:* Meeting a need (relational needs, physiological needs). A behavior designed to address a perceived internal state of need.

Nothing is harder to change than a survival behavior.	Behaviors that develop to support survival (by helping the child feel safer in his or her body, or by meeting a need) are often rigid and very hard to shift. Whether or not the behavior is actually helping the child now, it occurs because it is an attempt to manage overwhelming internal arousal.
The degree of internal and external resources a child has or lacks will contribute to the extremity of the behavior.	The more children have access to internal resources (strengths) and external resources (caregiver supports), the more easily a difficult behavior will resolve. In the absence of these resources, behaviors will continue to serve as the primary coping strategy for managing experience. It is for this reason that we target not just the behaviors, but the resources within and around the child that will ultimately make the behavior less necessary.

Skill #3: Identify Patterns of Behavior

Understanding why trauma-based behavior developed originally provides an important foundation for a behavior plan. Just as important is this next step: to understand, as much as possible, why this behavior is happening now. Teach and work with caregivers to identify the following, as concretely as possible:

Why Is the Behavior Happening Now?

Triggers	What leads to the behavior? When is the behavior most likely to occur? Concretely define the circumstances (emotional, relational, environmental) that typically precede the challenging behavior.
Function	What does the child appear to be trying to do (e.g., get attention, exert control, manage arousal, communicate frustration)? Without *agreeing* with the behavior, step back from it and consider what purpose the behavior is serving for the child.
Caregiver's typical response	When the child engages in this behavior, how do caregivers typically respond? Is this response consistent or inconsistent across caregivers? In particular, what is the caregiver's *emotional* or *arousal* response, and what is the caregiver's *behavioral* response?
Relational interplay	How does the child's response differ by caregiver? This area may provide information about *relational need* or about *effective and ineffective responses*.
Effective responses	What has the caregiver found to be effective in addressing the behavior? What makes things worse: a particular response (i.e., using a specific strategy) or a particular state (e.g., speaking in a calm voice versus yelling)?

Skill #4: Use Your "Go-To's"

Although the "best" or most effective behavior response strategy will vary by child, by situation, and by circumstance, there are two core strategies that apply across behaviors:

1. **Meet needs.** The single most useful strategy for addressing a negative behavior is to work to identify and meet the need that is driving a behavior. Consider the following example.

   > An adoptive mother of an 11-year-old girl reports to the child's therapist that her daughter is "too needy." When asked to describe what that means, the mother states, "She's always doing things to get attention, talking too loudly, trying to hang onto me, trying to climb onto my lap." When the therapist asked how the mother responded, she reported, "I don't want to encourage it, so I send her to her room." Further exploration confirmed that the mother's typical response style was to disconnect when her daughter's needs felt too overwhelming. The mother acknowledged that the behaviors have been escalating over time.

In this example, the mother actually has correctly identified the child's need: to get attention. The mother's response—of denying the need (removing attention)—is an attempt to manage the behavior by not rewarding it. However, for this child with a significant history of neglect, the denial of attention acts as a clear danger signal and escalates her arousal and her attention-seeking behaviors. As a result, her mother is frustrated, distressed, and overwhelmed, and the negative behavioral (and relational) pattern continues. Instead, the therapist works with the mother to do several things: (1) Look for opportunities to proactively provide attention (e.g., one-on-one time each evening), so that this time is predictable; (2) respond to need-fulfilling behaviors by naming them and providing alternatives: "It looks like you're needing some attention now. It's not comfortable for me when you sit on my lap, so let's sit together here on the sofa"; and (3) start to work toward understanding what might be driving highly needy behaviors (e.g., these behaviors escalate on days when the child has a difficult day at school), with the understanding that the behaviors are themselves a communication.

The following table provides examples of primary needs that may drive trauma behaviors and suggested strategies for meeting the needs. It should be reiterated that trauma-based needs are grounded, to some extent, in an overall sense of safety (or lack thereof) in relation to self, other, and the world.

Primary Needs and Strategies for Meeting Them

Need	Strategy
Connection: The need to feel seen, heard, and supported.	General goals may include building in predictable opportunities to connect, predicting disconnections, and/or developing strategies for reconnection. Some strategies include: ■ **Engagement.** As discussed in Chapter 8, engagement can often be the foundation for deepening connection. Engage in conversation, play, etc. ■ **Planned check-ins.** Work to identify specific times to connect throughout the day about positive and/or not-so-positive experiences, about emotions, etc. ■ **Supervision or presence.** Even when caregivers are not in direct contact with their children, they can assure them that they are "there" for them by being present and by providing adequate supervision. ■ **Communication routines.** As previously discussed, communication routines may provide children with a sense of belonging and connection and a felt understanding of their worth within the family context.
Control: The need to feel a sense of control over internal and/or external world.	Children who are impacted by trauma may struggle to gain and maintain an overall sense of control over their internal states and external experiences. In order to cultivate a growing sense of agency in these children, consider the following strategies: ■ **Offer choices.** This may include two desirable choices; a desirable versus undesirable choice, and/or a choice between action and inaction. ■ **Avoid power struggles.** When the need for control is driving child behaviors, it is unlikely that those behaviors will shift with control-based strategies (e.g., limit setting). Whenever possible, facilitate a child's sense of control by avoiding power struggles or authoritative or coercive styles of discipline. ■ **Support regulation.** See the second point (on p. 151) for specific strategies on supporting regulation and enhancing children's sense of control over internal experiences.
Containment: The need to feel a basic sense of safety internally and externally.	Containment is often about reducing the level of stimulation that a child is experiencing. Stimulation may be related to many internal and external factors. For example, consider the child who becomes overwhelmed in a noisy environment, in large groups, when boundaries are not clear, etc. Strategies for addressing containment needs may include the following: ■ Reduce exposure to stimuli (lights, noise, traffic, etc.). ■ Create quiet or comforting spaces in close proximity to others or more isolated from others, depending on individual preferences.

Need	Strategy
	▪ Develop and follow clear and consistent routines. ▪ Develop and follow clear boundaries and behavioral strategies (see the "Tools: Behavioral Response" section below for specific information).

2. **Support regulation.** When a behavior is out of control, before anything else can happen, you will need to apply safe, effective strategies for supporting regulation/de-escalation of the arousal and for managing the crisis. Pay attention to strategies for managing your own emotional responses, as well as those of the child/adolescent.

◆ **Use an adult regulation toolbox.** Link behavior plans back to the distress tolerance strategies identified in Chapter 7 ("Caregiver Management of Affect"). When working to address behaviors, caregivers should be able to identify how they will handle their own responses.

◆ **Contain and address unsafe child behaviors.** Safety is the top-priority goal in any behavior plan, and when a child gets highly dysregulated or out of control, it is important that behavior plans differentiate regulation strategies from limits. Consider the following example.

> A group home admitted a young boy (age 7) who became easily aggressive when dysregulated, spitting, kicking, and punching staff. Because his behaviors were so different when he was upset than when he was calm, staff members were becoming frustrated and typically reacted strongly to what they saw as "manipulative" outbursts. As a result, the boy's behaviors were leading to lengthy physical holds, and all privileges had been taken away.
>
> After a client review at a trauma team meeting, a different plan was put into place. Staff worked to understand typical triggers for his behaviors, and were able to identify that unexpected changes and any threats to the boy's perceived control led to strong reactions. Linking these triggers to his history of multiple placements, losses, and abandonment was helpful in staff feeling less frustrated. When the boy began to feel unsafe, staff shifted to helping him get to a small, contained sensory room, and then giving him space to calm down. A staff member remained available at all times, either in the room or just outside of it, reminding the boy every few minutes that it was okay to have big feelings, and that someone was available to talk when he was ready. One staff member stated, "He used to really aggravate me, but now I keep reminding myself that he's scared, and this is the only way he knows how to show it. I try to remember that he's a really good kid when he's calm, and I take a breath before saying stuff to him, so I don't say something I'll regret."

Skill #5: Use Your Behavior Response Tools Purposefully and with a Plan

In the following section on tools, several behavioral response strategies are outlined. Ideally, we are thoughtful about when and how each tool is used in every behavior plan. In reality, what often happens is that tools are used reactively and indiscriminately ("He shouted, so I put him in time-out; then he kept yelling, so I took away his favorite toy"). Keep in mind that multiple strategies can be used to address a single behavior, and that the best strategy for one child or family may differ from that for another, even when addressing the same behavior.

Tools: Behavioral Response

There are three primary behavior response tools we cover in this section: (1) praise and reinforcement, (2) behavior management strategies such as limit setting and ignoring, and (3) problem solving. Strategies and use of each, along with pitfalls and trauma considerations, are also described.

Tool #1: Praise and Reinforcement

GUIDELINES FOR USE OF PRAISE AND REINFORCEMENT

Guidelines		Trauma creates significant distress that impacts individuals and their caregiving systems. Over time, it is not uncommon for a negative pattern to build in which members focus almost exclusively on difficulties, stressors, and symptoms.
		When overwhelmed by distress, there may be a loss of awareness of the positives. Children (and their caregivers) may begin to identify primarily with the "bad": "I'm a bad kid," "I'm a bad parent."
		This same dynamic may build in milieu treatment settings, as staff begins to focus primarily on stress and pathology.
		This pattern may lead to helplessness and/or hopelessness: *This will never change!*
		The use of praise and positive reinforcement can: ■ Increase positive caregiver–child interactions. ■ Increase desired behaviors. ■ Increase attunement. ■ Increase felt safety. ■ Build self-esteem and self-efficacy for both child and caregiver. ■ Increase feelings of child and caregiver mastery.
		Praise and reinforcement must be a conscious choice. Surprisingly, the good things are often *much* more difficult to notice than the hard ones! Noticing the positives often requires effortful focus and selection of behaviors to target.
Selecting targets	Don't praise everything.	Work with caregivers to be selective. If they praise everything they see, it will feel false to them and false to the child. Pick things that are tangible, that are important, that are goals, etc., and focus on those.
	Start small.	Help caregivers pick one desired behavior to notice. They should consciously tune in to it and praise it whenever it appears. Have caregivers track their use of praise.
	Choose behaviors that are salient and desired.	Specifically select targets based on those behaviors that you are trying to build. For instance, if tolerating frustration without tantrumming is an important goal, then any sign that the child is doing this should be noticed and reinforced. Work with caregivers to specifically link the praise to the behavior or effort. For example, do *not say* "Good job," but rather: "Wow, I'm so proud of you. I just told you that you had to wait a few minutes before we went outside, and you said 'okay.' I know that can be hard, and I'm really proud of how you handled it."
		Help caregivers choose targets wisely. If the initial target is the one thing the child never does, neither the parent nor the child will experience success.
	Redefine "success."	Help caregivers think in terms of gradual shaping of desired behavior rather than overnight success. If the ultimate goal is for the child not to punch a wall when angry, for instance, then reinforce the first time the child yells and screams but doesn't punch.
	Beyond "being good"	Praise should not always be linked to actions. Praise is not just about shaping behavior but about building a positive sense of self. Work with caregivers to reinforce children's qualities and efforts.

Examples of praise statements	Behavior related	"You did a really good job at finishing your homework." "I like how well you're sharing with your sister." "I feel so proud when you find safe ways to tell me what you're feeling."
	Effort related	"I can see how hard you're working at that." "Thank you for trying to compromise, even though it's hard." "I can see how frustrated you are, and I'm really proud of you for not yelling."
	Child qualities	"I'm so proud of how kind you are." "You're so adventurous—I think it's great!" "What a great sense of humor you have."
	Open-ended	"You're such a great kid, I have such fun being with you." "I love it when we play games together." "It made me so happy to see you smile yesterday."
Reinforcers	Teaching point	One way to increase positive behaviors is to use concrete reinforcers.
	Adult attention is powerful.	Teach caregivers that adult attention is one of the most powerful reinforcers they can use. In building concrete reinforcement systems, don't lose sight of the power of praise.
	Reward charts	Work with caregivers to build concrete reinforcement systems. As with praise, choose one or two behaviors on which to focus initially. Develop star/sticker charts, point-reward systems, good job jars, etc. Work with caregivers to select developmentally appropriate methods (see Developmental Considerations on pp. 163–164). Help caregivers identify appropriate reinforcers. For young children, stickers, stars, and the like are often reward enough; older children will want to work toward concrete goals like the examples of concrete reinforcers listed below. The more children can be involved in defining what they are working toward, the more they are likely to be invested achieving their goals. Give, but don't remove. When using a reward chart or a reinforcement system, ideally children should gain something for positive accomplishments, but will not lose anything for negative behavior. The consequence of negative behavior is failing to earn a sticker (or whatever) rather than loss of previously earned ones. By not removing stickers, etc., children are sent the message that their previous positive behaviors still count.
	Examples of concrete reinforcers	Special time with caregivers. Extra privileges (e.g., computer/tablet time, television time, later bedtime). Getting to be the leader (e.g., choosing the family movie, choosing favorite food for dinner). Favorite activities (e.g., going to the park, playing cards, baking cookies, going out to eat). Concrete rewards (e.g., toys, games, books).

PRAISE AND THE TRAUMA RESPONSE

■ For some children who have experienced trauma, reward and positive attention can trigger a negative response. There are several reasons for this:

◆ Praise may be "ego-dystonic." For children who have a strong sense that there is something wrong with them, praise may not match their self-perception and may therefore feel frightening, like a falsehood or a trick.

◆ Positive statements can elicit attachment fears. Children who have been impacted by trauma have often experienced multiple losses—of caregivers, of places, and of other important figures in their lives. A positive relationship with an adult may elicit fears that the same things are about to happen. The fear in the child's mind is, "Why attach when someone could take this all away again tomorrow?"

◆ Praise can be a direct trigger or reminder of past abuse for children who were groomed by their perpetrator or for children who may have been rewarded following abuse acts. We recall some young people that we worked with sharing stories about being taken out for ice cream, shopping for clothes or toys, or going to the movies following their abuse.

◆ Finally, for children in group care success is typically rewarded with a move. Success means losing their home, the people that have been caring for them, and the predictability of their day-to-day life.

◆ It is important to note that providing praise can also be a trigger for caregivers with trauma histories. For example, for caregivers whose own childhoods were marked by a lack of positive attention and connection, encouragement to provide this to their children can feel uncomfortable or unsettling, and/or may elicit grief about what they themselves may have never received. Although we focus here on the ways that the *child's* trauma response may influence his or her experience of praise, it is equally important to be aware of and acknowledge the many reasons that adult caregivers may struggle with this.

Responding When Children Are Triggered by Praise

Don't take it personally.	Help caregivers be aware that praise may be a trigger their children. If a child responds negatively to being praised, help the caregiver separate the child's attachment fears from caregiver's experience of relational rejection.
Hang in there.	For many children, part of making meaning about trauma includes self-blame. Praise and reinforcement won't lead to immediate change in this area. Help caregivers build tolerance for the emotions (e.g., shame, guilt, frustration) that go along with witnessing negative self-statements by their children.
Don't argue it.	Help caregivers stand by their praise, without arguing. Teach them to keep the response simple. For instance, if the caregiver tells the child that the caregiver is proud of him or her, and the child rejects the compliment, the caregiver's response might be: "Well, *I'm* feeling proud of you, but it's okay for you to feel however you want."
Stay tuned in to child-affect.	If a child begins to escalate in response to praise, help the caregiver use attunement skills to name and respond to the underlying child affect. For instance, "I can see that was kind of scary for you to hear. Would a hug help you feel better?"

Tool #2: Behavior Management Strategies

GENERAL GUIDELINES FOR BEHAVIORAL MANAGEMENT

Guidelines	It is crucial that any behavioral strategies occur in the context of an attuned response that takes into account why the behavior occurred, as outlined previously. Acknowledging the emotion driving the behavior and working to address the pattern driving the behavior will ultimately decrease the need for limits.
	When developing a behavior management plan and identifying appropriate limits, work with caregivers to incorporate the full sequence of steps identified in the "Teach to Caregivers" section above (Skills 1–5), including in particular the "go-to" strategies (meeting needs, supporting child and adult regulation).

For many trauma-impacted children, limits in the past have been overly punitive, inconsistent, or nonexistent.

Children may use rigid control strategies to help them feel safer and therefore resist limits initially. However, over time, consistent limit setting will increase felt safety in the environment and ultimately allow children to let go of their tight control.

Caregivers may be hesitant to set limits with children who have experienced trauma. However, failure to set limits may inadvertently send many negative messages, such as:
- The child is incapable of controlling his or her own behavior.
- The child is too "damaged" to behave.
- The child is unworthy of the caregiver's attention.
- The caregiver is unable to handle the child's behavior.

Note that all of these messages increase the child's perception of powerlessness, which can *increase* negative behaviors.

In contrast, setting consistent expectations and limits sends a different message. It communicates that:
- Children *are* able to learn behavioral control.
- They have the ability to alter their behavior in a way that is appropriate to the situation.
- They are worthy of caregiver attention.
- Their caregiver can keep them safe.

Behavioral management strategies	Ignoring
	Applying consequences for behavior
	Employing a time-out

STRATEGY #1: USE OF PLANNED IGNORING

Definition	"Planned ignoring" involves actively *not attending* to undesirable behaviors that are not immediately dangerous. The goal of planned ignoring is to reduce the occurrence of these behaviors by not engaging actively with or about the behaviors, while simultaneously providing alternatives.
Appropriate targets	Examples of appropriate targets for ignoring include: - Whining. - Mild temper tantrums (unless they include unsafe expression for child or other). - Pouting/sulking. When a child engages in behaviors such as those just listed, the caregiver might: - Acknowledge the feeling. - Name the negative behavior. - Name a more appropriate alternative behavior. - Indicate willingness to engage with the child once the negative behavior stops.
How to ignore	Once the caregiver has engaged in these initial steps, it is important that the following happen: - Remove attention from the child's behavior. This does not necessarily mean ignoring the child completely, as to do so may be triggering. Do not continue to give warnings or engage extensively about the behavior once the initial statement has been made. - Immediately reinforce any positive alternative displayed by the child (e.g., if the child has been whining, immediately praise the child when the whining stops). - Set limits only if the behavior escalates and becomes dangerous to the child or others. If the behavior continues beyond several minutes, the caregiver may provide additional prompts (e.g., "I'd really like to speak with you, once you're ready to talk in a regular voice"). - If the behavior still continues to escalate, it may be an indication that the child is triggered and requires support for regulating.
Example	A 10-year-old boy has been told by his caregiver that he can't have a snack before dinner. He begins to yell and demand a snack. CAREGIVER: *(Acknowledge the feeling.)* I can see you're mad that you can't have a snack *(name the negative behavior)*, but yelling won't change my decision. *(Name a more appropriate behavior.)* You can tell me how mad you are, or go play with your basketball to help you feel less mad, but while

you're yelling I can't talk to you. *(Indicate willingness to engage with child when negative behavior stops.)* When you're ready to talk without yelling, I'll be in the kitchen.

BOBBY: *(Yells for another minute, which caregiver ignores. Then stomps off.)*

CAREGIVER: Good choice; I'm proud of you for listening and stopping your yelling. If you'd like to talk, come let me know.

Example 2	A mother has asked her 9-year-old to brush her teeth before bed three times with no response. The mother notices that her daughter hasn't responded, so she asks her an additional time, this time using a more assertive tone.
	DAUGHTER: *(Begins to yell at her mother.)* IIIIIIII KNOWWWW! You are the most annoying mother ever. I hate you!!
	MOTHER: *(Ignores daughter's behaviors and takes a very deep breath.)* I can see you're upset right now. I'm going to go into the other room to give you some space. Rather than remind you again, I'm going to set the microwave timer for 10 minutes so you have plenty of time to get your teeth done. Let me know if there is anything that you need.

Note: In this example it would have been easy for the mother to get pulled into addressing the disrespectful tone that her daughter was using toward her. A consequence may be needed if the behavior persists, but this mom chose to ignore the behavior and reinforce the need for space or distance.

STRATEGY #2: CONSEQUENCES FOR BEHAVIOR

Definition	This strategy involves naming and following through on consequences for undesirable behavior. Consequences may include removal of privileges, provision of natural or logical consequences, or an age- and child-appropriate version of time-out (described in the next table).
Appropriate targets	Behaviors around which limits should be set will vary according to family or system norms, but generally address those behaviors that are unsafe, aggressive, or violate familial/systemic rules. For instance, hitting, throwing toys at a sibling, yelling or screaming after being given warnings, name calling, and refusal to follow a directive may result in limit setting.
How to set limits/ consequeces	When initially working with caregivers to set limits, help them select targets and consequences that they can actually carry out. Help caregivers identify specific limits/consequences for specific behaviors in advance. The more caregivers are able to anticipate negative behaviors, work to understand them, and develop a proactive plan for addressing them, the greater likelihood that the limits/consequences will be appropriate.
	When a behavior occurs, teach caregivers the following steps: ▪ Acknowledge the feeling behind the behavior. ▪ Name the unacceptable behavior. ▪ Name the limit or consequence. ▪ Suggest an alternative behavior for current or future use.
	Be sure that this sequence occurs only after both child and caregiver are calm/in a regulated state.
Limits	Limits are most effective if they are: ▪ **Related:** Understanding the connection between limit and consequence increases when the limit is tied to the behavior (e.g., playing with a ball in the house after being told not to results in losing use of the ball for a period of time). ▪ **Age-appropriate:** Limits should be appropriate to the child's developmental stage. (See Developmental Considerations on pp. 163–164.) To the extent possible, pair the severity of the limit with the severity of the behavior. Mild behaviors should not be punished with excessive limits. ▪ **Calm:** Limits should be delivered in a calm tone of voice. Caregivers are less effective if they frighten their children. If necessary, caregivers should take the space to calm down before delivering a limit. ▪ **Timely:** Limits should be applied within a reasonable timeframe after the negative behavior, particularly for younger children. *Note:* In applying limits, it is important to be conscious of the child's state of arousal; help the child to modulate *before* applying a limit. Remember to use your "go-to's" and support regulation.

Suggested Sequence for **applying limits to a behavior that has already occurred** (e.g., unsafe actions).	Teach caregivers the following sequence for addressing behaviors that have already occurred:
	1. "I can see that you are feeling _____, but _____ is not okay" (e.g., "I can see that you are feeling angry, but hitting your brother is not okay").
	2. *Sample options:*
	  ▪ "You are showing me that you can't be safe right now, so you need to _____ ("go to your room," "sit on the steps," etc.) _____ ("for 5 minutes," "until I come get you," etc.)."
	  ▪ "You were told that if you _____, then _____" (e.g., "You were told that if you hit your brother, then you would lose PlayStation for the night. You chose to hit your brother, so now you will not be allowed to use PlayStation until tomorrow").
	3. "Next time you feel _____, I hope you choose to _____" (e.g., "Next time you feel angry, I hope you choose to come tell me instead of hitting your brother").

Suggested sequence of language for **eliciting behaviors that have not yet occurred.**	Teach caregivers the following sequence for eliciting desired behaviors: 1. "Please _____" (e.g., "Please pick up your toys"). 2. "I'm asking you again to please _____"(e.g., "I'm asking you again to please pick up your toys"). 3. "If you do not _____, then _____" (e.g., "If you do not pick up your toys by the time I come back into the room, then you will not be able to play outside after dinner"). 4. [If the behavior does not occur] "You were told to _____, and you chose not to. Now, _____" (e.g., "You were told to pick up your toys, and you chose not to. Now, that means you will not be able to play outside tonight").
Rationale	This sequence addresses the following: ▪ Provides child with a clear message of desired behavior, as well as consequences for failing to follow through. ▪ Allows the child an opportunity to connect actions with consequences, and to make a choice about behavior. ▪ Ultimately, the sequence removes the power struggle and places the responsibility on the child, as limits are clearly linked to the child's behavior.
Considerations	It is important to keep in mind what might be interfering with a child's compliance with a directive. Rather than assuming oppositionality, consider whether the child might be overwhelmed, shut down, confused, etc. Limit setting should be considered a final stage, after other options have been explored, rather than the immediate response.

STRATEGY #3: USING TIME-OUT

Definition	"Time-out" is a particular type of limit setting that involves the removal of the child from a physical location (and from the attention of others within that location) to a space where the child can spend a specified amount of time. For younger children, time-out often involves sitting in a specified place (e.g., on a chair, on a step); for older children, similar principles can be used (e.g., sending the child to his or her room for a specific length of time).
Appropriate targets	Time-out is useful for immediately stopping an unacceptable behavior, particularly those that are impulsive and/or unsafe. For trauma-impacted children, time-out may be useful for providing "space" to allow them to calm down from distressing emotion. Appropriate targets, in general, include those listed previously for limit setting.
How to	When a child engages in impulsive or unsafe behaviors, the caregiver should: 1. Provide a warning: "If you do not stop _____, you will need to _____" (e.g., "If you do not stop throwing things, you will need to take some space"). 2. If the behavior does not stop following the warning, restate the negative behavior and name the time-out location and the length of time. 3. If necessary, bring the child to the time-out location. 4. Once the child is in time-out, remove all attention until the specified length of time is over. Often, 1 minute per year of child age is used; caregivers can also specify, "Until you calm down," but the caregiver must clarify what "calm down" will look like. Keep in mind that these guidelines specify the maximum, rather than minimum, time; some children will

respond to very brief periods of taking space, and will become distressed if this time goes on for too long.
5. *Alternative:* See alternative descriptions below for holding time-outs in a safe space (i.e., time-in, safe space). For children with trauma histories, these alternatives may be more effective than classic time-out steps.

If the child refuses to go to time-out, the caregiver has two options:
1. Ignore the refusal, while reiterating the consequence. If the child is generally safe but refusing to go to the time-out location, the caregiver may state, "You have _____ minutes of time-out. which will not start until you sit in the chair [sit on the step, etc.]. Until you take that time as I've asked you to do, you may not play the game with us."
2. Use an if–then statement to name a consequence if the child does not follow through. (e.g., "Right now, you have a choice. You may go sit in time-out for 2 minutes, like I asked you to do. If you do not cooperate, then you will not be allowed to play outside any more today"). It is very important that caregivers *follow through* on these limits, once they are named.

Once the child has completed the specified time, the caregiver should:
1. Praise the child for following directives and remaining in time-out.
2. Elicit the child's understanding of why he or she was in time-out.
3. Acknowledge the feeling behind the behavior.
4. Give an alternative (or help child think of an alternative) for what he or she can do the next time, instead of the unacceptable behavior.
Optional: Request some reparation for the negative action.

Example

A 7-year-old girl, angry about having been told that she can't play outside, starts to yell and throw her toys.

CAREGIVER: *(Name the emotion and try to support regulation.)* Jemmie, I see that you are angry, but throwing toys is not safe. I am happy to help you calm down if you would like. Do you want to come sit with me?
JEMMIE: *(Ignores her and continues to throw toys.)*
CAREGIVER: *(Provide a warning.)* I'm sorry you're feeling so angry, but I can't let you be unsafe. If you don't stop, you will need to take some space.
JEMMIE: I hate you! *(Throws a doll at her.)*
CAREGIVER: *(Restate the negative behavior.)* I can see you're not ready to be safe right now. It is not okay to throw toys. Now you need to sit on the steps until you're ready to talk to me without yelling. *(Takes Jemmie's hand and walks her to the step. Jemmie continues to scream for a few minutes, which the caregiver ignores. After Jemmie has begun to calm down, the caregiver returns and praises the child for following instructions.)* Jemmie, you're doing a really good job. I can see that you're calming down because you're sitting on the step without yelling. *(Elicit the child's understanding.)* Do you know why I told you to sit on the step?

JEMMIE: No!
CAREGIVER: I told you to sit on the step because you were throwing things, which was unsafe.
JEMMIE: But I wanted to go outside!!!
CAREGIVER: I know you wanted to go outside *(acknowledge the feeling)*, and it made you mad that you couldn't, but throwing toys wasn't a safe way to tell me. But now, you're doing a really good job of using your words to tell me. I'm sorry you're so mad, but it's too late to play outside now. Please help me clean up the toys that you threw *(requires reparation, with support)*, and then we can find something else fun to do. *(Give an alternative.)* Would you like to draw a picture with me instead?

Alternatives to time-out

Children who experience trauma often need a high level of connection, engagement, and support when distressed. Although the traditional time-out strategy may be effective for some children, others will likely become more dysregulated when they lose connection with their caregiver, their play objects, etc. Consider the following alternatives:

■ *Time-in:* The goal of time-in is to address and stop a negative behavior, while continuing to provide reassurance that the adult is limiting the behavior, not rejecting the child. Rather than placing the child in a space that is separated from others, use a "time-in" technique in which the caregiver remains available, perhaps by sitting next to the child, allowing the child to sit on the caregiver's lap, remaining in the room, etc. Particularly for children with histories of neglect or abandonment, time-in may be much more effective and less triggering than time-out. Note that it is important that this connected time be in the control of the child to some degree—that is, the adult should not force the child to remain near the adult; this proximity should be an offer rather than a requirement. As an example: When the foster mother of a 6-year-old girl set a limit on throwing, she stated, "We need to take some space, because everything is starting to get too heated up and someone could get hurt. Let's go take some space on the sofa. Do you want me to stay right next to you, or sit over here?"

■ *Safe space/comfort zone:* Rather than framed as punishment, the explicit goal of a "safe space" (or comfort zone, sensory space, calming-down corner, etc.) is to support the child in regulating. This type of space sends the explicit message that it is understood that the child's negative behavior is, to some degree, driven by strong emotions or out-of-control body states. A safe space may be simple (a corner of a room with pillows, stuffed animals, and a blanket) or more elaborate (a sensory room in a milieu program filled with safe sensory objects). It is important that this space be introduced in moments of calm, and that the child/adolescent have an opportunity to contribute to both the materials and the use. Because the presumption is that the space will be used at least some of the time when the child is very dysregulated, care should be taken that objects in the immediate environment are generally safe.

LIMIT SETTING AND THE TRAUMA RESPONSE

■ As with reward and praise, setting limits can elicit strong emotions in traumatized children.

■ It is important for caregivers to consider the following in setting limits.

Trauma Considerations with Limit Setting

Reduce the need for limits.	Children with trauma histories often feel the need to be in control. Power struggles may be avoided by providing limited choice (e.g., "You can do your homework in your room or at the kitchen table. Which would you like to do?"). This choice provides the child with the illusion of control, while allowing the caregiver to maintain limits around the behavior.
	Have caregivers use their attunement skills to determine the reason behind child noncompliance. Differentiate children who feel overwhelmed by a task from those who are noncompliant with it. Try the following: ■ Elicit from the child what he or she is feeling and/or name what you are seeing (e.g., "You seem really upset by having to clean your room. What's going on with that?"). ■ Break down large tasks into smaller ones. ■ Offer to help.
	Compromise. Help caregivers define which rules are essential, and on which they can compromise.
Prioritize behaviors	Help caregivers to prioritize behavioral targets for limit setting. Often caregivers equate limit setting with good parenting. Remind them about the other strategies for increasing/decreasing behavior outlined in this chapter and support them in identifying *one or two behaviors* that require limits.
Choose your moments.	When trauma-impacted children are in a high state of arousal, they are unable to access higher cognitive functions, including logic, problem solving, planning, anticipating, delaying response, etc. So when a caregiver addresses a child, asking, "What's wrong with you? Why do you keep yelling? Haven't we talked about how important it is to speak in a normal tone of voice when you're upset?," the caregiver is essentially talking to the part of the child's brain that is not "online."
	When children are highly aroused, caregivers should do the following: ■ Name the unsafe behavior, if any. ■ Help child to use affect regulation and/or containment skills (including caregiver support), as necessary. ■ Apply limits only after child has calmed down.
Be aware of triggers.	All types of limit setting can act as triggers. Time-out and ignoring can trigger fears of abandonment and rejection; setting limits and consequences can trigger fears of punishment, authority, and vulnerability. Although they should not avoid the use of limits for these children,

it is important for caregivers to be aware of these possible reactions. The impact can be minimized by:

- Always naming the rationale for a limit and linking it to the behavior (rather than to the child).
- Always naming the boundaries around the limit (e.g., length of time in time-out, amount of time privilege is lost).
- Moving on. Caregivers should not continue to scold, bring up the behavior, or manifest excessive affect after setting the limit and carrying through with it. Caregivers should let the child know, explicitly, if necessary, that they still love him or her.
- Making adaptations to limits for specific triggers (e.g., a child who has been previously punished by being enclosed in a small space might spend time-out sitting in a nearby chair, rather than in another room).

Tool #3: Supporting Problem Solving

Definition	Problem solving is a largely adult-scaffolded skill set that is used to support children and adolescents in building awareness of choices, growing their ability to consider alternatives, and taking on challenges rather than just reacting to them. When we use problem-solving skills, we work to define the challenge, the possible ways of addressing that challenge, and the potential consequences of our choices. When youth are supported in this process, they are sent the message that they have the power to exert some control over their lives.
Appropriate targets	Problem-solving strategies should be used when both child and caregiver are in reasonably calm states. They may be used in anticipation of a difficult situation, to support planning, or in the aftermath to understand alternatives for similar future situations. These skills are also important to use whenever a child asks the adult for help in managing behavior (e.g., if a child says, "I don't know what to do when my teacher yells at me!," rather than providing an answer such as "Just calm down and don't worry about it!," use this skill set to help the child learn to assess a situation and identify his or her own solutions).
How to	This skill set is described in detail in Chapter 13 on executive functions. A brief review is provided here, as problem solving is an important tool to include in any behavior response skill set. Adult steps include the following: Communicate willingness to support the child and the belief in his or her ability to find a solution ("Let's figure this out"). 1. Help the child identify what the problem is (what is the situation you are working to help the child address?) 2. Identify goals or outcomes: What does the child want to happen? What do you want to happen?) 3. Identify choices: What kind of things might you or the child be able to do? 4. Identify consequences, both good and bad, of the possible choices: What might happen if we do A or B? 5. Make a plan and troubleshoot it. Pay attention not just to the child's role, but also to the adult supports needed (including the adult's own affect management).
Example	Larry, a 15-year-old boy in a group care setting, has recently been struggling with his reactions in the classroom, becoming quickly angry and frustrated when his work is corrected by the teacher. After talking it through with his teacher and his therapist, his advocate (a direct care staff member) sits down with him during an afternoon open time when Larry is calm. STAFF: So I've got something I want to connect with you about. I know you mentioned school's been rough lately, and I talked to Ms. Linden a bit too. Are you in an okay space to talk this through with me? *(Provides choice and checks that youth is regulated.)* LARRY: Yeah, I guess, as long as you're not here to give me a hard time. STAFF: Nah, no hard time. Just hoping we can talk it through, because it seems like you're getting pretty frustrated lately, and it's getting you in some trouble. *(Names the problem.)* I know you're talking about what's going on with your therapist, but maybe we can figure out how to handle it in the moment, okay? *(Presumes solution is possible.)*

LARRY: Yeah, okay. Like, what do you mean?

STAFF: Like, right now, when Ms. Linden tries to help you with your work, it sounds like you're getting frustrated pretty quickly, and then it heats up and you end up having to leave school, which means you lose your afternoon free time. *(Identifies challenging situation in concrete terms that include what's at stake for the youth.)*

LARRY: Yeah, man, it just feels like she's always on my case lately.

STAFF: Thing is, that's sort of her job, right, at least when it comes to schoolwork? But maybe there's a different way she can talk to you that would feel better, or something you can do or we can help you do when you're feeling frustrated. Can we brainstorm a bit? *(Engages youth in identifying alternative solutions.)*

This initial lead-in to problem solving would ideally be followed by a consideration of ways to address the identified challenging areas: (1) the ways the teacher is providing feedback; and (2) ways to manage Larry's own frustration and resulting behavioral responses/escalations. In this scenario, any solution involving the teacher (a third-party not present for this conversation) would necessarily need to include a conversation with the teacher. When this is not possible, solutions would need to focus on the youth's response to the other party's actions, rather than changing that person's actions.

Considerations — Youth ability to engage in this process will depend upon a number of factors, including:

- State: Which part of the child's brain is online?
- Stage or developmental capacity: Problem-solving ability increases over time, and younger children will typically require greater support.
- Agency: The child's belief in his or her ability to make choices or be successful; keep in mind that the strength of this belief may vary by state.
- Adult affect: What is the adult's ability to remain calm and provide ongoing support?

Putting It all Together: The Case of Olivia[1]

Olivia is a 7-year-old girl of mixed ethnicity. Her biological parents used substances (primarily heroin, marijuana, and alcohol), and there was frequent violence in their relationship. The family moved four times during Olivia's first 2 years and was homeless once. Often Olivia's mother would leave her with friends or other relatives for brief periods. Olivia and her mother moved into a shelter when Olivia was 3 years old, but her mother returned to Olivia's father after 6 months. Two months later, Dad was incarcerated because of a domestic violence incident and multiple intent-to-distribute charges. He was arrested in front of Olivia. Olivia was removed from her mother's custody when she was 4 years old after allegations of neglect and physical abuse.

In the past 3 years, Olivia has lived in five different foster homes. She has been in her current home for the past 5 months.

Overall Olivia has made significant progress while in foster care, although she continues to steal small items and hoard food in her new foster home. She can be affectionate with her foster parents, but gets overwhelmed, clingy, and demanding when asked to do small tasks. At times, her anger increases and she throws things at her foster mother. She appears to be settling into her routines but has a hard time separating at bedtime and can escalate, which can spur a lengthy tantrum.

---

[1] The material in this section is drawn from the ARC Reflections curriculum, developed in collaboration with the Annie E. Casey Foundation.

Every Behavior Has a Function

The possible needs that underlie Olivia's problem behaviors include the following:

- **Hoarding:** Possible needs include fear of not having enough to eat and/or the substitution of a physical need (food) for a relational need (connection).
- **Bedtime separation:** Possible needs include relational reassurance due to fear of nighttime, fear of being alone, and/or fear of foster parents not being there when she wakes up. Olivia may also have difficulty with state transitions.
- **Throwing objects:** Possible needs: The high-arousal response suggests a survival-based behavior. Is Olivia trying to regulate? To engage attention or connection? To elicit help with task completion? To gain control?

Use Go-to Strategies to Meet Needs

Every time Olivia's foster parents cleaned, they found old, uneaten, often rotten food in drawers and behind the bed. Establishing consequences was not effective. Working with Olivia's therapist, her foster parents:

- Identified a kitchen drawer and filled it with healthy snacks. They made it Olivia's drawer; only she could take food from it. They regularly made sure it was full.
- Put a food-safe garbage can in her room for any food-related products.
- Stopped talking about the issue.

The biggest power struggle that Olivia's foster parents encountered was around Olivia's completion of simple chores and self-care strategies. When she escalated to the point of throwing objects, the parents often escalated themselves. Olivia's therapist guessed that the throwing might actually be a request for support rather than a distancing strategy. As an experiment, Olivia's foster mother began to do simple chores with Olivia. For instance, she would say, "Olivia, let's pick up these toys. Which ones should we pick up first?" When she engaged with Olivia, she found the opposition decreased dramatically and Olivia was able to actively participate. In fact, Olivia was actually able to complete many tasks independently when her foster mother remained in the room and available.

Examples of Behavioral Response to Olivia's Challenging Reactions

- **Behavior:** Throwing things at foster mother when overwhelmed completing tasks.
- **Problem solving:** Olivia's foster mother sat with Olivia when she was calm, during their evening chat time. They talked about how everyone in the home was an important part of the family and contributed to keeping the house running smoothly. The foster mom noted that chores were hard for Olivia and asked if they could figure out a way to help Olivia feel more successful at them. When Olivia had a hard time generating ideas, her foster mother suggested that the two of them practice doing chores together. She also talked about ways Olivia could tell her that she was feeling overwhelmed
- **Praise and reinforcement:** Olivia's foster parents worked hard to notice whenever Olivia helped around the house or engaged in self-care (cleaned up her toys, put clothes in the

laundry, did age-appropriate self-care such as brushing teeth) and made sure to comment on it. They also began to tune into and name moments when Olivia got upset but didn't become aggressive, praising her for using her regulation tools.

■ **Limit setting:** When Olivia escalated to throwing and hitting, whichever adult was present quickly stopped the activity and tried to mirror her affect or energy (e.g., saying, "I see you are upset," or "Your energy just got really big") and cue Olivia to take a break. If this did not work, her foster parent would carry her to the regulation corner (a special corner set up with blankets, pillows, and comfort objects) and either sit with Olivia in his or her lap or wrap her in a blanket. They remained in the corner until it was clear that Olivia was calmer. Once she was calm, they talked about what had happened, reminded Olivia that it was okay to be angry but not to throw things, and put any thrown toys in toy time-out for 10 minutes.

■ **Praise:** Whenever Olivia went to her corner when cued, used coping skills, or completed chores successfully, her foster parents gave her a high-five or verbal praise.

■ **Problem solving:** During the established evening chat time, Olivia's foster parents would talk with her about any incidents, their observations of Olivia's behaviors and feelings, and discuss ways to handle things differently the next time. Over time, they were able to identify early warning clues that Olivia was having a hard time and use a special silly code phrase ("purple spotted dinosaurs") to cue Olivia to use her regulation corner. They also made chore times predictable.

The case of Olivia provides an example of strategies that her foster parents tried. In is important to acknowledge, however, that many children and adolescents who have experienced trauma struggle with behaviors that challenge us, push our buttons, and are very difficult to redirect or shift in a given moment. It is common to feel that strategies have maxed out, especially when what works with one child or teen does not work with another, and what worked yesterday doesn't work today. It is important to continue to experiment with strategies and to engage in ongoing assessment about the effectiveness of a strategy within each specific context in which behavior emerges.

Developmental Considerations

Developmental stage	Consistent response considerations
Early childhood	Young children rely strongly on external markers of success or failure. Because their internal sense of self is not yet well developed, they look to the cues of others to understand whether what they have done is "right" or "wrong." Unlike adults, young children have very little "filter" through which to interpret experience, and they will directly internalize the feedback the environment gives them. The more that feedback is (realistically!) positive, the better.
	Preschoolers are very concrete and have limited capacity to hold information over time. Therefore, reinforcement and limit setting both need to be immediate (if tied to specific events).
	Particularly for young children, praise and adult attention are the most powerful reinforcers.
	Consequences should be mild and immediate. Young children do not retain awareness of the links between behaviors and consequences for a lengthy period of time. Long time-outs or excessive punishments are counterproductive because the child will lose awareness of the rationale very quickly.

Developmental stage	Consistent response considerations
Middle childhood	Because industry is such an important developmental task, it becomes important to reinforce successful signs of a child's initiative. Pay attention to efforts outside of the home; caregivers should not just reinforce what they see but also what they hear from others. Encourage caregivers to build communication with teachers, Scout leaders, after-school people, etc.
	At this age, it is important to begin to elicit self-praise and self-reinforcement: What does the *child* feel good about? Of what is he or she proud? Reinforce the child's positive sense of self.
	Because older elementary school–age children have some capacity to delay gratification, this is a good age to start using point-reward systems.
	Consequences and limit setting become more salient at this stage as children are becoming more aware of the link between behaviors and outcomes.
	Limits can be slightly longer or more involved than for younger children (i.e., a child can receive a consequence at home for something that happened at school, or a consequence that lasts for a longer period of time). However, consequences should remain proportional to the behavior and age-appropriate.
Adolescence	Balance in limit setting is key. Help caregivers pick their battles.
	Natural consequences are increasingly important; the goal is for an adolescent to learn to make appropriate choices and to take responsibility for the consequences of those choices. Therefore, consequences should always be linked, either verbally or through the natural flow, with the choices the teen has made.
	Adolescents are moving toward independence, identity development, peer relations, and accomplishments/individual competency. Help caregivers reinforce adolescents' efforts in these areas.
	Because a goal for adolescence is increasing independent control over behavior, it is particularly important for caregivers to reinforce those moments when adolescents pay attention to their own actions and the outcomes. For instance, a teen describes a conflict with a peer that led him to lose his temper. Rather than placing a limit on the action (i.e., loss of temper), reinforce the *self-awareness*.

Applications

Individual/Dyadic

When working with primary caregivers (biological, foster, adoptive, or kinship), behavior management strategies are often a priority request. Enough with the *concepts,* we hear routinely, "Tell me what to *DO!*" The wish from many caregivers, understandably, is for there to be some formula—an action, a consequence, a statement—that will shift the most distressing child behaviors and make the family's life easier. Although the precise formula does not exist, the one formula to which we can attest is this: REPETITION. Behavioral strategies are most effective when applied over and over, in a responsive and attuned way. Remind caregivers that this is a very complicated skill and ensure that they are ready to take on the work that you are asking of them. Many caregivers will need a significant amount of support with attunement prior to implementing behavioral strategies.

In all homes it is important for rules and values to be explicit and clear. Work with caregivers to discuss rules with children in age-appropriate terms, and, when appropriate, to post "Family Rules" somewhere visible. The visibility of family rules is particularly important for children who enter into foster or adoptive homes, and who may have had the experience that rules and consequences may be different in different settings. Gaining a clear understanding of the rules and consequences is often one of the pressing concerns children have when entering new environments. Keep the rules simple; it is better, in most cases, to have a single rule linked to an overarching value such as "Be safe," than to have 10 rules commanding "Don't hit," "Don't kick," "Don't throw things," and so forth; language can be used to link the behavior to the rule (e.g., "Throwing that toy was an example of not being safe"). (*Note:* There are always exceptions; for some children, it is important to be clear and concrete when naming rules. Caregivers and clinicians should use their judgment.)

When working with caregivers to build consistent responses, it is important to pay attention to their current behavior management strategies, to the context of the child and family, to the caregivers' own parenting histories and beliefs, and to the pattern of child behavior and caregiver response. Pay attention to the "building success" strategies noted previously (p. 147). Start small and build; work with caregivers to build success using one tool before moving to another. Practice in session; role-play anticipated child responses and troubleshoot predicted problems. Whenever appropriate, integrate children into this work. For instance, if a parent will be attempting to use a comfort zone or sensory space for the first time, explain to the child in advance (i.e., *not* in the moment it is to be used for the first time), in age-appropriate language, what this space is for and when and how it will be used. Also when appropriate, coaching in the moment (i.e., in dyadic sessions) can be useful in helping caregivers apply these skills with their children. Reinforce caregivers for their attempts to use these skills, just caregivers are asked to reinforce their children. Providing active homework is crucial to the success of behavioral response strategies: Integrating new skills depends on practice and consistency, and inconsistent application will increase negative behaviors and response cycles.

Support caregivers in collaborating with other significant adults in the child's life around responding to the child's behavior. Help caregivers to communicate their goals with teachers and other adults. Similarly, help teachers and other adults communicate any particularly important goals to the primary caregivers. Team meetings are often useful.

Group

Parenting groups are often effective ways to teach behavioral response strategies because caregivers are able to receive both support and concrete suggestions from other caregivers. It is our experience that caregivers of trauma-impacted children have had to learn to be creative in applying parenting strategies, and that a wealth of knowledge often comes from other caregivers who have "been there." Consider the following examples of parenting strategies shared by caregivers in a group education setting.

> An adoptive mother of an 11-year-old girl with a history of significant neglect, whose behaviors escalated whenever the mother attempted to enforce a time-out, described her use of time-in with her daughter: "She gets too upset to sit by herself in time-out, so I put her wherever I am—if I'm cleaning the room, she has to sit on the bed quietly for 5 minutes, or if I'm cooking, she has to sit at the table. It's still not what she wants to be doing, but she can see me and she knows I'm right there, so she's not yelling for my attention the way she does if she has time-out in another room."

A similar strategy is described by a parent of a 6-year-old boy with a history of significant neglect:

"We tried ignoring his behaviors, but whenever we did, he would get more and more upset. We think being ignored and being put in time-out was really triggering for him, but we didn't want to *not* respond when he got out of control, either. What we finally started doing was having him sit on the sofa, and then one of us would sit next to him. We weren't giving him our attention, but we'd sit with him, with one hand on his knee or shoulder so that he knew we were there, and we'd sit there together until either the time-out period was over or until he was able to be calm enough for the next steps."

A third example involved increasing the child's felt control even in the face of a consequence:

"We built a 'chill-out' space under the table—it was really just a bunch of blankets and pillows, and one of her 'stuffies,' but no other toys. She can use it in two ways: One is, if she just wants to take a break, she can go in there whenever she needs to and take some space. The other is, if she's starting to get in trouble, and we need to set a limit but we can see that she's getting out of control, we give her a choice: 'You can either go to time-out for 5 minutes, or you can go into your chill-out space.' It's really cut down on a lot of the battles, because she gets some control, and she knows it's about helping her calm down."

What these examples have in common is a caregiver's understanding of the role of dysregulation in child behaviors: In each example, limits are balanced with a goal of helping the child achieve a modulated state. Furthermore, caregivers use their attunement skills to select behavior management strategies that decrease, rather than increase, their child's feelings of distress.

🏠 Milieu

Residential and other milieu programs often have expansive and sophisticated behavior management strategies; however, programs may struggle with ways to make these strategies trauma-sensitive and trauma-informed. A number of strategies may be useful for milieu programs to consider. Perhaps the most important consideration when applying limits with children who may be in highly aroused or shutdown states is the "three-stage approach," to which we refer to as the "observe, modulate, do" sequence. The sequence encourages caregivers to *observe,* first and foremost: to pay attention to patterns of behavior, get curious about the causes, tune in to child/adolescent regulation, and tune in to the caregiver's own regulation and reactions. Observing is an ongoing skill to cultivate as well as an in-the-moment strategy. The second stage, *modulate,* highlights the importance of managing physiological and emotional experience *before* engaging in action. Modulation applies to the experience of the adult caregiver, as well as to the experience of the child. The final stage, *do,* is the one in which "action" steps can take place: such as processing, problem solving, or limit setting. Because all of these require some degree of regulated state and the ability to reflect and self-reflect, none is likely to be effective when either the adult caregiver or the child is not regulated. This sequence can easily be taught to staff members as well as to youth in care. (One program we worked with renamed this strategy "Get curious, get calm, get busy!," and another used the Ice Cube lyric, "Check yourself before you wreck yourself!")

When applying limits in programs, it is important to work with staff to incorporate behavioral strategies that minimize power struggles. To increase youth felt agency and decrease feelings of helplessness (both of which decrease power struggles), teach staff to offer limited choice (e.g., "You can work on your processing sheet now or after therapy—when would you like to do it?") and to use problem-solving language ("Here are your two choices: You can sit in your room, or you can go to school. If you choose to sit in your room, then you will not be able to have free time this afternoon in the rec room. It's up to you. Which choice would you like to make?"). Whenever possible, use positive reinforcement rather than limits to shape youth behavior.

In targeting limits to youth behavior, it is important to pay attention to long-term goals rather than simply to short-term outcomes. In other words, what is the system trying to teach? Although an immediate consequence may decrease a specific behavior in the moment, it is more important, in the long term, to teach and support a youth to make good choices. Work with staff to catch signs of intensification or distress early, prior to significant escalation, and then to coach children and adolescents in making choices that will help them achieve positive outcomes. Pair this skill with youth modulation strategies and executive function skills.

When applying behavioral management strategies in a program, it is important that staff members are in communication with each other, so that response is consistent across staff and across shifts. Consider the following example:

> Jamie, a 15-year-old girl in a residential program, had been increasingly dysregulated in recent weeks, and when upset, had destroyed property and made self-harm gestures. Her clinician and one of the staff members had been working with her to tune in to her feelings of distress and to ask for support when upset. Together, they developed a plan that when feeling upset, Jamie would ask for one-on-one support from a staff member, rather than hurting herself or destroying property. Jamie was able to follow through on the plan when she became upset during the day and had successfully sought time with her favorite staff member, Tricia, on two occasions; she was able to use the time appropriately, make use of coping strategies, and return to her routine. A week into the plan, Jamie became upset late at night, after both her clinician and Tricia had gone home for the evening. Jamie requested support, but the staff on the third shift did not know of the plan and told Jamie that she would have to stay in her room and wait until morning. Jamie escalated and, within 20 minutes, had destroyed a significant amount of property in her room before staff intervened. Because she destroyed property, she was given the consequence of being removed from her current privilege level.

In this example a lack of communication regarding a behavioral intervention plan led to escalating behaviors as well as to unnecessary—and unfortunate—consequences for Jamie. Although the number of "moving parts" in most milieu programs makes it difficult to communicate about everything, it is important for programs to find methods to realistically communicate *key facets* of every individual's behavioral intervention plans.

When the primary tool that is used to change behavior is praise, it is important to remember to prioritize one or two target behaviors, as discussed earlier in this chapter. We have found that it is common in milieu settings for programs to incentivize "safe behavior" (which may encompass behavior that programs want to decrease as well as behavior that programs want to increase) with multiple reinforcers. When the target behavior is too general and when there are too many incentives, it can be confusing to the child and often ineffective when it comes to behavior change. We recommend building a "praise" plan around behaviors that you want to increase rather than decrease.

Finally, remember that praise can be a powerful trigger. Milieu programs and particularly residential centers are often tasked with supporting children who engage in significant risk behaviors—behaviors that may be dangerous to the child and to the staff who support the child. Positive behavior change, as it relates to risk behavior, may provide an overwhelming sense of relief and pride for the staff involved. This relief and pride can, at times, foster the overuse of praise and reinforcement. It may be important to remember that the most at-risk children are often those who experience significant shame and vulnerability. As a result their praise "button" or trigger can be very sensitive and easily activated, leading to what appears to be behavioral regression. To prevent this, remember to be targeted and thoughtful about how praise can be used to reinforce and support sustained progress for these children.

Trauma Experience Integration: State-Based Skills Application

Distress Tolerance and Regulation

Many of the children and families that we see have made complex adaptations to their experiences that impact multiple domains of functioning and lead to extremely challenging behaviors to manage. It can be overwhelming at times for providers to determine when, where, and how to begin addressing behavior change. Many caregivers, however, are often very clear about where they want to begin. As discussed earlier in this chapter, challenging behaviors are often the primary presenting issue for many of the families with which we work. Caregivers are seeking support for effecting behavior change in their children and often are hoping for rapid results. During early stages of treatment and/or in more distressed states, a primary emphasis is on acknowledging and supporting the intense distress the caregiver may be feeling in response to child behaviors, acknowledging how challenging it is to parent or care for a trauma-impacted child, and emphasizing the role of basic caregiver affect management skills as a foundation to addressing child behaviors. Provider attunement to caregiver needs and support for caregiver-prioritized goals are crucial. Exploration of caregiver values ("Who do you want to be as a parent/caregiver?") and goals ("What is important to you? What behavior do you want to see in this child?") lays a key foundation for identifying intervention priorities. Education about, and exploration of, the range of possible intervention strategies are important parts of this process. For instance, while it may seem counterintuitive to use praise as a tool for reducing aggression, it can be very effective for some children; for others, however, limits are the tool of choice. It is important in this early stage to actively link caregiver modulation and attunement work to effective child response strategies.

Curiosity and Reflection

As the caregiver is increasingly able to engage in curious observation and "feelings detective" work, discussed previously, he or she can begin to identify what a child may need in a given context (e.g., tantrums at bedtime seem to pull for connection and nurturance; tantrums at homework time seem to be a strategy for avoiding shame) as well as specific strategies for meeting those needs (e.g., bedtime connection rituals; redefining and reinforcing "trying" as homework success) and ways to build in additional regulation support (e.g., rubbing child's back during bedtime ritual; allowing child to listen to favorite music during homework time). Over time, caregivers can begin to incorporate effective responses and strategies into their repertoire of skills for supporting child regulation and behavior change. As this happens, children may begin to internalize caregiver response and move toward a higher level of independence with regulation. In parallel, caregivers may begin to feel more regulated with increasing knowledge about, and skills to shift, challenging behavior.

Engaging Purposeful Action

Over time, as caregivers build mastery of attunement skills, they will begin to collaboratively engage their child in achieving a shared understanding about the needs that are being communicated, why they are important (e.g., "I need you at night because I'm afraid of the dark"), how they are connected to past experience (e.g., "Dad used to be really fun in the morning but not so much at night—at night he would get really mad and say mean things to me"), and how best to meet them (e.g., "I really like when you come in my room and sit until I go to sleep"). This collaboration is also supported by the provider in direct work with the child on relational connection. The caregiver and child can begin to try out new, more direct strategies for communicating experience, including wants and needs. Caregiver identity may begin to shift to incorporate a greater sense of confidence and competence in this role.

Tools such as problem solving, praising, and limit setting can be implemented by caregivers to intentionally shift the trauma lens. For example, a caregiver and child can develop problem-solving approaches to repair moments of misattunement or disconnection between them, or moments where needs go unmet, and/or to strategize about how to communicate needs and strategies to the surrounding caregiving system. Limits can be used to teach children boundaries as well as other relational skills needed to safely and effectively engage in relationships and the world around them. Targeted praise can be used to shift self-concept by supporting a child's ability to engage with others and to experience and tolerate pride, self-worth, and a sense of agency. In this stage the caregiver is purposely selecting strategies that shift behavior by shifting the lens through which the child filters his or her experiences.

🌍 Real-World Therapy

🌍 **Be realistic.** Behavioral strategies are often very effective, but they require consistent effort and follow-through by caregivers. For a many caregivers, shifting their behavioral management strategies is hard, and targeting even a single behavior or skill can feel like the straw that broke the camel's back. Caregivers often need a lot of support, encouragement, and understanding (as well as concrete guidance: Help them make the chart, keep a supply of stickers, etc.) to be able to add new tasks. Keep in mind that ignoring is probably the hardest of the skills and should not be the strategy caregivers try first.

◗ **Pay attention to your own feelings and be solution-focused.** All clinicians have toolboxes containing, among other options, certain interventions that we depend on as "standards." In child work, caregiver behavioral skills training is often one such standard, and we rely on it as a tool that can invariably help with identified behavioral problems. When a family is unable to use these techniques—particularly when we believe they can make a difference—it can be very frustrating. It is easy to fall into the trap of becoming angry at or blaming the caregiver. It is important to try to take the family's perspective; failure of these techniques is often less about caregivers' rejection of the techniques than it is about their feeling overwhelmed by the intensity and variability of the child's behavior, or about the complexity of environmental circumstances. Work to identify (with family members) the barriers to implementation and help problem-solve and adapt the techniques.

◗ **Predict the problems.** When new limits or rules are applied, children may rebel: Their behavior may get worse before it gets better. Predict this "worst case" for caregivers, and help them find strategies to deal with both the behavior and their own responses. Be a cheerleader for the caregivers.

Part V

Regulation

What Does It Mean to "Regulate"?

- *Regulation* involves the capacity to effectively manage experience on many levels: cognitive, emotional, physiological, and behavioral.
- Successful regulation of experience may involve many different things, including:
  - Some degree of awareness of internal state
  - The ability to tolerate a range of arousal and affect
  - The ability to engage in action or cognition to modulate arousal and affective state
  - An understanding of the interconnections among aspects of internal experiences (i.e., sensation, feeling, thought, behavior)
  - An understanding of the factors that influence internal experience
  - The capacity to effectively communicate experience with others

Developmental Shifts in Regulation

- The earliest regulation challenge involves basic physiological organization: patterns of sleeping, alert interaction, eating, and eventually toileting. This regulation is largely supported through the external or simultaneous regulation of the caregiver.
- Over time regulation of experience moves from being primarily externally structured (i.e., soothing as provided by caregiver[s]) to primarily internally directed, although we continue to use significant others as modulation resources throughout our lives.
- All skills involved in regulation develop from a very basic level to an increasingly sophisticated one. For instance, a young child's awareness of internal state may be as simple as "I feel bad," whereas an older adolescent may be able to identify such nuanced states as "I'm feeling disappointed and concerned."

The Important Role of the Caregiving System

■ The caregiving system plays a prominent role in the successful development of all aspects of regulation.

■ Many caregiver behaviors contribute to the development of healthy child self-regulation over time. Among others, these behaviors include:

   ◆ *Reflection:* Reflection of the child's experience can be verbal (e.g., "You look like you're getting sleepy now") or behavioral (e.g., the caregiver who responds to the child's laughter with a smile). The mirroring of the child's experience through the caregiver's facial expressions, words, and actions supplies the earliest lens through which the child learns to interpret his or her experience. When paired with appropriate affect regulation on the part of the caregiver, attuned reflection also communicates to the child that his or her affect is tolerable and that the child is acceptable.

   ◆ *Modeling:* Caregivers' own expression and modulation of feelings provide both a visual language for understanding affect as well as a model of coping. The child learns to "read" and understand verbal and facial expressions and other nonverbal cues of emotion, along with their associated experience, by observing the ways in which caregivers' expressions pair with actions (e.g., the appearance of a loving expression paired with soothing) and experience (e.g., an expression of pain after touching a hot pan). Caregivers' actions in the face of distress serve as a demonstration of modulation strategies and affect tolerance (e.g., the caregiver who appears frustrated and then takes a deep breath and smiles). Through modeling, the child learns that even intense affect is normative, that there are strategies that can be used for managing and tolerating it, and that it does not last forever.

   ◆ *Stimulation and soothing:* When provided in an attuned manner, the caregiver is able to support a child in achieving optimal levels of arousal by alternatively providing stimulation and soothing. By responding appropriately when energy levels become overwhelmingly high (i.e., intense distress) or low (i.e., sleepiness), the caregiver's words, vocal tones, and behaviors become a source of physiological organization. Gradually, the young child internalizes these skills and begins to be able to independently maintain a comfortable state of arousal.

■ When caregivers are unresponsive, inconsistent, or abusive, infants and young children must rely on primitive modulation skills (e.g., rocking, thumbsucking, dissociation) to soothe their own affect. Lack of reflection and modeling leave children with no emotional language with which to interpret their own or others' experience. In the absence of reliable supports, and particularly in the face of ongoing stress and distress, children will either guard against affect or continue to rely on primitive coping, which leaves them unlikely to develop more sophisticated self-regulation strategies.

Working with Regulation in Historical Context

■ Shame, isolation, secrecy, and feelings of damage are often central to the trauma experience.

■ Children and adults who have experienced trauma may believe that there is something wrong with them, that they are different from others, and that strong emotions signal "craziness," "being bad," or a loss of control.

■ The elephant in the room:

   ◆ It is not uncommon for treatment to target specific areas of "deficit" or "pathology" (e.g., oppositional behavior, anxiety) in the absence of an organizing frame or context.

   ◆ Well-intentioned clinicians and other providers who do hold an awareness of the role of trauma in a child's presentation may hesitate to name it. This hesitancy often stems from a belief that a child must be fully "safe" before approaching historical experiences.

  ◆ When treatment occurs in the absence of an understanding of the role of history, the link between past and current experience is not addressed, and the self-perception of shame, damage, isolation, and secrecy may actually increase.

■ Naming the elephant: When working with the child who has experienced trauma, consider the following:

  ◆ Acknowledge the child in his or her entirety: past experiences, current reality, strengths, vulnerabilities, possibilities, interests, etc. Although it is important to understand the child in context, every child is more than the sum of his or her experiences. It is important to communicate from the start that we are interested in the whole child.

  ◆ Validate the adaptive nature of (often distressing) behaviors. Identify the role these behaviors may have played in the child's life. For instance, for a child who engages in frequent aggressive behaviors with peers, we might say, "It seems as if it's pretty important to you to show other kids how strong you are."

  ◆ Educate the child about the trauma response, triggers, and the links between past experience and current response. Understanding the human danger response and its current role in dysregulated or self-protective behaviors is a vital step toward providing the child with some measure of control and also decreasing the child's sense of stigma. Links to past experiences can be kept simple, especially early in treatment (e.g., "When kids have really hard things happen, like what happened to you with your dad . . ."). In Chapter 10 ("Identification") this topic is discussed in depth.

  ◆ Differentiate past and present. In working with children to understand, be aware of, and manage their current emotions and behaviors, it is important to engage their curiosity about the ways in which behaviors that were protective and adaptive in the past may not be as helpful in the present. Explore these behaviors with the child and family. For instance, keeping feelings from showing may have helped protect a child from a violent caregiver, but may currently be keeping the child from getting his or her needs met. Examine the role of context: There may still be situations in which the child needs to engage in self-protective behaviors.

Targeting Child Needs: Understanding the Functional Nature of Modulation Attempts

■ Many of the distressing behaviors and symptoms that lead to a child's referral for treatment can be understood as the child's attempts to cope. For instance, oppositional behavior may be a preemptive strike to cope with anticipated rejection or to gain control; self-injury may be an attempt at self-soothing; and sexualized behaviors may be attempts at control or connection.

■ Behavior and "symptoms" often provide a window into the child's experience of affect and arousal. All symptoms have many possible origins, and understanding the function underlying a child's behaviors is critical to successful treatment. The child's typical approach to managing emotion and physiology provides important information about his or her tolerance for arousal, his or her available repertoire of coping strategies, and the "emotional intensity" range within which the child is able to function versus feel overwhelmed. In Chapter 11 ("Modulation") we discuss the concepts of a comfort zone (the level of arousal that feels comfortable in the child's body). a safety zone (a more rigid range of arousal a child requires to feel safe within his or her body), and a danger zone (the level of arousal that leads to disorganization and overwhelm in the child). Because these patterns differ greatly across children, addressing regulation will be most successful when the provider begins by understanding the child's needs and current strategies.

■ Although it would be impossible to capture all possible child presentations, three common presentations are offered here to serve as examples.

Presentation #1: The Overly Constricted Child

Presentation	Overly constricted children are often quiet and have difficulty initiating conversation, activities, and interactions in general. They are not oppositional and, in fact, may be overly compliant. These children have difficulty describing any emotions; a typical response to "How are you doing?" is "Fine" or "I don't know" (which, for these children, is a realistic response). Constricted children appear defended against emotional experience in general, and often lack an understanding of how to connect emotionally with others. A common adaptation to overcome this limitation is to engage in "other-pleasing" behavior: Constricted children may appear to subordinate their own needs, opinions, etc., to others. In younger children this difficulty with self-expression may include failure to engage in imaginary play. At times these children may show explosive outbursts of emotion in response to what appear to be minor stressors, as their intense control becomes overwhelmed or challenged. In the aftermath of this intense emotion, however, these children return quickly to a constricted state and have difficulty acknowledging or processing the emotional experience.
Primary skills deficits	■ Limited emotional vocabulary ■ Limited awareness of internal experience ■ Restricted range of tolerance for arousal ■ Limited skills to cope with and manage emotional experience, including positive emotions ■ Deficit in ability to seek social support, particularly in the sharing or management of emotional experience
Safety and danger zones	The constricted child often has a very slim safety zone at the frozen/numb end of the arousal scale (on a scale of 0–10, this child prefers to live between 0 and 1).
Function of this adaptation	Constriction represents a child's strategy for coping with overwhelming emotion. In the absence of regulation skills and/or social support, the child relies on denying and withdrawing from emotional experience and physiological arousal.
Therapeutic considerations	■ Initial work should be displaced; gradually shift from external to internal (e.g., help child identify affect in a television show or book character). ■ Help child identify cues associated with affect. Behavior is often a good starting point, and it is less threatening than the feeling itself. Other children may respond to identification of body states or thoughts. ■ Because constriction is an attempt to disconnect from internal experience and external stimulation, clinical strategies that heighten arousal may be overwhelming. Down-regulation strategies (i.e., learning to calm arousal) may be important targets of intervention to build the child's sense of agency over managing internal experience.

Presentation #2: The Highly Aroused Child

Presentation	Children who present with predominantly high arousal often rely on a "front" to prevent others (and often themselves) from awareness of their vulnerability, perceived damage, and an often deep sense of shame and self-blame. These children generally have access to the "powerful" emotions—anger, frustration with perceived injustice, blame—but little ability to acknowledge more vulnerable feeling states such as fear or sadness. They may readily acknowledge being angry at someone or upset about something that has happened that day, but will deny feeling hurt or worried about the incident. These children frequently externalize; emotions are generally connected to outside events rather than to the impact of those events on them. Perceived

injustice is often a powerful trigger for these children and will likely be perceived frequently. Their presentation may be oppositional or argumentative toward people in authority, although they are often able to build relationships with people they perceive as less threatening or demanding. These children appear to desire connection but seek it in ineffective ways (e.g., as the "class clown," through negative behaviors). They have a profound sense of mistrust in relationships and have difficulty believing that others truly care about them. Because of this stance, these children may "test" relationships to see if others will abandon or harm them. This relational reenactment may represent their attempt to control anticipated negative interactions as well as to confirm their perceived sense of self and other.

Primary skills deficits	■ Acknowledging and coping with vulnerable emotions ■ Modulating intense emotion, particularly in the face of key triggers such as injustice, shame, etc. ■ Accepting responsibility for actions in social conflict ■ Engaging empathy and perspective taking in difficult relationships
Safety and danger zones	The highly aroused child often has a very slim safety zone at the hyperaroused end of the energy scale (on a scale of 0–10, this child prefers to live between 8 and 10). Lower levels of arousal may increase feelings of vulnerability or unease. Because the child is already at a high level of arousal, even minor stressors can lead to surges of distress and disorganization/impulsivity/reactive responses.
Function of this adaptation	Externalizing emotion and responsibility allows children who feel intensely shamed or damaged to protect themselves from those overwhelming feelings. Heightened arousal provides children with a sense of readiness and empowerment in the face of often-perceived danger. With limited skills to cope with intense affect, these children are unable to tolerate any feelings that threaten their already fragile sense of self.
Therapeutic considerations	■ Forcing these children to acknowledge difficult emotions before they are ready is likely to lead to power struggles and increased shame. ■ Normalizing denied emotions is a key intervention with these children. Often, this is done via displacement (e.g., "I could understand how someone might be very worried if happened to them"). ■ Providing psychoeducation about triggers and the trauma response may be very important for normalizing the anger response and may serve as a foundation for helping children learn to differentiate "true danger" from perceived danger. ■ Modulation strategies that move toward the child's arousal level (i.e., high-energy gross motor activities) may be more readily tolerable than those that work against the child's natural arousal state. It may be important to explore and practice high-energy activities that provide the child with control and organization.

Presentation #3: The Labile Child

Presentation	The labile child's presentation is changeable. These children are strongly affected by environmental triggers, others' emotions, and internal states. Clinical assessment is often complicated, because their presentation can vary from day to day and hour to hour. Their emotional reactions appear unpredictable and may be disproportionate to the apparent stressor; they may go from 0 to 60 in a matter of moments, or completely shut down just as quickly. Presentation in therapy is therefore inconsistent: On some days these children may appear very well put together, whereas on others they are reactive, withdrawn, or overwhelmed. Distress is experienced as diffuse, with difficulty differentiating both the type of emotion and its source. In addition, they have difficulty judging degree of emotion: Irritability feels like rage, for example, and sadness feels like despair. Emotional states are disconnected, and it is difficult for these children to access an emotional experience when no longer in the midst of it. When they are in the midst of it, however, they are unable to think past it. These children's lives are driven by emotion, but they have little cognitive framework for understanding it or ability to cope with it in healthy ways. These children may rely heavily on dissociative coping. As a result, their sense of self—and therefore of their emotional experience—is fragmented and may appear to shift rapidly.

Primary skills deficits	▪ Inability to modulate emotional experience (rapid escalation or numbing, with difficulty returning to baseline) ▪ Misreading of environmental cues; low threshold for perception of threat ▪ Inability to integrate experiences into a cohesive narrative and/or sense of self
Safety and danger zones	Children with a labile presentation often have a very slim safety zone, which may vary on the arousal scale (i.e., for some children it may be midrange, for others, higher or lower). Within their preferred range, these children are able to organize experience; however, in the face of even minor stressors or positive experiences that lead to increases or decreases in arousal, their ability to cope is compromised. As a result, very small gradations of experience can lead to rapid disorganization and sudden surges of arousal.
Function of this adaptation	These children have developed a heightened biological alarm system. In the face of *any* emotion-inducing stimulus (internal or external), their bodies provide them with the fuel they would need to survive if they were in true danger. However, this response has become as likely to occur presently with mild input as it did in the past with threatening input. Unlike constricted and highly aroused children, labile children may lack any organized strategy for coping with arousal states. As a result, their physically intense reactivity leaves these children at the mercy of their moment-to-moment experience.
Therapeutic considerations	▪ The goal with these children is not necessarily to alter their emotions, but to help them develop a range of modulation strategies for reducing the intensity to a realistic level, so that it is tolerable/manageable, and to help them identify its source. In this process, it is important to normalize children's emotions, teach them to recognize shifts in degree of feeling, and explore and identify a range of internal and external strategies for tolerating and managing emotional and physiological experience. ▪ Experience is state-dependent for these children; they may be able to discuss their emotions and alternative coping skills in the aftermath of an incident, but they will have a much harder time applying those skills in the moment, when their primary concern is survival. Because of this state-dependent aspect, repetition of skills and providing external cuing and support (co- or supported regulation) are essential.

10

Identification

> ## 🔑 THE MAIN IDEA AND KEY SUBSKILLS
>
> Work with children to build an awareness of internal experience, the ability to discriminate and name emotional and physiological states, and an understanding of why these states occur.
>
> ★ Increase youth ability to accurately identify, at an age-appropriate level, internal experience (emotions, energy/arousal), including:
> - ◇ *Language:* Developing a language for emotions and energy/arousal
> - ◇ *Connection:* Enhancing awareness of feelings, body sensations, thoughts, and behaviors; understanding the links among these and using these as clues to understand experience
> - ◇ *Contextualization:* Building understanding experiences that elicit emotions and arousal, including trauma-related triggers and responses
>
> ★ Increase youth's ability to accurately identify, at an age-appropriate level, emotion in other people.

★ Key Concepts

Why Target Affect Identification?

- Traumatic stress overwhelms the limited emotion management skill set available to developing children, often forcing them either to disconnect from their feelings and body sensations or to use rudimentary or unhealthy coping skills.

- Children who have experienced inadequate early caretaking and/or insufficient emotional support may have never developed adequate skills in identifying and expressing emotion.

- Other children may have developed limited skills that became overwhelmed and splintered in the aftermath of trauma, particularly if the trauma has had a substantial impact on the emotional functioning of the entire family unit.

- Because of these factors, children who have experienced trauma are frequently disconnected from, or unaware of, their own emotional experience.

work, the provider might begin to introduce known people. An example of this would be, "Why don't you act out how Mom looks when she is happy."

■ Visual cues:

 ◆ It can be very helpful to have visual cues (like emotion posters and character pictures, along with visual cues for energy or arousal) available in the therapy office, residence, classroom, or "toolbag" (home-based clinicians). Each child may need his or her own unique feelings face poster and energy scale. Some children will help to create visual cues for use in the therapeutic process. It may be important that nonverbal strategies such as these are a part of the therapy or intervention because many children either do not yet have language for their experience or do not have access to language when they are distressed. When such tools are available, children can simply point to the emotion or level of arousal that best illustrates how they are feeling in a given moment.

■ Caregiver/therapist modeling:

 ◆ We have always operated under the premise that the caregiver is the most important "tool" in this framework. As such, we suggest caregiver modeling as a particularly important tool for supporting youth identification. It is important that adults model affect purposefully and with appropriate boundaries. Consider the following example:

> A therapist is stuck in traffic on the way to work, and gets to the office in the nick of time for her appointment with a 9-year-old boy. The boy walks into the office and says, "Are you okay, Miss?" The therapist looks at him, takes a deep breath, and says, "Why do you ask that? What do you notice about me" "Well, you still have your coat on, you're breathing fast, your face looks angry, and you don't have my check-in out." The therapist then shares about her experience with traffic and labels her feelings. "I was frustrated and worried that I wouldn't get here on time for our visit because it is so important to me." The therapist then adds to the interaction by suggesting that they practice a modulation skill together: "Do you know what helps me to settle? I love to toss a ball back and forth. Will you do that with me for a minute?"

 ◆ In this example the therapist uses modeling to teach basic labeling of affect, mixed emotions, connection to cues/context, and modulation of affect.

Teach to Caregivers

■ *Reminder:* Teach the caregiver the Key Concepts.
■ *Reminder:* Teach the caregiver relevant Developmental Considerations.
■ Mirroring and other attunement skills, as described in Chapter 8, are an important support for emerging child identification skills. Work with caregiver(s) to actively practice and apply these skills in support of child awareness.

Tools: Identification

Teach to Kids: Psychoeducation about Feelings

■ Examples of how to speak with children about key teaching points are provided. Keep in mind, however, that psychoeducation should be provided in a developmentally appropriate way; thus language will vary from client to client.

■ The following table provides a guideline for speaking with children about affect identification. Not all teaching points will be relevant to all children.

Understanding Feelings

Teaching point	Important information as sample language
Everyone has feelings.	"Everyone—kids and adults—has a lot of different feelings. It's normal for things in our life to make us feel different ways."
	"There are no 'wrong' feelings—no one can tell you how you should or shouldn't feel about something."
	"There are lots of ways that feelings can show up, and if we don't know what our feelings are, they can come out in ways that hurt us or other people."
Feelings come from somewhere.	"Most of the time, feelings are not random—something causes them. Feelings can be caused by *thoughts, people, situations,* and *internal sensations.*" (Clinicians should provide concrete examples of ways in which each of the preceding domains can be linked to feelings.)
	"Special kinds of situations are the ones that feel dangerous. There are a lot of different kinds of situations that might feel dangerous to kids' brains. Once our brains decide that something is dangerous, our body gives us the fuel we need to deal with it. This fuel helps us react fast, move quickly, protect ourselves, and get to somewhere safe. When we go through danger over and over, our brains learn to recognize clues that danger might be coming (like sounds, smells, or things we see), so that we can react really fast. Sometimes these clues happen when there isn't really any danger. When that happens, we call these clues 'triggers.' When there is a trigger, our brain sets off our danger alarm to try to help us stay safe, even though there really isn't any danger around. It's important to learn to recognize triggers and our danger response, so that we can take the time to *think*, instead of just *reacting*."
	Note: Significantly expanded psychoeducation about triggers and the danger response appears in the next table.
It is not always easy to know what we feel.	Experiencing really hard things can interfere with kids' ability to know what they are feeling. There are a lot of reasons for this: ■ "A lot of kids learn about feelings from their moms or dads when they're babies or very little. [Can help to give examples—such as picking babies up and rocking them.] Sometimes, though, parents have a hard time helping their kids with their feelings. This could happen because . . . [may be useful to give examples or tie to kids' own experiences]. When that happens, kids have to learn all those skills later on." ■ "One of the ways kids may cope with trauma is to shut off or avoid feelings. This can help in the moment, but when kids do this often enough, they can start to lose touch with what their feelings are." ■ *Note:* It is important to use language appropriate to the client. The word *trauma* may be too abstract or triggering for some children. Use terminology that resonates with the child's and/or family's experience. ■ "Trauma can also create feelings that are so big, it can be hard to tell one feeling from another. So, for example, feeling mad can feel just like feeling excited." ■ "Sometimes feelings can come up so suddenly that it can be too confusing to know what they are or where they came from. This is especially true if something is triggering them."
There are cues that can tell us what we are feeling.	"Feelings show up in lots of different ways. They may show up in our behavior, our bodies, our facial expressions, our thoughts, our tone of voice, and in other ways."
	Behavior: "Sometimes our feelings come out in what we do, what we say, or how we act with other people. Feeling angry might make some kids hit someone, it might make other kids say mean things, or it might make kids act rude or refuse to do what they're told."
	Behavior: "Other times, feelings show up in what we *don't* do. For example, some kids, when they're upset, don't want to play or be with other people. They may hide out in their rooms or skip school."

Teaching point	Important information as sample language
	Body: "Feelings may show up in our bodies. We might get a stomachache when we're worried, or a headache when we're really angry or upset. We might notice that our muscles feel really relaxed when we're happy, or that we feel full of energy when we're excited."
	Facial expressions: "It's harder for us to see our own facial expressions, but what we feel will often show up on our face. We may smile, glare, curl our lip, show our teeth, or roll our eyes, depending on what we are feeling."
	Thoughts: "What we are thinking may give us information about how we are feeling. Sometimes our thoughts are about ourselves—for instance, we might think 'I did a terrible job at that' when we are sad or disappointed—and sometimes our thoughts are about other people—for example, we might think 'He's such a jerk' when we're mad."
	Tone of voice: "How we feel may show up in how we speak. Some people get really loud when they're angry, and others get really quiet. When we're really nervous, we might speak kind of softly, and when we're excited we might be louder."
It is important to be a "feelings detective."	"Knowing about our feelings can help us in a lot of different ways. When we know what we are feeling, it can help us to understand the situation we're in. For example, angry feelings may tell us we don't like something, and worried feelings may tell us we have a problem we need to try to solve. We can try to do something to manage or change the feeling if we don't like it or if it's too big or too small, and we can share the feeling with other people."
	"One of the things we are going to work on is becoming 'feelings detectives': We are going to work on understanding what different feelings are, how they show up, and what we can do with them."

Teach to Kids: Understanding Triggers

▪ It is important for children to understand the impact of the trauma response on their current emotional reactions. An important component of building affect identification and modulation skills is psychoeducation about the trauma response and its triggers.

▪ The following table provides key teaching points and sample language for speaking with children about triggers. Keep in mind that language should be geared toward the developmental stage and individual needs of the child client.

Understanding Triggers

Target	Description
The body's alarm system	*Teaching point:* The human brain has built-in systems that recognize danger and help to keep us safe.
	Sample language: "We all have a built-in alarm system that signals when we might be in danger. One reason why human beings have been able to survive over time is because our brains recognize signals around us that tell us that danger might be coming. This helps our bodies prepare to deal with danger when it comes."
Normative danger response	*Teaching point:* The human danger response is completely normal.
	Sample language: "When our brains recognize danger, they prepare our bodies to deal with it. We have four major ways to deal with something dangerous: We can fight it, we can get away from it, we can freeze, or we can submit.
	"What we pick to do sometimes depends on the kind of danger. So, for example, if a squirrel is attacking you, you might fight it, because you're bigger than it is. If a car comes speeding at you, and you're standing in the street, you'd probably run, because you can't really fight it, and if you stand still, you'll get hit. If you saw a big bear or some other animal nearby, you might freeze, because you can't really fight it, and you're probably not fast enough to run away. If someone much bigger said you had to do something or they would hurt you, you might go along with it to protect yourself."

Target	Description
Link between danger response and increased arousal	*Teaching point:* The fight–flight–freeze danger response is associated with an increase in arousal level. *Sample language:* "When it's time for our bodies to fight, run, freeze, or submit, we need a lot of energy to do any one of those things. So, when the brain recognizes danger, the "action" or "doing" part of the brain sends a signal to the body to release a bunch of chemicals, like fuel for a car. Those chemicals give us the energy we need to cope with the danger."
Overactive alarm	*Teaching point:* Overactivation of the alarm system occurs with chronic exposure or extreme exposure to danger. *Sample language:* "When the danger signal goes off, the 'thinking' part of our brains check out what is going on around us. If it is a false alarm, and there is no real danger, the 'thinking' brain shuts off the alarm, and we can keep doing whatever we were doing. If there is danger, the 'doing brain' takes over and gives the body fuel to deal with whatever is going on. "Sometimes, though, the danger alarm goes off too much. That usually happens when kids have had lots of dangerous things happen—like their parents hurting them, or someone touching them when they didn't want it, or someone yelling or fighting a lot. For kids who have had to deal with danger a lot, the 'thinking brain' has gotten tired of checking things out and just assumes that the signals mean more danger. So now, when the alarm goes off, the 'thinking brain' stays out of the way and lets the 'doing brain' take over."
Triggers	*Teaching point:* The false alarm goes off in response to reminders or *triggers*. *Sample language:* "False alarms can happen when we hear, or see, or feel something that reminds us of bad things that used to happen. Those reminders are called *triggers*. Our brains have learned to recognize those reminders, because in the past when they were around, dangerous things happened, and we had to react pretty quickly. "Different people have different reminders. So, if someone got yelled at a lot, hearing people yell might activate the alarm and make the 'doing' part of the brain turn on. If someone didn't get enough attention when he or she was little, feeling all alone or scared might turn on the alarm." *Note:* It is important to use examples that are relevant to the child.
How triggers manifest	*Teaching point:* The triggered response can be connected to dysregulated behaviors and emotions. *Sample language:* "Once our alarms turn on, our brains prepare our bodies for action. When that happens, the body fills with 'fuel' to prepare us for dealing with danger. This is really important if it's real danger—like a bear, or a speeding car, or a really mean squirrel—but it's not so helpful if it's a false alarm, and there isn't really any danger around. Imagine if you were in math class and something felt dangerous—suddenly, your body is filled with fuel. "Remember that the fuel gives us the energy to fight, or get away, or freeze. When our bodies have all that energy, we have to do something. So, some kids will suddenly feel really angry or want to argue or fight with someone. Some kids just feel antsy or jumpy. Other kids want to hide in a corner or get as far away as they can—and sometimes they don't even know why. Other kids will suddenly feel really shut down, like someone flipped a switch and turned them off. All of these are ways our bodies try to deal with something that seems to be dangerous. "Sometimes, though, what set off the alarm isn't really dangerous—it's just something that feels bad or reminds us of something bad that happened in the past. When kids have a false alarm like that, it can be hard for other people to understand what just happened and to help. Sometimes kids even get into trouble." (*Query:* "Are there times you've suddenly had a lot of energy, or felt really mad or upset or scared, and couldn't quite figure out what was going on?")
Recognizing triggers	*Teaching point:* Link to the skill of recognizing triggers. *Sample language:* "We're going to work on learning about what kinds of reminders might feel dangerous to you and how your body reacts when those reminders are around. Everyone has different triggers and different ways of responding when the alarm goes off. If we know what sets off your alarm and how you respond, we can get your thinking brain on board to help figure out when danger is real and when it's a false alarm."

- See child education handout **"The Body's Alarm System"** and child worksheets **"My Body's Alarm System," "My False Alarm Goes Off When . . . ,"** and **"Identifying Triggers"** in Appendix D.

Exercises for Building Identification Skills

- The menu includes activities in multiple modalities; choose activities based on child preference.

- Some activities may be more arousing than others; pay attention to helping children wind down before the end of session.

- When doing identification exercises, pay attention to identification of triggers and triggered responses.

- Consider ways that all activities described in the following material can be adapted to the child's current level. For instance, for a young child or a child with a limited feelings vocabulary, feelings flashcards might focus on "basic" emotions (e.g., happy, sad, mad, worried); with an older child, there might be exploration of nuance (e.g., angry vs. frustrated vs. enraged).

- There are numerous worksheets in Appendix D that may be useful for helping children learn to recognize and understand their feelings.

- The following activities target one or more of the skills involved in affect identification. The following key is used to identify potential targets:

  - **I-S** *Identification of emotion in self*
  - **I-O** *Identification of emotion in other*
  - **C-Bod** *Connection to body sensations*
  - **C-Th** *Connection to thoughts*
  - **C-Beh** *Connection to behavior*
  - **C-Ext** *Contextualization—external:* factors in the environment that precipitate the feeling
  - **C-Int** *Contextualization—internal:* internal factors (e.g., fatigue or hunger) that contribute to the development of different feelings

Affect Identification Exercise Examples

Activity	Targets	Description	
Feelings flashcards	**I-S, I-O, C-Ext**	Suggested materials	Create flashcards using drawings, magazine/book pictures, etc., that depict a range of emotional expressions. Cards can be created solely by clinician or jointly with the child.
		Techniques	■ Have the child identify and label what he or she believes that he or she is seeing in the picture. ◆ Progress from basic to subtle: ◆ Start with pictures that contain obvious affect. ◆ Start with a limited number of basic emotions (e.g., sad, mad, happy, worried). ◆ Expand to subtler emotions and/or variations on a single emotion (e.g., a series of cards that depict frustration, irritation, anger, rage).

Activity	Targets	Description	
		Techniques	▪ Have the child identify and label what he or she believes that he or she is seeing in the picture. 　◆ Progress from basic to subtle: 　◆ Start with pictures that contain obvious affect. 　◆ Start with a limited number of basic emotions (e.g., sad, mad, happy, worried). 　◆ Expand to subtler emotions and/or variations on a single emotion (e.g., a series of cards that depict frustration, irritation, anger, rage). ▪ Have child identify possible reasons for each emotion (e.g., "What do you think happened to make him [her] feel _____?"). ▪ Have child identify personal experiences that might elicit the same or similar feelings (e.g., "What kinds of things might make you feel _____?").
		Considerations	▪ *Pacing:* Build slowly and pay attention to child distress. Over time, moving from external to internal areas of experience may help the child develop comfort with this skill. ▪ *Relevance:* Use materials appropriate to the child's world. Consider issues of: 　◆ Cultural/ethnic background 　◆ Child likes/dislikes (e.g., sports figures) 　◆ Degree of displacement needed (e.g., photographs vs. cartoons)
Feelings charade	**I-S, I-O, C-Beh, C-Ext**	Suggested materials	Prompt cards may include: ▪ Feelings ▪ Scenarios (with three or more people) Some children prefer to use puppets, dolls, stuffed animals, etc.
		Techniques	Can be used one on one, with families, or in groups. Consider the following: ▪ Select feeling; one person (child, clinician) acts out feeling, and the other must guess. ▪ Person guessing the names cues that led him or her to identify specific feeling. ▪ Select scenario; two people act it out, and the third must guess emotion of each player. With larger groups, can be reenacted using different feelings. ▪ Use puppets, dolls, or stuffed animals to act out feelings and/or scenarios.
		Considerations	*Relevance:* Clinician should use scenarios appropriate to the child. *Reading level:* Assess child's ability to read card.
Word play	**I-S, I-O**	Suggested materials	None, or cards with neutral words. Suggested words include "Oh," "Really?," "Yes," "No," "Hmmm." May be helpful to have a list of feelings for prompting.
		Techniques	▪ Pick a word (e.g., "Oh"). ▪ Model saying the word in different states (e.g., "How does 'Oh' sound when it's angry? Excited?"). Pay attention to use of cues such as voice tone and volume, body language, eye contact, posture and muscular tension, etc. ▪ Have the child guess the feeling; point out or elicit from child the cues that led to feeling identification. ▪ Take turns identifying which feeling the other is showing.
		Considerations	None.

Activity	Targets	Description	
Feelings detective	I-S, I-O, C-Beh, C-Th, C-Ext, C-Int	Suggested materials	Paper or whiteboard writing tool
		Techniques	Help children identify connections among feelings, thoughts, behavior, and experience.
			■ On paper or whiteboard write a list of emotions (start with basic; if appropriate, move to advanced).
			■ Talk or write out ways that feelings may show up in behavior.
			■ Talk or write out different thoughts that might lead to a feeling. Note that thoughts are frequently harder for children to identify; provide general examples (e.g., "If I thought that no one liked me, I might feel sad or worried.").
			■ Talk or write out different situations that might lead to the feeling. Again, it is often useful to provide examples.
			■ As children become proficient with these skills, begin to apply them to real-world situations. For instance, if a parent reports that the child seemed angry last night, ask the child to use his or her feelings detective skills with you to identify what was going on.
		Considerations	*Introduction of technique:* Help children understand the rationale for this technique. Here is a sample introduction for younger children: "Kids are very good at telling grownups how they are feeling with their behavior. Words are sometimes harder for kids. You probably know a lot about kids because you are a kid. Maybe you can teach me some more. What kinds of behavior do you think kids use to show grownups that they are sad, mad, or happy?" Allow the child to be the expert.
Body awareness	I-S, C-Bod	Suggested materials	■ Large rolls of white paper *or* standard letter-size paper
			■ Markers or other drawing materials in a variety of colors
		Techniques	■ Provide basic psychoeducation about how feelings are held in the body. Help children understand that one way to identify and differentiate emotions is to learn how different feeling states are held in their body.
			■ Do a body drawing: On standard paper, draw a silhouette figure of a body *or* have the child lie down on large sheet of paper and trace the child's body.
			■ Make a key.
			◆ Have children identify emotions that they sometimes have; if they deny having a range of emotional experience, consider asking them to simply generate a list of emotions or to generate emotions that kids might have.
			◆ For each emotion on the list, have children assign a color that represents that emotion; create a "key" on the same or separate page.
			■ Locate the emotion in the body.
			◆ Provide an example of how emotions might show up in the body. For example: "Feeling worried might make your stomach feel funny, or feeling angry might make your fists clench." Elicit examples from children of where their emotions show up in their bodies.
			◆ Have children color specific areas of the body to indicate each emotion's location. Keep in mind (and name) that:
			● Some feelings may be held in more than one part of the body (e.g., "*Mad* might make your fists clench and your face hot").
			● More than one feeling can be held in the same place (e.g., "Both *scared* and *excited* might make your heart beat faster").
			◆ Work with children to expand details about the physical sensations associated with the feeling. For instance, muscles can be tense or loose, body temperature can be hot or cold, fists can clench or hands can be numb. Pay attention to feeling states marked by *lack* of sensation (e.g., for some children, anger may be marked by a sensation of numbing throughout the body).

Activity	Targets	Description	

			▪ Work with children to learn to tune in to and recognize these different physiological states. For many children, these body states will act as a "clue" in their feelings detective repertoire, as it may be easier for them to recognize physical states than thoughts, triggers, or specific emotions. ▪ Over time, incorporate this exercise into your feelings check-in (e.g., "What is your body feeling today?").

		Considerations	▪ Keep in mind that working with the body has implications for traumatized children. Consider:
			  ◆ The body may act as a *trigger*. In particular, a full-body tracing may not be appropriate for some children, depending on the degree of discomfort that they have with their bodies and/or the degree to which their history includes physical violations. Always offer a child a choice between using the silhouette or the full-body trace.
			    ◆ The body trace may also be an issue for children with sexualized behaviors and for those who have difficulty maintaining appropriate physical boundaries. For these children, the silhouette should be used.
			▪ Help children tune in to physical manifestations of emotions by commenting on them when they are visible in the therapy room. For instance, if, after a known stressor, a child appears hyperaroused (e.g., jumpy, fidgety, having a hard time sitting still), say, "I notice that your body has a lot of energy today [state your observation]. You've been pretty jumpy since you got here, and you've tried a bunch of different toys without being able to focus [be specific]. What do you think your body might be telling you? [elicit child's participation]." Help children draw on previously learned feelings detective skills.

What is in your head?	**I-S, C-Ext, C-Int**	Materials	Paper or whiteboard, markers or other drawing materials in variety of colors.

		Techniques	▪ Draw a silhouette of a large head. Do not include features; simply draw the outline.
			▪ Select a specific emotion to target. Classically, this exercise is done with *worry*, but it can be used with other specific emotions.
			▪ Provide psychoeducation. Teach children that all of us have many different things going on in our head at the same time. Some things take up a lot of space (and therefore a lot of energy), and other things take up less space. The goal of this exercise is to help identify what kinds of thoughts or experiences lead to a specific emotion (e.g., worry), and how much of our energy that emotion is currently taking. Note that this exercise both links experience to feeling and provides a foundation for affect modulation techniques.
			▪ Make a key.
			  ◆ Have children identify specific thoughts, experiences, or people who are linked to a specific emotion. Note that this may be simplistic and/or concrete: for example, "My mom," "School," etc.
			  ◆ Have children select a different color to represent each identified eliciting event.
			▪ Have children color in a portion of the head, with the amount of space colored used to represent the amount of energy or "space" that thought takes up. Using this technique, a big worry should take significantly more space than a small worry; something that makes a child feel very excited should take up more space than something that feels only a little bit exciting.

		Considerations	▪ This technique may be useful for initial and/or ongoing clinical assessment. ▪ Keep in mind that the representations of different "worries" (or other emotions) will likely change over time. This exercise is a useful tracking tool and can be used to help children tune in to and become aware of changes in their experience over time.

Activity	Targets	Description	
Feelings book	I-S, I-O, C-Bod, C-Th, C-Beh, C-Ext, C-Int	Materials	White paper, colored construction paper, pens or pencils, drawing materials, materials to bind book (e.g., file folder, binder clips, ribbon). Note that the book should be bound in such a way that it is easily altered/reorganized over time.
		Techniques	■ Introduce the exercise. Tell children that they will be creating a book that is all about them. ■ Create a front and back cover using two sheets of construction paper. Allow children to be as creative as they would like with their covers. Consider suggesting that they include things that represent their interests, personality, etc. ■ Insert blank pages in between the cover pages. Additional pages can be added over time or included from other therapy exercises. ■ The feelings book can be used in many ways. The following are some suggestions: ◆ Daily check-in. ◆ Emotion drawings. Have children generate a list of emotions and draw a picture about one emotion each week. ◆ Emotional experiences. Have children use feelings detective skills to write about one experience each week that elicited an emotion (positive or negative). Help them identify thoughts, behaviors, body sensations, etc., associated with the feeling.
		Considerations	■ Be creative in the use of the feelings book; tailor it to the child. ■ The book is most effective if it is incorporated into the therapy routine on a weekly basis. ■ Review the book with children on a semiregular basis. For instance, notice with children if their emotions are changing, if they have experienced the same feelings for weeks in a row, if the same experiences keep eliciting strong feelings, etc. ■ The book can be useful for ongoing clinical assessment.
Examples of other exercises	All	Books	Use child's favorite stories and/or books (available in the therapy room) to discuss the emotions of identified characters. Pay attention to thoughts, behaviors, somatic expressions, contexts, etc.
		Television shows	Use child's favorite television shows and/or television characters to discuss emotional experience. Again, pay attention to thoughts, behaviors, somatic expressions, contexts, etc.
		Modified board games	Incorporate affect tasks into board games. For instance, while playing Candy Land, assign a feeling a particular color space. Any time someone lands on that color, name an experience that elicits that emotion.
		Deck of cards	Create a deck of cards with four emotion faces, rather than four suits. Use numbers to represent intensity of emotion. Select cards from deck and act out situations, etc.

꙳ Developmental Considerations

Developmental stage	Identification considerations
Early childhood	Tasks at this age should be concrete. The focus is on differentiation of basic feelings rather than subtle variations. Initial exercises should use the four basic feelings (happy, mad, sad, scared/worried). A significant amount of affect identification work can be done via children's spontaneous play. Elicit from child and/or name what characters are feeling, doing, expressing, and why. Remember that the emotional cues of younger children are frequently somatic (e.g., stomachaches) and/or behavioral (e.g., irritability, opposition).

Developmental stage	Identification considerations
Middle childhood	During this stage, children are increasingly able to use words to describe their experience. Balance drawing techniques with those that help children put words to experience.
	Children are increasingly able to connect internal sensations, feelings, and experiences. Keep in mind, however, that this age group is less likely to play than younger children, and less able to hold sustained conversation like adolescents; therefore, structured tasks are often the primary therapeutic tool during this stage.
Adolescence	Adolescents have an increasingly sophisticated grasp over the nuance of language and affect. They can identify subtler types of feelings, as well as multiple feelings at the same time. They may have a particular preference for verbal and/or written techniques.
	It is common for traumatized children to vacillate between, or remain in, a single pattern of emotional constriction/avoidance and/or intense emotional expression. These extremes may be particularly heightened for adolescents.
	Some adolescents will rely on their newly developed verbal and analytical skills as an avoidance strategy. Rather than connecting to a feeling, they will invest their energy in discussing and analyzing it. It is important to continue to help these adolescents gently connect back to internal experience.
	Other adolescents will become easily aroused and overwhelmed by feelings and unable to access higher cognitive functions to explore emotional experience. It will be important to help these adolescents learn how to tune in to signs of intense emotion and utilize calming techniques.
	Adolescents may be able to self-identify typical behavioral patterns in response to emotions. Help them describe things they usually do if they're angry, upset, sad, etc. Use these as cues to help them identify emotions and triggering situations.
	Adolescents are more likely than younger children to use coping strategies (e.g., alcohol, substances, sex, cutting) in the face of emotion that adults find unacceptable. It is important that adolescents know that they have permission to talk about these matters in the therapy room. Link these less healthy (but often effective) strategies to underlying emotions, thoughts, and eliciting experiences.

🏠 Applications

🏠 Individual/Dyadic

Identification of emotions and internal experience is generally a cornerstone of our work with children who have experienced trauma. Because dysregulation of experience is such a prominent impact of trauma, learning modulation becomes a primary task. In order to modulate, however, a child must first be aware of the presence of a feeling or arousal state.

In our experience almost all individual sessions incorporate, in some way, the naming and exploration of internal experience. Particularly with younger children, consider building structured "feelings check-ins" into the session routine. It is often helpful to include a check of both emotion and energy/arousal, as this will support modulation work. With older children and adolescents, check-ins can be less structured while still exploring significant weekly events (e.g., by using a "thumbs-up" and "thumbs-down" event-of-the-week method). Consider, when appropriate, incorporating caregivers into weekly check-ins; this is particularly helpful for building an understanding of affect identification in others.

For children who have a limited feelings vocabulary due to age or deficits in self-expression, building a language for emotions will be a key component of the work. Incorporate activities such as the ones described above into sessions. Pay attention to the child's comfort level (e.g., initially use displaced figures, such as magazine faces, rather than exploring the child's own affect to increase tolerance for this work). Beyond structured activities, much of affect identification work happens in the moment. If affect identification is a goal for a particular child, pay attention to moments that lend themselves to naming, normalizing, and exploring internal experience. It is particularly important to pay attention to moments of mixed emotion.

Psychoeducation about triggers and triggered responses is often a key component of this work. Worksheets and educational handouts provided in Appendix D may be helpful. Keep in mind, however, that discussion of triggers and their origins is often affect provoking for both the child and the family. Pay attention to the child's response, normalize associated affect, and incorporate modulation strategies, as needed, into the work.

When appropriate, incorporate caregivers into sessions in some way. Support children in sharing emotional experience directly with caregivers. Work with caregivers to use their attunement skills, including reflective listening, outside of the treatment setting as a support for affect identification.

🏠 Group

Many identification tasks lend themselves well to therapeutic groups, either as a focus of the group or as part of session routine. Consider incorporating check-ins at the start of each group (e.g., by asking each group member to identify current emotion(s), level of intensity, or level of energy/arousal). Role plays and improvisation are a great group activity for identifying feelings, feeling clues, and feeling contexts. Group leaders can portray a scenario or invite group members to act out a situation; other group participants can identify players' feelings, possible thoughts, facial expressions, triggers, and behavioral responses.

When there is familiarity and safety among group members, they can support each other in identifying cues of emotion in self and other. For instance, group members can provide information about how they know when another participant is angry or happy. In addition, many of the tools described in the toolbox section can be used over time to support skill building. For instance, we have implemented 12- to 16-week groups that focus on building awareness of the connection between energy and thoughts by practicing the "What's in your head?" technique on a weekly basis. This routine facilitates skill practice and ultimately provides group members with the opportunity to build mastery.

Clips from movies and television shows offer a useful forum for teaching about and exploring triggers and triggered responses (along with other aspects of emotion). Look for moments of fight, flight, and freeze responses and explore the function of these responses. Pay attention to participant vulnerability in these discussions and to the importance of validating the range of responses. Consider the following example:

A group of adolescent boys in a juvenile justice facility were shown clips from a movie about a young teenage boy with an abusive father. In one scene the father enters the house, having clearly been drinking. The boy freezes on the stairs and remains still and watchful as the father yells and throws things at him, before exiting the room. After the group leader paused the clip, one of the boys stated, "Man, I would have punched that a**hole!" The group leader acknowledged the wish and asked the participants what they think would have happened if the boy had punched the father. The group agreed readily that the boy—small for his age and no match for his father—would have been beaten. After a discussion of why the boy would stay still instead and how that stance might have protected him, the group watched a second clip, shortly after the first scene, in which the boy is yelled at by someone outside the home and has a rageful response, destroying property and punching a wall. The boy who had made the first comment stated, "Bet he wishes that was his dad."

Through exploration of the danger response in film, these boys were able to tolerate a more vulnerable discussion than they might otherwise have been able to do. When possible, it is important to take the next step and to explore participants' own possible triggers and danger responses.

Milieu

Milieus such as schools or residential programs offer a natural forum to support youth identification. Work with staff at all levels to observe and reflect youth behaviors and emotions. Pay attention to positive as well as challenging emotions; it is equally important to observe and celebrate a child's positive affect as to notice and support a child in coping with distress. Set as a goal the identification of early cues of dysregulation (e.g., what a particular child looks like or does *before* the explosion), name these when they appear, and support the youth in using modulation strategies. Consider the role of affect identification in youth reactions to staff. Be aware of the potential for miscues; explore these using the modeling technique described earlier in this chapter (e.g., "What did you think my reaction meant?") and clarify them.

Consider incorporating check-ins into daily routines (e.g., at the start of class, during meals, at the end of the day). Create an environment that acknowledges affect, using visual cues, posters, and/or bulletin boards. It may be helpful to create "themed" bulletin boards (e.g., pictures of "happy moments," examples of activities that people might do when sad, etc.).

Affect identification work may play an important role in conflict resolution. Use identification skills to support perspective taking (e.g., asking, "What do you think Sean might have been feeling when he said that?"). It is important to pay attention to timing in this work; it is difficult to have perspective (a skill requiring the "thinking brain") when a child is not modulated. Once calm, use reflective listening skills (attunement) and problem-solving skills (executive functions) to support children in understanding their reactions, associated situational precipitants and triggers, and potential solutions.

Trauma Experience Integration: State-Based Skills Application

Distress Tolerance and Regulation

During early stages of treatment or when children/adolescents are experiencing more intense stress, identification work will emphasize basic identification or recognition of distress, and may be highly dependent on the attuned responses of the provider and/or other caregivers. For instance, a goal may be to support the child in building basic awareness that feelings are "going into the red" and that there is a need to seek support from others or to take space; or to support adults around the child in recognizing and naming early cues of emotion or dysregulation. Because high levels of distress or dysregulated arousal are often "wordless," attempts to engage using language may backfire; during this state, language labels may simply act as a cue to support engagement in modulation practice, as described in the next chapter, or to support the child in feeling attuned to and mirrored.

Curiosity and Reflection

As the child or adolescent is increasingly able to engage in reflection, and during more regulated states, identification work can focus on a wider range of goals, including identification of triggers ("When people hassle me, it just makes me feel on fire, like I want to punch someone"); recognition of patterns ("Every time my mom and I argue, I just need to take space. I think it's just that I feel so shut down, I can't handle being around her for a while"), and building awareness of the function of behaviors ("It's not that I hate my teacher, it's just that sometimes I start to feel kind of trapped or closed in when I'm in that class, and when I take off, I feel like I can breathe again").

Engaging Purposeful Action

Over time, as children and adolescents are increasingly able to tolerate connection to internal experience and have developed awareness of and language for a range of emotions and internal states, identification work can be utilized to support development of self-narratives and the processing of traumatic experience. These more advanced processes involve a more focal identification of the range of internal experiences associated with both specific identified traumatic events and with self-narratives.

Increasingly, clinicians and other caregivers should also work to support youth in engaging their curiosity in the moment by building and supporting their capacity to notice—at a developmentally appropriate level—shifts in self-states as they occur both within clinical settings and in daily life. This capacity ultimately will serve as the foundation for the development of youth's active ability to modulate internal states.

Real-World Therapy

Kids have their own agendas. Some children reject structured feelings activities. Keep an eye on the goal, even if you can't do the specific activity you had planned.

Be true to the context and to provider and child preferences. This section has provided an array of sample activities as a way of stimulating ideas about possible useful techniques. Keep in mind two points:

1. There are no limits to the number of potential exercises you can create. Use your imagination and create feelings-relevant activities that will match the interests of the child with whom you are working.
2. A lot of this work happens in the moment, and in conversation, rather than through structured therapeutic activities. Tune in to opportunities to explore affect in the material children are already bringing to you.

11

Modulation

🔑 **THE MAIN IDEA AND KEY SUBSKILLS**

Work with children to develop safe and effective strategies to manage and regulate physiological and emotional experience, in service of maintaining a comfortable state of arousal.

★ Build an understanding of *comfortable* and *effective* states.

★ Build an understanding of degrees of feelings and energy.

★ Support children in exploring arousal states and in developing a sense of agency over tools that allow them to manage emotions and energy.

★ Support and facilitate strategies that effectively and comfortably lead to state changes.

★ Key Concepts

★ Why Target Modulation?

■ The ability to safely and effectively modulate emotional and physiological experience is often a key challenge for children who have experienced trauma. Two primary historical factors influence this difficulty with modulation:

 Attachment disruptions and challenges. Young children initially rely on their caregivers to act as "external modulators" by providing comfort and soothing at predictable times in the day (e.g., bedtime) as well as during times of distress. Often this modulation is accomplished through positive sensory experiences such as rocking, swaddling, sucking, or singing. Over time, young children internalize these experiences and develop skills for self-soothing, which in turn supports the development of "felt safety" (in relationship, in the world, and in the child's own "skin"). Children who experience unresponsive, inconsistent, or abusive caretaking may fail to develop healthy age-appropriate skills, and instead must rely on primitive regulation strategies, such as self-harming behavior, inappropriate or risky sexual stimulation, or substance use.

 Traumatic stress response. When children are exposed to overwhelming stress, particularly chronic stress, they must cope with high levels of arousal. In the face of

197

overwhelming emotion and in the absence of adequate external soothing via attachment experiences, children attempt to employ whatever modulation skills are immediately available. Often these strategies do not adequately reduce arousal. As a result, children either fail to regulate or regulate to the extremes (e.g., constriction).

■ In the face of current stressors and triggers, children often move rapidly into "danger mode." Even minor stressors may derail children because their early experiences provided insufficient support for the development of physiological organization. Their ability to remain regulated is impacted by sudden surges of arousal, shifts in neurological control from cortical (frontal) to subcortical (limbic) areas, and desperate—and unconscious—reliance on rigid and often primitive strategies to manage internal and external experience. In other words, the child's capacity to engage his or her "thinking brain" is derailed by the activation of the "survival brain."

⭐ How Does Trauma Impact Modulation?

■ Children who are unable to modulate may attempt to (1) overcontrol or shut down emotional experience, (2) manage their arousal through physiological stimulation or behavior, or (3) rely on external methods to self-regulate. Often, children are not aware that they are engaging these strategies to manage emotions or arousal.

   ◆ Some children **overcontrol or shut down** emotional experience via:
      • Constriction/numbing
      • Avoidance
      • Isolation
      • Distraction
      • Fantasy/daydreaming
      • Rigid control of the environment or others
      • Selective mutism

   ◆ Other children **manage arousal through behavior or physical stimulation:**
      • Physical movement: jumping, climbing
      • Primitive self-soothing: rocking, thumbsucking, hair twirling
      • Aggression
      • Sexualized behaviors
      • Escape or running behavior

   ◆ When emotion management strategies fail, children/adolescents may **rely on overt methods to alter or control physiological states:**
      • Substance or alcohol use
      • Eating control/dyscontrol
      • Self-harm
      • Sensation-seeking activities
      • Relational reenactments

▪ Note that these methods are not mutually exclusive; coping strategies used by a child may vary over time (e.g., depending on developmental stage) and within different contexts. This is true for most of us. Individuals rarely rely on one strategy for every internal state that they experience. For instance, you may employ one strategy when sad and a completely different strategy when angry. There are some strategies that an individual may use at home but would never use at school or at work.

▪ It is important to note that children and adolescents often engage in high-risk behaviors because they "work": They support regulation in the moment. In addition, these strategies often shift arousal very quickly. Modulation work focuses on finding "replacement" strategies that can be as effective in shifting internal experience *and* that are safe.

🧰 Therapist Toolbox
🖐 What's the Stake?

Difficulty with modulation (of emotion, of behavior, of relationship) is often one of the primary reasons that a child or adolescent is referred to a clinical provider. These challenges may affect the child's functioning in multiple settings. Interventions to address modulation are often framed around the dichotomy of "bad" and "good," and as an absolute: "You're getting too angry, you need to stop reacting so much"; "She needs to stop getting in trouble and do a better job listening"; "His behavior at home is really bad"; "She needs to stop exploding and just relax." Not surprisingly, youth—particularly those who struggle with more explosive or labile affect and arousal—may be defensive and guarded around interventions designed to help address their energy and, in turn, behavior and emotion: The interventions may feel shaming and controlling, and, whether explicitly or implicitly, designed to disempower the youth and invalidate their experience.

In order to engage in learning how to modulate their emotions, behaviors, relational functioning, and bodies, youth need to have a stake in that work. The core goal of building the child's or adolescent's awareness of comfort and effectiveness, described below in the section "Skill #2: Teach to Kids—Understanding Comfort Zone and Effective Modulation," is largely designed to build youth's stake in this process. Our goal is not (directly, at least) to support the young person in behaving, getting along, acting nicely, and not exploding; it is to support him or her in having a body that feels bearable or even positive to live in (comfort), and to feel powerful in navigating his or her world (effectiveness).

Many children who have experienced trauma feel at the mercy of their emotions, which they experience as overwhelming, unpredictable, and powerful. Emotional experience is intricately linked with arousal; modulation (and dysregulation) typically occurs on a physiological level. For many reasons, it is often helpful to focus on the concept of arousal or energy, rather than on emotion per se. It is easy to make the mistake of suggesting that the goal is, for instance, to help a child "feel less angry." In using this kind of language, we invalidate the child's experience of anger ("Your anger is not important/appropriate/correct"). The alternative is to help the child *be* angry, but at a level of arousal or energy that is tolerable, comfortable, and controlled—which in turn allows the child to do something more productive with his or her anger. For this reason, many of the modulation interventions described in this chapter focus on ways to access awareness of the body and body states, and on methods to support the child in shifting these states toward increasingly comfortable and "in-control" levels of energy, rather than reducing emotions per se.

Behind the Scenes

- **The complexity of modulation:** If any of our readers have ever been told to "just calm down," then it is likely that you understand that it is not that simple! Modulation, or the ability to move toward optimal levels of arousal, involves a number of different strategies and skills:

  - First, you have to know that you are feeling something—which requires the ability to identify an initial emotional or physiological state and the degree to which it is comfortable and/or effective. *Awareness of current arousal level, whether high or low:* "I'm feeling really charged up." "I'm feeling really shut down."

  - Second, you have to stay connected to what you are feeling. This includes the ability to tolerate internal states that may be experienced as uncomfortable. It is important to note that modulation involves the ability of the child to *tune in to, tolerate,* and *sustain connection to emotional states or arousal.*

    - Often, children will appear to have the ability to modulate, because they are able to talk about emotions in a calm manner or are observed to shift from high arousal to calm.

    - However, constricting or shutting down affect suggests that the child is unable to tolerate it rather than using healthy modulation skills. Similarly, verbalizing emotion without any felt connection to it may indicate a lack of tolerance for the internal experience of that emotion.

    - For example, it is common to work with an individual who presents content that is clearly distressing. We may see a glimmer of emotion such as the watering of eyes. Then, as quickly as it appears, it disappears because the individual shuts it down and is unable to stay with the emotion.

  - Third, you have to be aware of changes in state. This includes the ability to identify and connect to subtle changes in state. *Awareness of shifts in arousal:* "I just started to feel a little calmer." *Recognition of the cues of state changes:* "I can tell I feel calmer because my stomach is churning a little less."

  - Fourth, you have to differentiate emotional experiences and their impact on arousal. This includes the ability to *recognize the link between emotions and energy or arousal changes:* "Whenever I get mad, I get really revved up."

  - Fifth, you need to have the *ability to identify and use strategies to manage those state changes:* "When I breathe really deeply, it helps my stomach start to feel better."

- Modulation is a very complicated skill set, and intervention and support for each of these steps—often over an extended period of time, and in many different affect and energy states—may be necessary to build the child's or adolescent's capacity to regulate or coregulate in the moment.

- **Modulation is bidirectional:** It may involve increasing arousal (i.e., up-regulation) or decreasing arousal (i.e., down-regulation). Every child will have a different *comfort zone,* or range of comfortable arousal. It is important to partner with children in learning about and exploring their own preferred arousal state.

▪ **The dual goals for modulation: comfort and effectiveness.** What is *comfortable* for a child may be different from what is *effective*. In teaching and supporting modulation skills, both of these constructs will need to be explored.

◆ *Comfort zone.* One key goal of modulation is to help a child feel comfortable in his or her body. Many of the children and adolescents we work with have different "safety zones," or range of arousal, in which they tend to settle and in which their bodies feel safe. Trauma can have a significant impact on a child's safety zone. For instance, some children may feel safest at very high states of arousal because long-standing "danger readiness" and hypervigilance have allowed them to feel "ready for action" and therefore less helpless or vulnerable. For other children, a highly constricted state may feel safest. For these children, who often have few effective coping strategies, arousal in their bodies may feel quickly overwhelming, and they may expend significant energy to keep their emotions and arousal state at very low levels.

Because of this impact of trauma, our work often involves (*sloooooooowly* and carefully) *expanding* a child's safety zone so that the child is increasingly comfortable in a range of arousal states. Be cautious as you go: If you try to bring down the arousal too quickly of a child who lives in the upper ranges, he or she may feel unsettled and engage in some behavior designed to increase arousal back to comfortable levels. Similarly, if you try to increase the arousal of a constricted child before he or she has the tools to manage the arousal, the child may shut down further in an attempt to manage these feelings. Consider the function of a child's safety zone in your selection of modulation activities. For example, begin with activities that allow a child to stay within that safety zone and then slowly modify and/or change the activity to expand the zone.

◆ *Danger zone:* Energy/arousal can be a very complicated thing to work with. Attunement skills, including in-the-moment assessment of energy, are critical. Because arousal is directly linked to the trauma response, it can, at times, act as an internal trigger or reminder of past abuse. We have observed this linkage numerous times. Consider the following example:

> Austin is a 16-year-old male who resides in a residential care facility. One afternoon the staff was engaging Austin in a dance activity. Because Austin enjoyed dancing, this was a strategy that had been used on a number of occasions. On this afternoon, many staff observed that Austin was enjoying the activity as evidenced by smiles, laughter, and engagement with staff. What happened next was unexpected: Austin's affect changed in an instant from happy to rageful. He ran outside, found a shovel, and returned to the residence threatening harm to staff and peers.

◆ In the above example, Austin's arousal appeared to increase to what we refer to as the *danger zone* creating an unsafe situation for all involved. This process can also occur if the arousal becomes too low. Consider the following example with the same young man:

> Austin was participating in group treatment. The content of the group that day involved themes related to loss of a caregiver. This was a difficult topic for Austin, whose mother had died 6 months prior. Austin was prepared for the group process

in advance of the group and had demonstrated a number of the skills described in our previous chapter. He appeared calm throughout the whole group. His arousal decreased over time, but the therapist running the group did not want to push him to engage. Again, in an instant Austin shifted into an apparently unconscious state. He did not respond to attempts at engagement, he was drooling, and he could not be immediately regulated up from this completely shut-down state.

♦ *Effective modulation.* A second key goal is to help children achieve a level of modulation that will help them navigate their world most effectively. Effective modulation often requires an awareness of context. An appropriate level of arousal in a classroom, for instance, is different from an appropriate level of arousal on a playground. Additionally, for children who live in dangerous communities, arousal levels connected with vigilance to danger may be essential to their safety. It is important that skill building in modulation incorporate an understanding that no level of arousal is "wrong"; however, the ability to manage arousal may help children effectively navigate the current moment (e.g., modulating in service of effectively relating or communicating, effectively getting needs met, and effectively and safely completing tasks). If a child's comfortable state of arousal is higher or lower than situations routinely require (e.g., the highly energetic child who must frequently work to bring down his or her energy), it is important that the child have alternative places or moments in which to safely experience the preferred energy state.

♦ *Exploring arousal states:* In order for children to tune in to variations in arousal, clinicians need to concretely support them in eliciting changes in their states. Achieving state changes can be done through fun activities (e.g., tossing a ball, dancing) or through more targeted regulation (e.g., deep breathing). Work with children to notice their own physiological reactions to these activities. A key teaching point is that children have the power to change their own physiology. Over time, the goal is for them to be able to autonomously implement these strategies.

♦ Not all modulation activities will be effective or enjoyable for all children. Frame the activities as **experiments** and allow children space to actively explore their own reactions. What may be down-regulating for one child may be up-regulating for another. It can be helpful to routinely emphasize this point when introducing modulation activities. For example, "We are going to play ball toss right now. This activity might bring your energy up, it may bring your energy down, or your energy may stay the same. It can feel comfortable or uncomfortable. We can check in about what it was like for you after we're done." Consider concrete measures of children's reactions: Have them practice appraisal skills, including monitoring heart rate, pace of breathing, body temperature, and level of muscle tension, both before and after activities. Providers can practice their own self-monitoring skills to model this process. Additional techniques include using charts, scales, and the like to track degree of arousal, positive versus negative experiences, and so on. Be mindful that even referencing "the body" may increase vulnerability in some children.

♦ *Building comfort zones:* When exploring and experimenting with arousal, it may be helpful to create actual *comfort zones* for children and teens to use. In program and therapy settings a comfort zone could be set up in a room or designated space with sensory tools. For instance, one residential program developed "comfort corners" in each resident's rooms. Each corner was uniquely tailored to the specific modulation needs of each individual teen. Another example came from an individual provider who created a space underneath his desk for one client. When the client had "cozy" time, she would go under the desk with a preferred stuffed pal that came to her meetings with her, and the provider would play lullabies on the computer. Cozy time was practiced during each meeting and could also be requested as needed. In homes we have seen a range of possibilities, including comfort zones in bedrooms, closets, under dining room tables, or simply areas of the home where modulation tools could be found, including in the laps of caregivers. When possible, we want to create real-life examples of "comfort" that are concrete and accessible to our children and teens. The important point is to bring the concept of a child's own unique comfort zone to life by providing the necessary resources.

Practice modulation regularly, and not just during times of distress. It is often helpful to incorporate modulation activities into the session or daily routine. For instance, a modulation activity can be incorporated into the session opening and/or closing, start or end of classtime, before bedtime, and at other key points in a child's day. The regular integration of modulation strategies into daily routine is likely to increase *baseline* regulation (i.e., the capacity of the child to be comfortable and effective); in turn, the more the child has a level of baseline comfort and control, the less likely the child is to head into the danger zone during moments of distress.

■ It is particularly important for children to practice modulation techniques when they are calm to gain mastery over the skills and internalize an awareness of how their body feels in different states of arousal. Initial practice of these skills should not be paired with significantly distressed or constricted emotional states.

In thinking about why routine practice of regulation strategies is so important, it may be useful to think about how the capacity to soothe develops in the infant or young child. Children learn self-soothing capacity through repetitive and consistent exposure to positive sensory experiences at times that are often associated with safety. For example, a caregiver often reads, sings, rocks, or moves. Over time, these skills can be actively applied in the moment (distress) to manage arousal. It is generally difficult for any individual to learn a new skill in a moment of distress, *and* the skill is unlikely to "feel safe" internally if it is *only* associated with distressing experiences.

■ To apply these skills successfully in the moment (e.g., when upset or shut down), children will often need cuing (from caregiver, clinician, teacher, etc.). Essentially, the caregiver (or whoever) will need to act as the "external modulator" by modeling, cuing, and **actively participating** in the modulation activity with the child. Over time the goal is for children to apply the skill independently.

■ **Use of attunement to support modulation:** When connecting modulation skills to emotion, build on the vocabulary developed with the child during affect identification exercises. For instance, if a child talks about getting "really hot" when angry, think together about ways to "cool down."

■ In addition to formal exercises, affect modulation work can often be done in the moment.

   ◆ In session, tune in to and notice signs of state modulation or state shifts. When appropriate, build on reflection by engaging the child in active attempts at modulation.

◆ In play:

  ● Play behaviors

  (The child comes into session calm, but when asked about her day, starts pulling out multiple toys, and is now slamming figures around the dollhouse.)

  THERAPIST: Wow, all of a sudden your energy got really big—there's lots of toys on the floor, and those dolls are really looking busy. It seems like being asked about your day might have kicked up some feelings.

  (If distress continues)

  THERAPIST: Let's you and I take a big, deep breath and stretch before we keep playing.

  ● Displaced in play

  (The child has an action figure and a toy lion. He shows characters interacting, then suddenly begins slamming figures together, having lion growl, etc.)

  THERAPIST: Boy, that lion just got really mad all of a sudden. It seemed like they were playing calmly, and then the lion started growling. I wonder what's going on with him?

◆ In interaction:

  (The adolescent comes in appearing angry and shut down, arms folded, no eye contact. When the therapist initially notices and comments on his appearance, the adolescent rejects it, stating, "Everything's fine." After several minutes of interaction, the adolescent starts to appear more relaxed.)

  THERAPIST: It looks like you're starting to calm down a little bit. I can see that your muscles aren't as tense, and you're looking at me more.

◆ In statements:

  (The child talks about her relationship with her mother, which has always been a highly triggering subject. In previous conversations, the child's statements were accompanied by a high degree of distressed affect [loud tone of voice, fists clenching, arms crossed, etc.]. Today, the child still has apparent anger in her voice, but is less intense, and her body appears more relaxed [e.g., arms uncrossed].)

  THERAPIST: I'm noticing that when you talk about your mom today, you seem a little less angry.

◆ When observing your clients during various interactions, tune in to their attempts to modulate and to their preferred strategies. For example, you may have clients who come into the office and immediately reach for a stress ball or other manipulative to squeeze, or move. Other clients may gently rock back and forth in their seats or begin tapping on their legs when their arousal starts to increase. Kids will often give us clues about which modulation activities are likely to be most successful for them.

Teach to Caregivers

■ *Reminder:* Teach the caregiver the Key Concepts.
■ *Reminder:* Teach the caregiver relevant Developmental Considerations.
  ◆ Teach caregivers to identify modulation strategies.

- Teach caregivers to use their detective skills to identify the strategies that their child or teen may be using to modulate. All of us use strategies every day to manage experience. Many of us are unaware of modulation strategies that we are using because the process of engaging them is often unconscious. It is not until we intentionally focus on building our awareness of these strategies that we recognize them. For instance, one provider noticed that she touches and then presses her ear when she needs to focus a bit more; another provider realized that he rubs his fingertips together when he needs to calm; a caregiver noticed that she looks away when overwhelmed, and another caregiver noticed that her child hums when trying to engage and increase the energy he needs to begin his day. The strategies that people use to modulate are often subtle but effective in shifting arousal in the moment.

- In addition to learning to recognize their own strategies (caregiver affect management), caregivers will need support to identify the range of strategies that their child/teen is using. Some strategies may be obvious, such as physical activity, listening to music, and engaging in art, whereas others, less so. One teen learned that she decreases her arousal by biting on her bottom lip. When teaching about modulation it can be helpful to engage the caregiver in attuning to this specific skill set.

- In addition to the strategies just described, it is important to teach caregivers about the role that self-harming and risk behaviors play in modulation.

  - Self-harm is a complex topic; safety should be prioritized in any treatment.

    - A number of authors have developed interventions that include detailed modules for working with individuals who self-harm (e.g., Linehan, 1993; Miller, Rathus, & Linehan, 2006). Therapists are encouraged to familiarize themselves with the array of techniques for evaluating and intervening in the case of self-harming behaviors. In the following table we offer some teaching points on self-harm as they relate to modulation work with children impacted by developmental trauma.

Self-Harming Behaviors and Modulation: Key Concepts

Self-harming behaviors generally represent the child's or adolescent's attempt to modulate emotional experience. Although it is not healthy, self-harm is used because it is—in the moment, at least—effective.

When intervening in the case of self-harming behaviors, it is important to (1) understand the function of the behavior and (2) provide safer alternatives.

Be aware that, as with any modulation strategy, self-harm may serve dual functions. It may act as:
  - A *down-regulation* strategy, helping the child turn off overwhelming affect.
  - An *up-regulation* strategy, helping the child come back from a numb or constricted state.
Note that children may use self-harm to serve different functions at different times.

Replacement strategies should attempt to match the original function of the self-harming behavior.

Since trauma often occurs within a relational context, social support may not be a viable option for children and adolescents in times of significant distress. Therefore, to the degree possible, it is often useful for replacement strategies to include the ones that can be implemented independently.

It is important to provide psychoeducation about the function of self-harm. Help children and adolescents (and their caregivers) understand the role that self-harm has played in their attempts to modulate their own experience. Involve them in developing alternative strategies.

It is important that there be a balance between addressing imminent risk and providing a safe environment in which to discuss and address self-harming behavior. Self-harm often involves shame and secrecy, along with extreme reactions from caregivers (and, at times, clinicians). If every instance of self-harm is met with threats of hospitalization or extensive increase in services, the client's ability to actively participate in learning new skills will be reduced. Pay attention to your own emotional responses to a client's self-harm and work with caregivers to both understand and tolerate their own emotional reactions.

Teach Caregiver to Support Modulation

▪ In Chapter 8 on attunement, we discussed the caregiver's important role in supporting the child's modulation and the steps toward doing so. We briefly revisit those here.

Caregiver Role in Child Modulation

Teaching points	Caregivers play a key role in helping their children regulate emotional experience.
	It is often helpful to teach caregivers to identify their child's current modulation strategies. This step overlaps with attunement in that we are explaining the modulating function of various behaviors. Strategies may be positive and effective, such as art, writing, athletics, etc. They may also be concerning, as indicated earlier in this chapter.
	It may be important to remind caregivers that the initial goal is for their child to practice strategies *with* support. Early in treatment we are not asking children to practice modulation independently. Often, the best regulation is *coregulation:* in addition to verbal cuing, caregivers can engage in many of the exercises described above *with* their children. For instance, rather than cuing a child to stretch, teach the caregiver to stretch along with the child, take deep breaths together, etc. We have found that strategies are often more successful if caregivers have opportunities for experiential learning specific to modulation. For example, we have parenting programs in which caregivers practice modulation strategies independent of their child to enhance their comfort with a tool (see Chapter 7 on caregiver affect management) prior to asking them to engage directly. They can practice in caregiver meetings, dyadic sessions, and in their home setting.
	Teach caregivers to use their attunement skills to identify *variations* in their child's emotional experience and/or arousal level. What does the child look like when escalating? When shutting down? Develop a list of cues specific to the child.
	Teach caregivers the distinctions between *up-regulation* and *down-regulation*.
	Teach caregivers to support appropriate modulation strategies in the child (i.e., down-regulation strategies when hyperaroused, up-regulation strategies when constricted). Develop a menu of strategies that caregivers are comfortable supporting.

For in-the-moment support for coregulation, teach caregivers the following steps:

Caregiver steps to support modulation	*Pre-step:* To the degree possible, try to be proactive in development of "modulation support plans." Use your attunement skills to identify common "clues" that your child is having difficulty regulating, common situations that may be challenging to manage, and strategies that may be helpful to use for various child/adolescent states. When an episode of dysregulation happens, use this as information to help with the next episode. The more a caregiver feels "ready," the easier it will be to try a strategy in the moment.

1. Pay attention to signs that your child is having difficulty modulating emotional or physiological experience. Name (very simply) what you see. For example:
   - ▪ "It looks like your body is starting to have really high energy."
   - ▪ "Wow—you just started yelling—it seems like you're getting pretty upset."
   - ▪ "I'm not sure what happened, but it looks like you just kind of shut down."
   - ▪ Be careful that the language used for labeling is not judgmental or blaming. It is important that your child is given permission for the feeling; your language should separate concern about modulation from concern about the emotion itself.

2. Pay attention to your own state, and use your in-the-pocket strategies if necessary. It's common and typical for a child's surge of dysregulation to lead to the caregiver's own arousal surge.
   - ▪ In putting together a modulation plan with your provider, you should consider what tools you might need in the moment to be effective. For instance, do you need to . . .

take a deep breath? Use a self-statement? Step out for a moment if the situation is safe enough? Ultimately, the goal is to support you and your child in achieving a comfortable and effective arousal state, and the more in control you are, as the caregiver, the more feasible this will be.

3. Support the use of modulation techniques. Cue your child to use already learned skills and/ or practice the skills with your child. For example:
   - "Let's try some breathing like you learned in therapy—then we can talk about what's upsetting you."
   - "Do you want to come cuddle for a moment to help calm down?"
   - "You just got really quiet and still when we were talking about school. I think it would help if we got up and shook it off, before we keep talking about this."

4. Reinforce the use of modulation techniques with your child. For example:
   - "You just did a great job using your breathing to calm down."
   - "I'm really proud of you for trying to practice using your stress ball."

5. After he or she has regained some degree of comfort and control, help your child identify and process what precipitated the difficult emotion. Use attunement skills and reflective listening skills.

Teach Caregivers about Building Comfort Zones

It can be helpful to review the concept of real-life comfort zones with caregivers. Work with them to:

- Identify possible spaces in the home or milieu that could be used as a comfort zone.
- Collaboratively assess the feasibility of using each space as a comfort zone. Identify the strengths and challenges of each selection prior to identifying the comfort space.
- Encourage caregivers to take an "inventory" of the modulation resources that they currently have in the home or milieu. If there are barriers to accessing or enhancing modulation resources, work with caregivers to problem-solve around this area.
- Support the caregiver and child in identifying resources that are most likely to be comfortable and effective in a given context.
- Work with caregiver and child to incorporate their comfort zone into the modulation plan described previously.

✏️ Tools: Modulation

Skill #1: Understanding Degrees of Feeling and Energy

- An important step in modulation is to understand that feelings and arousal/energy come in all sizes and to be able to tune in to those subtle differences.
- Modulation is often about gradation: Most children can tune in to extreme states more easily than to subtle shifts. This is particularly true for children whose cognition has been significantly impacted by trauma.
- All of these techniques can be incorporated into opening and closing check-ins, as well as used during the session to help the child track changes in observable affect. Beyond formal exercises, use these concepts in the moment to help children build awareness of the range of feeling and arousal states.

■ This concept may be applied to build awareness of the varying sizes or degrees of emotion states and of energy and physiological regulation in general. Use this skill to help children identify not just their emotions, but how their bodies feel.

■ Once children are able to use these techniques to identify their current feeling, the techniques can be used to:

◆ *Link to past experience.* For example: "When that argument happened, how mad were you? If this circle was all the mad in the world, color in how much would be filled to show how mad you were."

• *Help the child tune in to changes in affect.* For example: "What about 5 minutes later?"

• *Compare across experiences.* For example: "I remember when we talked about how revved up you were when your brother hit you. Do you think you're *more* revved up this time, *less* revved, or about the same? How can you tell?"

• *Link to specific modulation strategies.* For example: "Color this circle for how high your energy was when you first had that argument, then let's color this one for how you felt after you listened to your music for a little while."

• *Generate ideas for modulation.* For example: "Right now you said your energy is at a 10. What would we need to do for you to go down to a 9?" *Note:* Do not try to reduce affect from a 10 to a 0; it is better for the child to successfully modulate small degrees of affect or energy than to feel overwhelmed by the expectation of fully shifting an arousal state.

■ You can modify language as needed. For example, some children like to refer to energy in numbers; some use "high, medium, low"; some refer to high energy as a "roadrunner moment" and low energy as a "turtle moment." Another common term that we use with kids to identify moments of distress is "Big Feelings." Language use is one of the places where individual needs and provider creativity comes into play.

Activities That Build Understanding of Degrees of Feeling and Energy

Activity	Description
Number scale	Have children identify current emotion on −1 to +10 or −10 to +100 scale. Use concrete markers to indicate what a −1, a 5, or a 10 might look like or feel like. Note the use of bidirectional number scales: For children who feel really frozen or shut down, it is important to have numbers or other markers that acknowledge that state.
Thermometer	Draw outline of thermometer. Have children color in how much of the identified feeling they are experiencing. Use concrete markers to indicate high, moderate, and low levels of feeling.
Circle	■ Have children color in a portion of a circle to indicate how much of a single identified feeling they are experiencing. ■ Have children create a key of different feelings by using different colors. Color each in a circle, in proportion to how much children are currently feeling (in relation to identified event, last week, etc.).
Poker chips	Have children select a number of chips to indicate how strong their current emotion is (e.g., "If these chips were all the mad in the world, how mad are you right now?").
Clay	Identify chunk of clay as containing all the "[identified emotion]" in the world; have children tear off from the clay how much they are currently feeling. You can implement the same technique with paper, M&M's, markers, etc.

Activity	Description
Paper	Replicate the above example using pieces of ripped-up paper. Ripping paper may also support in-the-moment regulation.
Color	Have children develop a color scale that corresponds to different levels of mood, energy, or control. Use the colors to check in at various moments or to link to concrete modulation strategies.

Skill #2: Teach to Kids—Understanding Comfort Zone and Effective Modulation

- Building a language around, and an internal awareness of, energy or arousal level are key foundational components for doing modulation work with children.

- Developing a shared understanding of energy involves both an educational and an experiential component. Beyond just teaching the concepts in this section, consider, for instance, (1) mapping a child's energy onto a scale like those used in the "Skill #1: Understanding Degrees of Feeling and Energy" activities (p. 208); (2) tossing a ball, jumping up and down, jogging in place, or dancing at different energy levels (low, medium, high); and (3) checking on energy level at various points during the session or before and after key activities.

- Educational points and sample activities in the following table can be modified to meet the needs of children at different developmental levels. Keep in mind that distinctions for children at earlier stages of development will be broader (e.g., "low, medium, high"), whereas older children/adolescents can often grasp more nuanced distinctions, such as those implicit in number scales.

- The psychoeducation that is embedded in this skill frequently serves as the foundation for the more experiential modulation work that takes place over time, and may be introduced explicitly or woven into ongoing interaction as part of supporting the child in experimenting with modulation strategies.

Managing Feelings Comfortably and Effectively

Target	Description
Normalizing and teaching the concept of energy	*Teaching point:* We all have different levels of energy in our bodies at different times. *Sample language:* "Everyone has energy in their bodies. Sometimes our energy is really low, like when we're sleepy; sometimes our energy is somewhere in the middle, like when we're feeling really focused and calm—such as doing homework or playing a board game; and sometimes our energy can be really high, like when we're running around with friends or playing sports. "Energy helps us do what we need to do, and all kinds of energy are important. Low energy is important, because sometimes we need to sleep and rest, and high energy is important, because sometimes we need to be really active. "A lot of things can affect our energy, like whether we've slept enough, or eaten enough, who we're with, where we are, and what time of day it is." *Possible activities:* Create an "energy scale" with the child (using numbers, high/medium/low, etc.). Elicit from and list with the child different activities that need different energy levels, or different clues that show someone's energy is high, medium, or low. Cut out pictures of people engaged in different activities from magazines and label their energy. Use your created scale and engage in different activities—tossing a ball, dancing, jumping—at different levels of the scale: How does dancing at a 3, for instance, look and feel different from dancing at a 7?

Target	Description
Linking energy with feelings	*Teaching point:* How we feel has an impact on our energy/arousal.
	Sample language: "One of the really important things that can affect our energy level is how we feel. For example, being excited or angry or scared can make our energy get really high; being sad or lonely can make our energy get really low. "This is especially true for 'danger energy'; when our brains think that something is dangerous, our energy can change really quickly. *(Refer to Teach to Kids section on triggers in Chapter 10, p. 186.)* Sometimes, having our energy change can be an important clue that something is going on with our feelings."
	Possible activities: Make a list of different feelings and have children label the feelings according to their own energy level: Do they have high or low energy when mad, sad, happy, etc.? Think about different kinds of energy levels within a feeling: "mad," for instance, comes in lots of sizes. Think of a range of feeling words that goes with a particular feeling (e.g., for *mad:* annoyed, irritated, frustrated, angry, enraged) and plot the words on an energy scale. Elicit the differences in situations that may lead to those feelings, ways they feel in the body (e.g., "Does *frustrated* feel different from *enraged*? How?"); how in control—or not—they feel when experiencing each feeling; different behaviors that might go with each feeling; etc. Have children act out the different feelings: "What does it look like when you walk into a room *annoyed* versus *enraged*?"
Understanding "safety zone" and "comfort zone"	*Teaching point:* Some energy levels feel more comfortable than others.
	Sample language: "All of us have different bodies and different brains. That means that each of us feels most comfortable with different kinds of energy. Some people really, really like it when their energy is high, some people really like it when their energy stays low, and some people like their energy to stay somewhere in the middle. Sometimes, the reason we like our energy to be high or low is because it feels safe to us—it's what we're used to, or it's what has helped us out when things felt hard. Sometimes it's because that level of energy feels really good in our bodies—and in that case, we might call it our *comfort zone.* If our energy gets too far out of our safety zone or our comfort zone—like if someone who likes low energy gets too heated up—it can feel really uncomfortable. Sometimes we try to do things to change our energy, to get it back where it feels good."
	Possible activities: Help children explore their comfort zones. Using your developed energy scale, have them plot what they think their most comfortable zone is. Pair each child's comfort zone with the different modulation activities with which you experiment: Have children check in on their energy level (e.g., "Where is it? Did it go up or down from where it started?") and whether or not they like how their body feels. Explore whether their safety or comfort zone is wide ("Do you like to have high energy sometimes and low energy sometimes? Where? When?") or narrow, and how this preference might affect them ("What is it like when things feel too high/too low? What kinds of things do you try to do to manage that?").
Understanding the role of context	*Teaching point:* Context will affect how effective our energy level is.
	Sample language: "Where we are and what we are doing can make a difference in whether our energy level helps us or gets in our way, and in whether our energy is safe or not safe. Having really high energy may feel really good, but there are places that high energy can get in our way. *(Elicit examples from the child, e.g., the library, in class.)* When high energy starts to get out of control, like if we're really mad or really upset, it can get in the way of getting our needs met, or it can make us do things that aren't safe. "The same thing is true for low energy. Low energy can be really good when we're sleepy, but it can get in the way if we need to do something like chores or homework. Shutting down our energy when we're feeling scared or upset can sometimes feel safer, but doing that can also get in the way of asking for help or doing something that feels good."
	Note: It is important to use examples that are relevant to each child and to involve him or her in the discussion.

Target	Description
	Possible activities: Make a list of concrete activities relevant to the children. Include both relevant daily activities (e.g., sleeping, eating, playing football, taking a dance class, doing homework) and relational activities (e.g., asking for help, telling someone they're angry). Explore what they think the "effective zone" is for each activity: At what energy level do they think engaging in that activity will be most effective? Why? Explore what might happen if energy were too low or too high. Pay attention to the ways that the child's own comfort or safety zone helps him or her to be more effective in some situations, but less effective in others.
Understanding the many strategies we may use to change our energy.	*Teaching point:* We do things to change our energy all the time. *Sample language:* "We all do things during the day to try to shift our energy. For instance, one child might change the way that she is sitting in her seat during class to try to bring her energy up so that she can pay a little more attention to what's going on; another child might take a deep breath to calm himself just before going in front of the class to present a project; still another child might look away from someone who is bringing her energy up to try to manage that experience. Bottom line: We are all trying to manage energy much of the time. If we think together about this, there are probably things that you are doing to bring your energy up, down, or to keep it the same—and generally to keep it comfortable. Sometimes we know what our strategies are and sometimes we are totally unaware of the fact that we have and are using strategies already! Part of our work is to figure out what you are already doing to change your energy and whether or not what you are doing is comfortable and effective. *Possible activities:* Help children explore their current modulation strategies. Building on work described previously (identifying comfort zones), ask them to share activities or behaviors that they engage in to bring their energy up, down, keep it the same, etc. Ask them to identify activities or behaviors that help them to feel more comfortable. They can list these, draw them, and/or find pictures that represent their current strategies. If you have additional ideas about strategies the child is currently using (e.g., self-harm, aggression, withdrawal), it may be important to frame those behaviors as strategies and include them in the activity.
Building a sense of agency over modulation	*Teaching point:* There are ways that we can purposefully shift our energy. *Sample language:* "There are a lot of different things we can do to change our energy when it doesn't feel comfortable or when it's getting in the way of something we want to do. We can think of these things as 'energy tools.' An energy tool helps us move our energy up or down. Not every tool works for every person, and not every tool works every time (just like sometimes you need a hammer, and sometimes you need a screwdriver). Because of that, we're going to practice different tools, and figure out which ones you like, which ones feel good in your body, and which ones feel like they might work." *Note:* Expanded education about this point appears in a later section, "Building a Feelings and Energy Toolbox." *Possible activities:* A wide range of activities is described later in this section.

Skill #3: Exploring Arousal States—Exercises to Modulate Arousal

- Much of the work of modulation is experiential: It involves engaging actively in physiological experiences that shift or sustain arousal and emotional states, with a goal of supporting children in becoming increasingly comfortable, effective, and organized in their internal states. Following is a series of exercises that may be used to address this goal. Work with each child to "experiment" with different activities. For each activity, notice and track with the child:

- ◆ Whether and the extent to which the activity changes the energy level to higher or lower, and how it affects the body (e.g., in terms of heart rate, breathing, temperature, muscles)
- ◆ Whether and the extent to which the activity feels comfortable or uncomfortable
- ▪ **The language of experimentation:** It is important to frame each activity as an experiment and to collaborate with the child/adolescent to determine his or her response to it. The language of experimentation is critical for two primary reasons.
    1. Due to the unique make up of each of us, we really do not know which techniques will lead to desired changes in energy. Every time the therapist (or caregiver) engages in an activity, it will be important to prepare the child for the possibility that something uncomfortable (and potentially frightening) may happen. This can prevent the kind of triggering that often occurs when children are sent to adjunctive activities (yoga, athletics, karate, etc.) without such preparation.
    2. If the therapist suggests an activity with the premise that it will "work" or be helpful, then the child may potentially experience shame or a sense of personal failure when he or she does not feel better.
- ▪ Techniques that are effective in shifting negative arousal states or sustaining positive arousal states and that feel comfortable to the child can then be added in to the child's toolbox.
- ▪ The exercises described in the tables below provide examples of how to implement classic techniques with different age groups. Use your imagination to create new ones!
- ▪ **The external modulator:** Work with caregivers to cue the child in the use of these skills outside of the therapy room. Consider incorporating caregivers into dyadic practice of these activities in the session, both to build attunement and to increase generalization. In milieu or community settings, the range of caregivers may play a role in providing cuing, support, and co-participation in modulation activities.
    - ◆ Beyond the caregiver role in *activities,* keep in mind that the act of engaging with another person (whether a primary caregiver, a helping adult, or a peer) is often a primary source of modulation (as well as, for some children, a source of dysregulation). Like any other activity described, dyadic engagement can be up-regulating or down-regulating. Work with children to identify modulation resources (see Chapter 12, "Relational Connection," for expanded information) and work with caregivers to tune in to the ways that interaction with their children increases or decreases arousal.
- ▪ **Mirror, match, and modulate:** Although this approach may feel counterintuitive when using formal exercises, it is often useful to start with an activity that mirrors the child's arousal level and modulates *toward* a child's extreme before modulating away (e.g., for a child who is already hyperaroused, "turn the volume up" before turning it down; this allows expression and engagement and normalizes affect).
    - ◆ For exercises that involve cuing or guiding by the therapist, it may be useful to create an audiotape for the child to bring home.

- **Reminder about safety zone/danger zone:** With all activities, keep in mind the role of the child's safety zone: A highly aroused child may feel uncomfortable becoming too relaxed, and a highly constricted child may feel discomfort with too much arousal. Move slowly in shifting arousal states, emphasize the child's control, and check in often with the child.

  ◆ It is important to be particularly cautious when working with children who are in a constricted or numb state. Some children who become overwhelmed will shut down as a way of managing the affect. While in this "turned-off" state, children are able to tolerate, but unable to directly cope with, the immediate stressor or related affect, because the numbing effectively disconnects them from the situation.

    • Initial modulation strategies are used to help children reengage with their own experience (both internal and external) and tolerate emotional and physical sensation. Once children are reengaged, they can then make use of more sophisticated coping mechanisms (e.g., modulation strategies to reduce affect, identification strategies to understand affect, and expression strategies to communicate experience).

    • Keep in mind that constriction or numbing suggests the presence of underlying distress. Therefore, it is important to pace the use of these exercises and to be on the lookout for signs of distress.

DIAPHRAGMATIC BREATHING

- Diaphragmatic breathing is a particularly valuable skill for a child to gain, because breathing is the easiest and quickest way to have an impact on physiology. Use of deep, steady breathing will often need to be paired with other activities (e.g., learning to take three deep breaths before engaging in movement, muscle relaxation).

Diaphragmatic Breathing

Developmental stage	Technique variation
Early childhood	■ *Bubble breathing* (real or imaginary): Teach children to blow a very big bubble without letting it pop; to do this, they must blow slowly, evenly, and then release. ■ *Pillow breathing*: Have children lie on the floor with pillow or stuffed animal on stomach. Teach them to breathe so that pillow/animal rises and falls with each breath.
Middle childhood	■ *London Bridge:* Have children raise arms (as in the game "London Bridge"). Breathe in as arms go up; breathe out as arms come down. See how slowly they can move their arms up and down. ■ *Imagery:* Have children imagine taking a deep breath and blowing out birthday candles; have them try to paint the opposite wall with their breath; have them smell the flowers and blow a dandelion puff.
Adolescence	■ *Diaphragmatic breathing:* Teach adolescents the principles of diaphragmatic breathing. Have them try to breathe in through their noses to a slow count of 3, pause, and then exhale slowly out through their mouths. Their abdomens should move out as they breathe in, and in as they breathe out. Their shoulders and chests should remain steady. Have them practice by placing a hand on their stomachs and observing their hands rise and fall. ■ *Pair with visual imagery:* Have adolescents imagine calm/peace coming in as they breathe in through their noses, and the tension exiting as they breathe out through their mouths.

GROUNDING

■ We have found adaptations of grounding techniques, as originally described by Marsha Linehan (1993), to be extremely useful for helping children and adolescents shift energy states.

■ Grounding techniques can be used both for decreasing arousal and for increasing arousal, or reengaging from a constricted state. Keep in mind the following:

   ◆ When used for down-regulation, grounding may involve self-soothing and internal engagement (e.g., mental lists). When used for up-regulation, it is important to focus children on reengaging with self and the environment.

   ◆ Once children have learned the techniques, external cuing may continue to be important.

   ◆ Verbal grounding techniques (e.g., lists, naming the days of the week, naming things in the office, "I Spy" for younger children) may be particularly useful for children who are disconnected.

   ◆ The shift from numb to embodied may be triggering for some children; to minimize this possibility, the grounding strategies should not overload the senses (e.g., use subtle vs. strong scents).

■ As children become re-embodied, it is often helpful to incorporate movement (covered in the next section).

Grounding

Developmental stage	Technique variation
Grounding techniques appropriate for down-regulation	
Early childhood	Have children tune into their senses, using concrete, easy-to-hold stimuli, such as: ■ Magic wands ■ Magic rocks ■ Worry stones ■ Piece of velvet cloth ■ Small stuffed animals ■ Glitter cream ■ Pleasurable smell
Middle childhood	Similar to early childhood, at this age children like to have something tangible that they can carry with them and manipulate, such as: ■ Stress balls ■ Wikki Stix ■ Lanyard string ■ Grounding stone
Adolescence	Adolescents can use similar techniques as those above, but they can also use more sophisticated and abstract techniques, such as: ■ Mentally listing simple information (e.g., days of the week, months of the year, favorite animals) ■ Listening to music ■ Writing or drawing ■ Noticing what they see, hear, and feel (i.e., they focus on physical sensations, not emotions)

Developmental stage	Technique variation
	Grounding techniques appropriate for up-regulation
Early childhood	▪ Play "I Spy," tuning in to things in the immediate environment.
	▪ Have children describe a known (safe) environment.
	▪ Have children tune in to a feather being run up and down their arms (by self, therapist, or caregiver, as appropriate).
	▪ Have children rub hands with glitter cream.
	▪ Have children do butterfly self-hugs (arms crossed across chest).
	▪ Pretend the floor is sand and have children "dig a hole" with their toes.
Middle childhood	▪ Have children name 10 things they see in the office.
	▪ Have children describe their favorite person (or book, movie, television show, food, etc.).
	▪ Have children squeeze a stress ball.
Adolescence	▪ Ask the adolescents to tune in to and describe physical sensations (e.g., body in the chair, feet on the floor).
	▪ Describe four, then three, then two, then one thing the adolescent hears, sees, and feels (physical sensations) to gradually increase focal awareness of surroundings.
	▪ Have the adolescent describe something step by step (e.g., what he or she did when waking up that morning).

MOVEMENT

- ▪ Almost any kind of movement can be used to experiment with energy. In order to increase engagement, be creative, consider the child's interests and comfort level, and have fun. Examples are offered in the following table.

- ▪ Many activities can be tailored to different developmental stages. For instance, although "yoga poses" are listed in adolescence, many yoga activities are geared toward younger children as well (e.g., games such as Yoga Pretzels [Guber, Kalish, & Fatus, 2005] and Yoga Bingo [distributed by Spiraling Hearts, n.d.]).

Movement

Developmental stage	Technique variation
Early childhood	▪ Hop like frogs: Start slowly and gradually speed up.
	▪ Play (and sing) *head, shoulders, knees*, and *toes* (*knees and toes*).
	▪ Play the Hokey Pokey.
	▪ Play a follow-the-leader game using movement, "animal walks" (e.g., move like a horse or elephant), drumming, etc.
Middle childhood	▪ Challenge children to do as many jumping jacks as they can (or give a number: e.g., "I wonder if you can do 10 jumping jacks in a row").
	▪ Put on music and have children dance; start with slower music and speed up.
	▪ Play Simon Says.
Adolescence	▪ Play door- or garbage-can basketball.
	▪ Toss a ball back and forth.
	▪ Turn on music and dance.
	▪ Drum or play another musical instrument.
	▪ Go for a walk.
	▪ Do yoga poses.

MUSCLE RELAXATION

▪ Muscle relaxation exercises are generally used to help children release stress or tension, either in the moment or as an ongoing relaxation strategy. Exercises that target muscle relaxation can help children feel a sense of control over their bodies, and are useful for exploring and recognizing the contrast between states of tension and relaxation. When using these exercises, help children tune in to and notice variations in muscular/physical experience before, during, and after engaging in the activity.

Muscle Relaxation

Developmental stage	Technique variation
Early childhood	▪ *Robot/rag doll:* Teach children to walk stiffly like a robot, then melt into a rag doll. ▪ *Spaghetti:* Have children move like uncooked spaghetti, then cooked spaghetti. ▪ *Caterpillar/butterfly:* Have children move like a caterpillar still in the cocoon, then spread their wings like a butterfly. ▪ *Turtle/giraffe:* Have children act like a turtle going into a shell, then turn into a giraffe stretching for a leaf.
Middle childhood	▪ *Curl and release:* Teach children to crouch and curl up like a football player getting ready for a play. After crouching for a moment, yell "Hike" and have children stretch up to catch a throw. Have them also do it in slow motion for instant replay. ▪ *Doorway stretch:* Have children push with both arms against doorframe, hold for count of 7, then release. Have children notice the difference between pushing and releasing. Variations can include pushing against a wall or against the therapist's or caregiver's hands.
Adolescence	▪ *Tense and release:* Have adolescents move through different muscle groups in the body, tensing and then releasing. Have them tune in to and notice the difference between sensations when muscles are tensed versus relaxed. ▪ *Pair with breathing:* Have adolescents tense muscles while breathing in, then relax while breathing out.

IMAGERY

▪ Visual imagery, whether self- or other-guided, can be useful for increasing felt safety, decreasing arousal, and (re)gaining control when feeling out of control. Techniques should be geared to children's developmental stage and personal preferences.

Imagery

Developmental stage	Technique variation
Early childhood	*Safe place:* Imagery is difficult for young children and therefore must utilize concrete cues. For instance, rather than imagining a safe place, have children draw it and/or have them and caregivers create a concrete safe place within the home to which children can go when distressed. Similarly, designate a section of the office as each child's "safe place."
Middle childhood	Use images and concepts that are relevant to children. For instance: ▪ Have children identify favorite superhero or superpower (tuning in to strength, bravery, etc.); have them imagine being with that figure or having the power themselves. ▪ Identify favorite television, movie, or book character with which children associate a sense of safety or admiration; have them visualize being friends with that character. ▪ Have children draw a favorite place, real or imaginary, and guide them through imagining it (e.g., "What do you see? Hear? Feel? Taste?"). Have them practice this at home.

Developmental stage	Technique variation
Adolescence	Adolescents can utilize imagery techniques independently or with cuing, depending on preference. Concrete cues become less important. For instance: ▪ Have adolescents imagine a peaceful, healing light entering their bodies and erasing areas of tension. ▪ Have adolescents imagine a protective force field surrounding their bodies to keep them safe; adolescents can choose the color of the force field, who is in the field with them, physical sensations they are experiencing, temperature, etc. ▪ Have adolescents imagine a positive future self, including the qualities they might have, the feelings of calm and strength, etc. ▪ Have adolescents create an imaginary safe, peaceful place. Teach them that they can use this image for brief visits (e.g., if feeling stressed in class) or for longer periods (e.g., to calm down before bed).

OTHER MODULATION STRATEGIES

▪ Many modulation strategies do not fit neatly into the preceding categories, and many more possibilities exist than can be described in this book. We salute the occupational therapists and other professionals from whom we have learned about myriad ways to support children in achieving physiological organization. Note how many of these strategies resemble the soothing techniques naturally used in earlier developmental periods; for many children, these techniques may continue to assist them with modulation. *An important note:* It is crucial that children remain in felt control of any modulation strategy; any strategy into which a child is forced or coerced will ultimately be retraumatizing. Given that important caveat, we offer the following as examples:

Blanket Wrap. Some children may respond to the containment and organization provided by wrapping themselves in a blanket, whether weighted or standard. Blanket wraps offer a child a way to seek nurturance, soothing, and physiological organization without the arousing qualities of more relational soothing (e.g., a hug). Blanket wraps may be an alternative for children who are reluctant to accept physical affection in the face of distress or who struggle with appropriate boundaries.

Deep Pressure. Some children will respond to sensations of deep pressure. Pressure can be self-applied (e.g., using a "self massager") or other-applied (e.g., with the child's consent, using pillows above and below the child to make a "child sandwich"). Application of pressure by others should be done carefully and at the child's direction.

Tactile Engagement. There is a range of tactile sensations that children may find naturally modulating. Rinsing hands, molding clay, sifting through marbles, and tossing bean bags may each appeal differently to children. Explore (and observe) the tactile sensations toward which a child is naturally drawn.

Activity Engagement. Many of the natural activities of childhood can be modulating and organizing for children. Pay attention to the way a child's energy changes when engaging in crafts or artwork, listening to a story, playing a board game, or playing with peers. Any activity can be organizing for one child but disorganizing for another. Similarly, an activity that increases arousal for one child may decrease it for another. Explore and track each child's responses.

Appraisal and Control. A number of activities require children to both focus and exert control. A popular one at our center is balancing peacock feathers (with a nod to the colleague who first shared this activity with us; Macy, personal communication). Other activities may include rolling Chinese Baoding balls (also known as medicine balls) without allowing them to clink or chime, balancing on one foot, or walking across a low balance beam or in a straight line. We have found these activities to be most effective when paired with breathing (e.g., teach the child to breathe deeply, three times, before engaging in the activity). We have also found it useful to frame these as a "challenge" for younger clients: "Let's see how many tries it takes to balance the peacock feather for 10 seconds." Remind children to take their breaths, then let them go . . . even if it takes seven (very active) tries; by the seventh, successful effort, the child will typically be more organized and calmer.

Sound. For some clients, the use of sound may provide either up- or down-regulating experiences. Consider experimenting with different music, sounds, and so on, to elicit desired changes in physiological/emotional states.

STRATEGIES FOR PRACTICING ALTERNATING STATES

- *Alternating-states regulation* involves helping children learn how to flow through and tolerate increasing and decreasing levels of arousal.
- Many of the following techniques involve using fun activities to teach children how to tune in to and change arousal level on cue.
- These techniques are often particularly useful in dyadic work.
- Each technique can be adapted to the needs and preferences of a particular client or age; some may be more appropriate for younger or older children.

Regulation of Alternating States

Technique	Technique description
Turn up the volume	This exercise uses music or a symbolic "knob," "controller," or "slide switch" to cue faster or slower movement. It may be helpful to allow the child to be the controller first, while the therapist models faster or slower movement. Description: 1. Decide what will be used to control movement. 2. Agree on ranges (e.g., hands in the middle means medium movement, hands up in the air means fast, softer music means slow). 3. Designate who the first controller will be. 4. As the controller shifts (music level, hand position, etc.), the other person moves faster or slower.
Slo-mo	This exercise uses slow-motion movement to teach children how to slow themselves down. Once children have gained skill in moving in slow motion, they can be cued to shift into it when in a hyperaroused state. Description: 1. Teach children to move in slow motion by first modeling a typical movement (e.g., yawning, running):

Technique	Technique description

THERAPIST: Have you ever seen someone move in slow motion before? It's like moving through Jell-O, or through really, really thick water. Moving in slow motion looks really funny, but it's really hard to do. Watch: What if I ran in slow motion? It might look like this . . . (demonstrate moving in slow motion).

2. Invite the child to join you in a slow-motion movement; the child can pick the action. If it is an older child (e.g., 10- to 14-year-old boy), it is often helpful to make this a challenge: "Let's see who can move the most slowly from here to there."
3. Practice shifting to slow motion in response to cues; walk around the room normally with a child and take turns yelling, "Slo-mo." When the cue is given, each person has to immediately shift to slow motion until the "Slo-mo-off" cue is given or until a "freeze" cue is given.
4. If the child becomes practiced in this technique, the cue can be incorporated into daily routine by caregivers, teachers, etc. (e.g., if child is running through the halls, the teacher cues "Slo-mo").

Stop–start   These exercises involve games that shift children's actions from movement to immobility (e.g., freeze). Many classic children's games fall into this category (e.g., Red Light/Green Light, Musical Chairs).

Description:
Note: Use adapted versions of classic children's games. Example here is given for "Freeze Dance."
1. Frame the game for the child:
THERAPIST: We're going to play a game that helps you practice being in control of your body. *(Elicit from child, "When is it okay to move and be silly?" For example, at recess. "When is it important to slow your body down?" For example, in class.)* This game is kind of like Musical Chairs. When the music plays, we can jump around and be as silly as we want. When the music stops, we have to freeze.
2. One person should be selected to be the controller (in a therapy group, the leader is typically the controller). In individual therapy, the controller should still move after turning on the music.
3. The controller should turn the music off without warning; everyone freezes. The therapist should provide reinforcement for the child's ability to freeze on cue.
Note: Variations can include verbal cues ("Freeze," "Go"), visual cues (red stop sign, green go sign), etc.

Big–small   Big–small techniques are used to help children connect all the parts of self through movement (big, medium, small) and to identify appropriate situations for each style. This technique is useful for children who have difficulty with gross motor control and with awareness of self in space.

Description:
1. Help children identify all the ways in which their bodies physically expresses themselves (via voice, movement, speed, posture, etc.).
2. Start with the child's preferred way of moving. For instance, for a child who typically runs instead of walks, shouts instead of talks, etc., start with "big."
3. Select a day to be "Big Day" in therapy (or a portion of the therapy session). On that day, select an array of ways to move *big.* For instance, do a body trace on a life-size piece of paper, run and jump, talk loudly, etc. *Note:* It is often useful to do "Big Day" outdoors or some other place where it is appropriate to talk or move loudly.
4. During or after Big Day, help children identify places where they usually are "big"—for instance, at a park, at a swimming pool, on the beach, with their friends at recess, etc.
5. Follow up Big Day with Small Day (this is typically much harder for children). Draw on teeny pieces of paper, talk in a whisper, tiptoe, etc. As with Big Day, identify places where children are typically "small"—for instance, in the library, in a classroom, at night, etc.
6. Integrate concepts of big, medium, and small into therapy. For instance, if a child typically runs down the hall, cue him or her to "Walk small"; in therapy, shift from moving "small" to "medium" to "big."

Drumming   Drumming (with actual drums or tapping on the knees, desk, etc.) and/or the use of other musical instruments may help children modulate through faster/louder and slower/softer movements. This technique is particularly useful for children who have difficulty slowing down. Drumming also is an excellent attunement exercise.

Technique	Technique description

	Description:
	1. Select the instrument. Actual hand drums can be used, or children can thump on their knees or a table.
	2. Provide ground rules: For instance, drum sticks may not be used to hit anything other than the drum.
	3. Both clinician and child should use the same instrument.
	4. Possible variations:
	   a. Follow-the-leader. Take turns tapping out a pattern. The second person must copy the pattern. Be conscious of incorporating faster and slower patterns.
	   b. Simultaneous follow-the-leader. One person is designated as "leader"; the other person must match the first person's rhythm and/or pace. Take turns as leader and follower.

Skill #4: Building a Feelings and Energy Toolbox

▪ The goal of building a "feelings and energy toolbox" is to identify, for specified emotions and energy states, safe skills children can use to cope with their experience. Because not every skill will work every time, it is important that children have a repertoire of available skills. This subtarget of modulation is typically a process that takes place over time, as children become increasingly aware of various arousal states; aware of their own safety, comfort, and danger zones; and have opportunities to experiment with a range of strategies.

▪ When toolboxes are developed, they become a concrete way to cue children in their use of identified skills; the toolboxes may be actual boxes, or, for older children, lists or menus of skills.

Creating Feelings and Energy Toolboxes

How to build a toolbox	Suggested materials	*Box:* Shoebox or other container (e.g., lunchbox), materials to decorate box (e.g., magazines, stickers, construction paper), writing materials *Tools:* Possibilities are wide; may create symbolic tools with children using, for instance, clay, drawing, etc.; may also include actual tools (e.g., stress ball). *Alternatives:* ▪ Set of index cards labeled by tool/activity on one side and set of energy or emotion states on the other; or by energy/emotion state on one side and list of possible tools/activities on the other ▪ Paper list ▪ For older children/adolescents, electronic list on tablet/smartphone

	Techniques	▪ Building a Feelings and Energy Toolbox is a technique that should be implemented only after children have an understanding of:
		  ◆ What feelings are and at least a basic language for them
		  ◆ The concept of energy and arousal
		  ◆ Current actions (safe and unsafe) when experiencing strong emotion
		▪ Frame the rationale for the Feelings and Enegry Toolbox with children:
		  ◆ **Normalize feelings.** For example: "We've talked about how everyone has different kinds of feelings, and that no feeling is wrong."
		  ◆ **Differentiate safe versus unsafe expression.** For example: "Sometimes when people feel things really strongly, they do things that aren't all that helpful or safe." *(Give relevant examples from child's life, for example*: "Like, sometimes when kids are mad, they can get into fights and get in trouble at school, or when kids are really excited, it's hard for them to sit still and focus.")
		  ◆ **Highlight importance of feelings.** For example: "Feelings are important—they tell us a lot about what's going on and what we need. It's not healthy just to turn them off, because eventually they're going to build up or show up somewhere else."
		  ◆ **Provide rationale.** For example: "Since feelings are so important, we're going to build a toolbox [or, "create a menu"] of different things you can do when you're having different feelings."

■ Help children identify key emotions. Emotions addressed should include both (1) basic emotions (e.g., mad, sad, worried, happy) and (2) emotions that are difficult for children to cope with (e.g., embarrassment).
■ Alternatively (or in addition), identify different energy states. Again, pay attention to those that children find comfortable, as well as those that are more distressing or that interfere with their lives.
■ Work with children to create physical boxes or alternative strategies for capturing the tools they identify over time. They can label their box, decorate it, etc., as desired. Older children can choose to keep a list in a journal, notebook, etc. It may be useful to have a separate page for each emotion or energy state, so that children can add new techniques as they are identified.

Considerations	■ When working to create a repertoire of skills, be wary of overdoing. Children should develop mastery over a small number of skills before adding new ones. ■ Keep in mind that creation of these boxes is a process. New techniques and skills can and should be added as they are identified. ■ It may be important to reevaluate identified techniques over time (e.g., as child enters a new developmental stage; with life transitions). What worked at one point in time may not work at another. ■ In creating tools, consider the **energy of the emotion.** Often, anger, excitement, and fear are **externally directed "action" emotions,** and effective tools involve *releasing and focusing the energy.* In contrast, sadness and worry are often **"frozen" or internally directed emotions,** and effective tools involve self-soothing and reengaging. *Note:* The following are provided as examples; be creative and involve children in identifying helpful cues to include in their boxes.
Examples of tools for the toolbox	
Excitement	■ Small objects that children can manipulate in hands to channel energy (e.g., Wikki-Stix) ■ Small container of bubble liquid with wand ■ Doing specified number of jumping jacks (*cue for toolbox:* picture of child doing a jumping jack) ■ Butterfly hugs (folding arms across chest, and tapping shoulders like a butterfly flapping its wings) (*cue for toolbox:* picture of a butterfly)
Anger	■ Pushing against a wall or doorway (*cue for toolbox:* drawing of a doorway) ■ Stress ball to squeeze ■ Small ball of clay (to flatten)
Sadness	■ Picture of a favorite person or animal associated with comfort ■ Favorite or comforting object (e.g., teddy bear) ■ Soothing sensory object (e.g., piece of velvet) ■ Drawing materials or journal
Worry	■ Small box or container and pad of paper on which to write down worries and put them away ■ List of five distractions (i.e., activities child can engage in and/or positive things to think about) ■ Index card with stop sign on one side and positive statement on the other (e.g., "I can handle this") ■ Blank index cards and black marker; child can write down worry and then black it out.
Fear	■ Picture of a safe place ■ Picture of a strong person whom the child associates with safety ■ Small object from the therapy room or home (i.e., a transitional object) ■ Small tube of glitter cream or nice-smelling lotion for self-soothing (for younger children, can be "magic safety cream")

It is also possible to include music that you've listened to or pictures of the child doing specific activities. There really is no limit to the possible tools that can go into the toolbox. The important point to normalize and model is the idea that we all have and use strategies all the time. It can be helpful to provide concrete examples from the therapist's or caregiver's toolbox!

Skill #5: Supporting and Facilitating Modulation Strategies

■ When treatment has focused on addressing modulation in children and adolescents, it is not uncommon in moments of distress for providers and caregivers to communicate, either explicitly or implicitly, the message, "You're upset! Go use your tools!" In fact, in moments of calm, if a provider was to ask an adolescent in a residential program (for instance) what he or she is supposed to do when upset, it is likely that young person can rattle off a list of skills ("Go to my room, talk to a staff, journal, take a breath"). This *cognitive* awareness of the link between distress and tool use is very different from the ability to actually *use* tools in moments of distress or dysregulation. In fact, moments when the young person is mostly highly dysregulated are perhaps the least likely times that he or she will realistically be able to access those skills, at least at first. It is for this reason that we identify the role of building external supports for modulation as a primary skill.

■ In order to support and facilitate modulation plans, consider the following:

Supporting and Facilitating Modulation

Engage caregivers.	Consider the specific locations and situations in which a child/adolescent may be struggling with arousal or emotion. Identify and specifically engage key caregivers in each setting (parents, teachers, after-school providers, mentors, direct-care staff, etc.). With the youth's permission, share information about tools that appear useful for the child. Brainstorm ways that the caregiver can support the child in utilizing skills or can provide space/permission for the child to access tools when needed. In "Teach to Caregivers" starting on page 204, we review key education points to help caregivers support modulation. Integrate this education into the engagement process.
Develop a plan.	In order to be effective, it is likely that modulation plans need to be *proactive* (i.e., to anticipate challenging situations instead of just reacting to them) and *specific* (i.e., identifying appropriate tools, supports, limitations, stressors, etc.). Work with both the child and the surrounding system to target specific plans in response to specific patterns of dysregulation.
Practice and troubleshoot.	Engage the child/adolescent as well as the caregiver(s) in practicing the plan when calm. Consider not just what might go well, but what might go wrong. For instance, if the plan is, "Mom will remind Janae to use her calming space when she gets upset," what will Mom do if Janae yells at her and refuses to go to the calming space? What alternatives might there be utilized to give each of them space in the moment and to prevent escalation? Incorporate both the child's and caregiver's stake in outcomes into conversations about modulation plans.
Provide a range of context-appropriate tools.	Consider the context when developing plans. It is likely that the child may need access to different tools or strategies when at school than when at home, in one classroom versus another, with peers versus with a parent, etc. Consider what the child has access to, permission for, and the degree of supports and external resources needed to realistically engage in various strategies.

ꤧ Developmental Considerations

Developmental stage	Affect modulation considerations
Early childhood	At this stage the role of the caregiver in affect modulation is crucial. Young children depend on caregivers for support and nurturing, and it would not be developmentally appropriate to expect them to modulate all on their own. Involve caregivers, as much as possible, in affect modulation work. Physiological regulation provided by caregivers (e.g., cuddling, rocking, back rubs) is often important for young children. However, keep in mind that some children may have built

Developmental stage	Affect modulation considerations
	defenses against touch. It is important to normalize this response for caregivers and to help them find acceptable ways to interact physically with their children, while respecting the children's need for boundaries. Teach caregivers to ask even young children for permission to touch—allow some control.
	Younger children normatively view degrees of feeling in terms of extremes (e.g., big vs. small), rather than in nuanced increments. Match their level when teaching degrees of feeling and use concrete markers wherever possible. For instance: ■ Use arm gesturess to show how big a feeling is ■ Use concrete anchors: for example, "feelings as big as this room," "feelings as small as a penny" ■ Coloring in circles (thermometers, etc.)
Middle childhood	During this stage, children are increasingly able to identify degrees of emotion. Help children tune in to subtler variations of their own emotional experiences.
	Help children stop arousal *before* it hits crisis level. Children at this age can be taught to recognize internal cues of escalating arousal (e.g., changes in body state) as well as external cues (e.g., people saying, "Shhh"). Pair this recognition with modulation techniques.
	Increase child's involvement in modulation strategies at this stage. For instance, if a child identifies being "50 poker chips mad," ask, "What would it take to get you down to 45 poker chips?" Put children in the position of power/knowledge about their own affect state.
Adolescence	Adolescents may be increasingly sophisticated in their capacity to understand changes in emotional experience. However, when triggered, adolescents may regress to earlier emotional stages and have difficulty making use of developed skills.
	Continue to provide external cuing and reinforcement, but be aware that adolescents may resist supports.
	Adolescents are at particular risk for use of dangerous modulation strategies, such as self-harm and/or substance use. It is particularly important that an adolescent have a repertoire of modulation skills that can be implemented independently.

Applications

Individual/Dyadic

Modulation activities are often an important focus of individual therapy, as dysregulation in its various manifestations is a typical reason for referral. We view the building of modulation abilities as a process that involves many components, including the caregiver's own affect management, attunement, and support, as well as the child's awareness and understanding of his or her own physiological and emotional states and a slow building of skill in managing these.

An essential foundation of this work is developing a common language with a child and caregiver to serve as a cue for future attempts at modulation (e.g., "I see that your energy is getting really big . . .") as well as in depathologizing child behaviors and responses. Similarly, engaging the caregiver and child in the building and using of feeling and energy "tools" supports agency on both sides and creates an expectation that the child and caregiver are collaborators in observing and managing arousal. In addition to finding that foundation, much of modulation work hinges on what we refer to as "the hook." As in all other therapeutic work, it is important to have a full understanding of a child's likes, dislikes, interests, and talents, to help guide your exploration of arousal. For example, we often tell the story of an Alaskan Native youth who took great pride in a tribal culture that values hunting and fishing. The therapist working with him was able to talk about modulation through that lens, with an emphasis on being in a calm state of mind—staying still and quiet in order to be successful in these acts. They used the peacock feather (described in a previous section) to practice down-modulation.

We have found it useful to build modulation practice into our session routine; for instance, children who typically enter the session with a great deal of energy may need a quick up-regulation activity to meet them where they are at, and then a focusing or down-regulation activity to help them engage. Many modulation activities are perceived by younger children as games; by adding a reflective or curious layer to the game (e.g., noticing the child's energy shift or asking about the child's experience), the clinician can help the child build awareness of his or her body's energy and control.

Many modulation activities can be applied in the moment to help a child navigate difficult moments like session transitions. For instance, an older child can be cued to walk up the hall at an energy level of 3 instead of 7; a younger child can be cued to walk up the hall as a turtle or in slow motion. Modulation strategies for adolescents can be practiced and planned for negotiating anticipated challenges. For instance, prior to inviting a caregiver into a session for a difficult conversation, explore and practice with the adolescent strategies (e.g., holding a grounding stone, squeezing a stress ball, doing deep breathing) that will help him or her maintain an effective level of modulation. Any attempts at modulation (whether successful or not) should be noticed and reinforced by the clinician and (ideally) by the caregiver. Effective tools should be shared with caregivers, so that they can be practiced and reinforced in the home setting.

Beyond session tools, work with caregivers to notice and incorporate into daily life activities that naturally modulate and organize a child (e.g., drawing, cuddling, listening to music, singing) as well as to pay attention to the events and activities that seem to disorganize a child. When these events/activities are unavoidable (e.g., transitions), consider ways to build modulation exercises into the routine. For many children, adjunctive activities such as participating in sports, martial arts, yoga, or the performing and expressive arts provide natural forums for learning how to control, manage, and express arousal and emotion.

Group

Many of the skills, exercises, and psychoeducation described in this chapter can be incorporated into group activities. As in individual therapy, modulation activities can be incorporated into group session routine (e.g., a starting "warm-up," opening "energy check," closing "cool down"). Consider paying attention to group modulation as well as individual modulation: For instance, at the start of a group, plot all members' energy levels on a magnetic or paper thermometer. Notice differences in group dynamics when all group members are at high energy versus low or diffuse energy levels.

Many modulation activities work particularly well in a group format. For instance, drumming, turn-up-the-volume games, and follow-the-leader activities all work well in groups, and can be adapted to apply to younger children as well as adolescents. In addition, we have also developed groups that focus primarily on modulation. For example, we have run "toolbox" groups with children and adolescents who create tools for their boxes such as "find its," like wave machines or stress balls. Each week focuses on the development of a new tool to practice together. Other groups have emphasized specific modulation skills such as movement and focus groups, like music groups or yoga groups.

🏠 Milieu

Building an awareness of and support for modulation is essential to supporting the experience of children and adolescents who struggle with management of arousal and emotion within a milieu environment. A primary first step for many milieus (schools, residential programs, hospital settings, etc.) is learning to differentiate the need for limits from the need for modulation. Note that these are not mutually exclusive; however, it is often helpful to consider these as a two-step process: When a child or adolescent is dysregulated, noncompliant, or overly shut down, the *first step* is to support the child in modulating him- or herself (including ensuring physical safety); the *second step* is to apply limits and consequences, when appropriate. It is our experience that for many milieu programs, application of consequences in moments of significant arousal leads inevitably to escalation, as the child or adolescent feels increasingly helpless and triggered; ultimately, this arousal and mutual escalation may lead to a need for physical restraint. In programs in which we worked to build an increased awareness of modulation strategies, along with support for staff members and awareness of their own affect management needs, restraints dropped to almost zero, *despite a complete lack of focus on restraint reduction as a target.*

⊞ Modulation can be supported via daily routines. Consider, for instance, use of focusing activities at the start of the school day; relaxation and yoga groups as youth are making significant transitions or schedule shifts; energizing activities such as sports to help youth discharge energy after lengthy periods of focused time; and down-regulating activities in the evening. It is particularly important to pay attention to decreasing highly arousing activities in the evening, given the particular difficulty of trauma-impacted children in navigating the transition from wakefulness to sleep.

Many modulation tools can be made available throughout a milieu. We have worked with programs that have (1) incorporated baskets of handheld manipulatives into the classroom (allowing children to squeeze stress balls or twist Wikki Stix to manage arousal); (2) built and filled Feelings and Energy Toolboxes for each child to keep in his or her room; and (3) added blankets, pillows, and other self-soothing materials into classic time-out rooms. Our favorite example is the "Sensory Room" built by one program to replace one of their time-out rooms. The room is lit softly, lined with blankets and pillows, and contains baskets of materials designed to appeal to the five senses (e.g., a range of tactile objects, various lotions, pictures of peaceful scenes, different kinds of music). Rather than simply being placed in a time-out area, adolescents in this program are given the option of requesting time in the sensory room.

Individual planning is often another area in which modulation can be integrated. Many programs offer "coaching breaks" at known "trouble spots" throughout the day for a particular child or adolescent. Consider "the hook" discussed above when thinking about how to structure "coaching" or "modulation breaks." We worked with one young man who loved to listen to a pop star. He was able to take dance breaks listening to her music at various points throughout his day to support his overall success. Another child who struggled with transitions during the day had the opportunity to go on "Mission I'm Possible" trips during that time that involved movement and chores. Creativity and "outside-the-box" intervention often goes hand in hand with modulation work.

Addressing modulation is one of the domains in which programs can be the most creative, given the "buy-in" and understanding of the staff. Psychoeducation and support for staff—and the parallel active practice of modulation by team members at all levels—are essential for successful change in this area. The culture of modulation in a program can often involve what many program directors refer to as "calculated risk." Consider a program's decision to have frozen oranges available to its youth as a modulation tool. The young women in this program primarily used oranges as a grounding tool (tactile and olfactory sensations). One young woman also liked to toss the orange with a staff member. Many would worry that the orange could be used to harm someone else, specifically that it could be used as a projectile. This is a calculated risk that requires significant education about why the tool is available, when to offer this tool and when not (i.e., not at moments of full-blown escalation), and how to support youth in using it effectively.

○ Trauma Experience Integration: State-Based Skills Application

Distress Tolerance and Regulation

During early stages of treatment and in distressed states, the primary focus of modulation is often that of *supported* modulation: engaging the attunement skills of the entire caregiver system—whether primary, therapeutic, or milieu—in recognizing and understanding patterns of distress, and supporting and facilitating increasingly regulated states across settings. A primary goal is to identify triggers for and cues of dysregulation, and to develop targeted and proactive plans to support youth in accessing and engaging in distress tolerance and safety plans when overwhelmed. Modulation strategies can be practiced in calm states, and should be built into daily routine whenever feasible. Youth who struggle with frequent episodes of overwhelm can be supported in engaging their curiosity outside of those moments, but in-the-moment modulation will largely be facilitated by the caregiving system.

Curiosity and Reflection

Youth who have gained some degree of safety in the therapeutic relationship, and/or who are in calm-enough states to be reflective outside of the distressed moment, can often begin the work of developing greater attuned understanding of their own patterns of dysregulation, and particularly of the role of triggers and the trauma/arousal response in that dysregulation. In addition to experimenting with and practicing the range of modulation skills described previously, clinical work can integrate a growing awareness of ways that moments of dysregulation may be about more than "the moment," and link these states to historical or ongoing experiences of danger. In turn, youth can be supported in identifying both internal cues of danger and internal and external resources and strategies that support felt safety.

Engaging in Purposeful Action

As youth are increasingly able to build their awareness of shifts in arousal states and impending dysregulation in the moment, a goal becomes to increase their capacity to use—at age-appropriate levels—active and increasingly independent modulation strategies that prevent rather than respond to hyper- or hypoaroused states. This capacity will rely on integrating and supporting the youth's curiosity about and awareness of his or her own affect states, an understanding of what drives these states, and motivation to recognize and "catch" the states in the moment.

In addition, as a child or adolescent develops an increasing capacity to tolerate distress and make use of both internal and external resources, it is increasingly feasible to integrate modulation skills in service of supporting trauma or life narrative work.

Real-World Therapy

Practice, but be realistic. Children will not be able to apply modulation skills in the moment immediately; it takes time for these to translate from the intervention setting to the real world. Help kids stick with it. Allow time each week for children to practice these skills.

Why should I? Admit it—sometimes it feels good to get angry, or sad, or over-the-top excited. Don't be too quick to modulate—a child may need time to engage in a feeling or energy state before working to change it. As long as a child is safe, don't rush the state shift.

Part VI

Competency

Why Target Developmental Competency?

- Development is a dynamic process, and each developmental stage is associated with key tasks that children must negotiate, drawing on emergent assets such as growth in cognitive functioning, as well as on past successes.

- Tasks at each stage build on tasks from previous stages. So, for instance, successful establishment of peer relationships in middle childhood builds in part on the early childhood success in developing secure attachment relationships.

- Throughout childhood, competencies emerge across domains: cognitive, interpersonal, intrapersonal, emotional, and physical/motor.

- Many developmental competencies are, in themselves, associated with resilient outcomes in future life stages. It is therefore important that intervention with children whose development has been impacted by trauma targets achievement of key developmental tasks as a primary goal. Given the impact of trauma on developmental course, targeting developmental competency should be considered an integral component of, rather than an adjunct to, "trauma-focused therapy."

How Does Trauma Impact Achievement of Development Tasks?

- As detailed in previous sections' Key Concepts, there is extensive evidence that trauma has the potential to derail developmental competencies across domains of functioning and across developmental stages.

- Exposure to trauma is implicated in the impaired development of:

  - *Interpersonal competencies,* such as building early secure attachment relationships, positive peer relationships, and mature relationships in adulthood.

  - *Intrapersonal competencies,* such as positive self-concept, awareness of internal states, realistic assessment of self-competencies, and capacity to integrate self-states.

229

◆ *Cognitive competencies,* such as language development; school performance and achievement; and growth of executive function skills, including problem solving, frustration tolerance, sustained attention, and abstract reasoning.

◆ *Regulatory competencies,* such as the ability to identify emotional states; realistically interpret others' cues and expression; regulate physiological and emotional arousal; manage, organize, and coordinate physical/motor responses; and share emotional experience.

A Three-Part Model, Revisited

■ In Chapter 2, we highlighted a three-part model for understanding child behaviors through the lens of (1) impacted systems of meaning, including a prominent assumption of danger; (2) activation of functional danger-avoidance and need-fulfillment strategies in the face of relevant cues, leading to dysregulation of emotion, behavior, and physiology; and (3) interference from developmental challenges, with reliance on alternative adaptations to regain equilibrium.

　◆ In the *Attachment* section of this framework, we target the first level of this model by seeking to build safe-enough surrounding systems and to strengthen or repair child–caregiver relationships.

　◆ In the *Regulation* section of this framework, we target the second level of the model by working with children and their caregivers to foster a healthy understanding of internal experience, and the acquisition and use of strategies for tolerating and shifting emotional and physiological states.

　◆ In this, the *Competency* section, we highlight the importance of targeting the third level: the range of additional developmental competencies relevant to successful navigation of life experiences.

■ Given the number of key developmental tasks, we focus more intensively on three key domains identified as particularly relevant to resilient outcome among highly stress-impacted youth: the capacity to build and sustain meaningful relationships over time, the ability to engage executive functions in the service of making active choices, and the healthy development of personal identity. In this introductory section, we briefly highlight additional domains that may be important to target in work with trauma-impacted youth.

　◆ In assessing and selecting relevant developmental tasks to target, keep in mind the importance of considering *developmental stage* rather than *chronological age.* Children vary in level of developmental competency across domains (e.g., consider a cognitively advanced child with earlier developmental interpersonal competencies) and across time or setting (e.g., consider a child whose emotional competencies vary by level of stressor, or a child who regresses when placed in a new home).

Early Childhood

A primary task of early childhood is the establishment of a secure attachment and development of basic self-regulation skills. In addition, consider addressing the following target domains:

Social Skills

■ Work with caregivers to build children's ability to interact with others in appropriate ways. Teach and model cooperative play. Set limits around negative behaviors in interaction.

■ Involve children in natural forums for social interaction. Consider the use of playdates, preschool, Head

Start, community centers, playrooms, and so forth. Caregivers should remain present and involved in these contexts with young children.

■ Balance structured with unstructured activities. It is important that children develop the ability to follow the rules as well as use their imaginations. It is also important that children be able to play both cooperatively and independently.

■ Help children develop an early understanding of empathy. Teach that different people have different feelings. Encourage children to respond to others' emotions in appropriate ways. It is important to differentiate between taking *undue responsibility* for others' feelings and *caring* about those feelings.

Motor Skills

■ Involve children in activities that build gross and fine motor skills.

■ For gross motor, consider the use of sports, dance, martial arts, gymnastics, and the like. Focus on cooperative rather than competitive play during this period.

■ For fine motor, consider the use of arts-and-crafts projects, puzzles, tracing objects and letters, or sensory inputs of various sizes.

■ When possible, caregivers should be involved in activities with their children; doing so fosters positive dyadic experience along with motor skill development.

Learning Readiness

■ Work with caregivers to facilitate and motivate children's interest in learning. Primary at this stage is an interest in exploring the surrounding environment.

■ Encourage caregivers to explore *with* their children. Tap into natural forums: Take a walk, go to the park, read a book, go to the library. Pay attention to asking and wondering together.

■ Work with caregivers to help their children apply new information. For instance, if the child has developed interest in how spaghetti is made, suggest that child and caregiver cook a dish together. If a child is learning a new game, play it together at home or in the session.

■ Work with caregivers to challenge children. Encourage children to try tasks just above their comfort zone. Normalize the reality that some tasks are more difficult than others. Use regulation strategies to help children build frustration tolerance. Identify/articulate frustrations when they happen and encourage continued effort. Help children achieve cooperatively what would be just above their grasp individually.

Elementary School/Middle Childhood

Industry is increasingly important in middle childhood, as children explore the world outside of their homes. At this stage it is important to target both individual achievements and connections to others and to the larger world.

Social Skills

■ Peer relationships become increasingly important throughout the elementary school years. To be successful, children need to accurately read others' intentions; negotiate interactions; experience empathy;

and tolerate delay, disappointment, and frustration. Ability to work cooperatively and tolerate compromise are particularly important. Pay attention to deficits in these areas and work with children to build appropriate skills.

■ Help children become increasingly involved in adjunctive activities. Encourage participation in sports, clubs, arts activities, after-school programming, and so forth. As children become involved in competitive activities, emotion regulation skills become increasingly important.

■ Many other skills highlighted in this framework, such as problem-solving and affect regulation skills, are often important to successful peer interaction. Pair those skills when helping a child navigate real-life interactions.

■ Traumatic triggers are often prominent in social interactions. Help children identify when "old" feelings get in the way of new relationships.

School Connection/Achievement

■ School is a primary domain of competency in middle childhood. It is more important that children be invested in and feel positive about school involvement than that they be academically successful.

■ Work with school systems to support children in experiencing success. Create a team. Identify school personnel who can serve as resources for the child in the school setting. Collaborate in treatment planning.

■ Work with caregivers to reinforce effort and to show interest in children's school accomplishments. Build lines of communication with the school setting. Balance encouragement and praise with limit setting.

■ Work with caregivers to provide a structure that accommodates changes in routine. Pay attention to transitions and create appropriate routines, as needed. Help structure the home setting in a way that supports children as they strive to accomplish school goals (e.g., homework).

■ Help caregivers balance prioritization of goal accomplishment with unstructured time. It is important that children have opportunities for rest and play in addition to work.

Personal Responsibility

■ It is important for children to have clear and reasonable expectations. They need to know what the rules are, what the expectations are, and to know that people believe that they can accomplish their relevant goals. Children will often live up—or down—to our expectations of them.

■ Children are increasingly able to understand the rationale for rules. Help them differentiate rules in different locations (e.g., home vs. school) and the reasons for those rules. Involve them, to some degree, in setting household rules.

■ Encourage children to take increasing responsibility. Work with caregivers to build age-appropriate chores in the home setting. Because it is important that children experience success in completing chores, work with caregivers to designate appropriate tasks and to monitor and reinforce task completion. Caregivers should provide support, as needed, with an ultimate goal of independent task mastery.

Adolescence

Primary tasks of adolescence include exploration and establishment of a coherent identity, beginning stages of separation and individuation from caregivers, and building a foundation for independent functioning. Many of these skills are discussed in other sections of this framework; additional considerations are highlighted here.

Social Skills

- Adolescents must increasingly be able to negotiate a variety of social interactions independently. These include peer interactions but also interactions with teachers, potential employers, community members, and the like.

- Create opportunities for adolescents to come into contact with a range of people in different contexts and work with them to practice effective communication skills.

- Work with caregivers to balance involvement with the adolescent need for privacy. Caregiver involvement may shift toward expressing interest, rather than knowledge, per se.

- Work with adolescents to maintain individual opinions, thoughts, and goals even in the midst of peer influence. Pair social skills with identity work.

- For teens who have experienced harm in interpersonal relationships, social connections can trigger fear as well as either premature intimacy or rejection of intimacy. Help adolescents define positive relationships and then develop them.

- Help adolescents develop effective conflict resolution skills. Note that this area involves many of the same skills previously addressed in identification and modulation, along with skills that will be covered in the coming chapters. Work with adolescents to use the following steps in addressing conflicts:

  - *Know your own cues:* Tune in to cues of self-distress. (identification)

  - *Choose your moments:* Calm down before approaching a difficult situation. (modulation)

  - *Identify goals:* What does the adolescent want to accomplish? (executive functions, identity)

  - *Take perspective:* What might the other person be experiencing? (identification of other's internal state)

  - *Evaluate outcomes:* Be flexible—what has/has not worked? (generate alternatives; executive functions)

Community Connection

- Work with adolescents to expand their involvement in the world outside of the home. This may include extracurricular activities, participation in community programs, or employment.

- There are many ways for adolescents to contribute to the larger community. Community involvement develops agency, efficacy, and social connection. Keep in mind that community involvement can be formal or informal. Help adolescents define the ways in which they currently make a difference, and/or how they want to make a difference.

- It is normative for adolescents to develop relationships with people from an expanded social circle, including other adults. Work with caregivers to tolerate these connections; although caregivers should stay aware of those with whom their child is interacting, it is important to allow some latitude as adolescents struggle to gain independence in their interactions.

■ Community connections are a key forum for exploring interests as well as building or expanding individual skills and attributes.

Independent Functioning

■ Throughout this developmental stage, adolescents are moving toward increasingly independent functioning. It is important that tasks and activities begin to reflect this independence.

■ School accomplishments are increasingly important to future functioning. Work with adolescents to connect current achievements with current and future goals.

■ Work with caregivers to involve adolescents in discussion about and establishment of household rules, roles, and structure.

■ Jobs can be an important forum for building self-efficacy, self-reliance, and responsibility. However, it is also important to help adolescents establish realistic expectations and goals, job-wise, and to make sure that jobs do not interfere with adolescents' ability to continue to participate in other important domains of their lives.

■ Personal responsibility is an essential value for adolescents, and it is strongly associated with resiliency. Help adolescents explore their own actions and the natural consequences of those actions. Bring the language of "choice" into conversations.

■ Pay attention to fostering the range of life skills relevant to future independent functioning. Work with adolescents to learn to do such things as open bank accounts and budget money, navigate appropriate interaction in a range of settings, manage basic household tasks, and identify and access external resources. A focus on these key areas is particularly important for those adolescents who will have less of a caregiving "buffer" as they transition into young adulthood (e.g., adolescents who will be "aging out" of substitute care). Whenever possible, work to connect adolescents with individuals and other social resources who will be able to provide support through and beyond this transition.

Young Adulthood

Although this book primarily focuses on youth through adolescence, the children and adolescents of today are the transition age and young adults of tomorrow, and our work in the field has increasingly included this vulnerable and often overlooked population. As they increasingly enter into the world of "independence," young adults face a range of life challenges that must be negotiated, in the absence of the external supports that are (ideally) provided to their younger counterparts. We have found in our work that the vast majority of constructs covered in this book apply equally to transitioning young adults as to children and adolescents, and we briefly highlight key competencies and targets here.

Identity Exploration

■ Young adults are often still exploring many facets of identity. Encourage continued exploration of areas of interest (sports, arts, computers, cooking, etc.) as well as other aspects of identity (culture, values, gender and sexual identity, group affiliation, etc.) that contribute to a comprehensive understanding and narrative of self.

- A key part of identity is our understanding of self in relation to our family—whether family of origin, family of choice, or otherwise. Services for young adults, particularly those services that are designed to support independence, may not primarily focus on family connection, and may in fact ignore the role of this important aspect in the young adult's ongoing development of sense of self. We have encouraged providers who work with young adults to continue to support exploration of and connection to family identity and, when appropriate, to include family members in the work.

Social Connection

- Intervention with transition-age youth and young adults often emphasizes (necessarily) those skills and capacities needed for *independence*. However, this stance may lead to neglect of the equally important goal of *connection*. Support young adults in identifying and building a social network that may include family as well as additional social supports and relational resources such as mentors, spiritual leaders, coaches or sponsors, as well as peers. Consider identifying a range of needs (emotional, recreational, logistical) and working with young people to identify, access, and expand environments and relationships that connect them with individuals who can support those needs (e.g., therapists may help with emotional needs, peers may share similar interests, family members may be able to provide basic logistical supports). It may be important to support young adults who have had historical relationship losses and failures in recognizing the limits of any single individual's capacity to meet all needs comprehensively.

- Young adults may begin to engage in increasingly intimate relationships. Support young adults in exploring special challenges that emerge within this context (e.g., pregnancy and/or parenting; reenactment of past experiences; traumatic triggering related to perceived rejection, loss, abandonment; triggers related to physical/sexual contact) and the meaning of intimacy as it relates to future family identity (e.g., "What will my family identity be in the future?"). In addition, explore the strength and resilience that can emerge within the context of intimate and/or long-term relationships.

- Young adults impacted by trauma may need support with social engagement and/or social skills. It may be necessary to provide concrete education and strategies for effective ways to relate to and communicate with others within a particular context. The skills discussed in Chapter 12, "Relational Connection," can support this work.

Vocational Functioning and Life Skills

- Work with young adults to identify key domains of life functioning relevant to successful independent living (i.e., vocational, housing, financial, relational) and support them in honestly assessing and identifying their own personal areas of strength and vulnerability.

- Support young adults in identifying and setting both short- and long-term goals, and then in identifying key skills, resources, and relationships that might be needed to reach those goals. For instance: "Having my own apartment" may require a job that provides enough money to pay rent and an ability to set and keep a budget, to organize and pay bills, and to prepare food. In turn, "Having a job" may require an ability to identify open positions, develop a résumé, learn interview skills, reliably manage a schedule. Working toward smaller steps and short-term goals can be embedded in the context of the "pathway" toward longer-term goals.

- Develop and maintain awareness of available vocational support resources in your community: for instance, vocational training programs or job placement services. Provide concrete support to young people in accessing and negotiating these resources.

Developmental Toolbox

■ As much as for younger children and adolescence, successful navigation of the challenges of early adulthood requires a range of developmental capacities that may have been compromised by developmental trauma. It may be important to carefully assess strengths and challenges in all domains of functioning. It continues to be important to attune to "stage, not age" with this population. Young adulthood can be a particularly stressful time as demands for independent functioning increase. This added pressure places young adults at risk for engaging regulation strategies that may be harmful (e.g., substance abuse). Support young-adult clients in developing the range of developmental capacities described in this book, including the capacity to regulate a range of emotional and physiological experiences, the ability to identify and work toward goals, and a coherent sense of self.

Each core domain of this framework emphasizes key developmental competencies for trauma-impacted youth and their caregiving systems. Given the dynamic nature of development and the impact that trauma has on developmental processes, it is essential that the treatment of chronic trauma include assessment and intervention focused on the myriad of developmental strengths and challenges. As we move forward in this section and the next, we focus on helping children (1) move beyond survival so that they are consciously *acting,* rather than reacting; (2) establish a sense of self that is coherent, strengths-based, and future-oriented; and (3) understand and transform early traumatic experiences so that they are able to establish a coherent life narrative.

12

Relational Connection

 THE MAIN IDEA AND KEY SUBSKILLS

Help children build the skills and tolerance for effectively engaging and sustaining connection with others.

★ Explore the goals of connecting with others; build comfort and safety in relationship.

★ Identify/establish resources for safe connection.

★ Create opportunities for connection via structures that support communication.

★ Support communication by coaching and modeling effective skills, including:
  ◇ Effective nonverbal communication skills
  ◇ Effective verbal communication skills
  ◇ Alternative communication strategies

★ Key Concepts

★ Why Target Relational Connection?

■ A significant proportion of children who have experienced traumatic stress have, as part of that experience, been through attachment losses, betrayals, or harm in the context of relationship. As a result, many children struggle to build safe and lasting relationships, and any "failures" in this domain prevent them from having many different kinds of needs met.

■ Sharing internal experience is a key aspect of human relationships. An inability or unwillingness to effectively communicate with others prevents children from being able to form and maintain ongoing healthy attachments and subsequently from mastering developmental tasks that rely heavily on this skill. There are several reasons why communication and connection may be impacted in children who have experienced trauma:

◆ *Early attachment.* In a healthy attachment relationship, children's experiences are validated by reflection, mirroring, and appropriate responses by caregivers to shared information. When children's attempts to communicate their emotions, needs, and thoughts are met with anger, rejection, and/or indifference, they learn two things:

237

1. **Shame.** "My emotions and needs are wrong, bad, or unimportant."
2. **Need for secrecy.** "If I share what is happening inside of me, something bad will happen."

◆ *Vulnerability.* Emotions and other internal experiences are an aspect of human existence associated, in many ways, with vulnerability. Sharing what is happening inside of us allows others a window into the internal self. Acknowledging fear, sadness, anger, or joy involves risk for everyone, but particularly for a child who has experienced harm. In the mindset of a child who has been exposed to family violence, for instance, acknowledging joy raises the possibility of it being taken away; expressing anger may increase the potential of threat. For children whose lives have been organized around survival, minimization of risk is often a primary adaptation. Learning to hide their experiences may help children feel more in control or less vulnerable.

How Does the Impact of Trauma Affect Relational Connection?

There is an intricate connection between attempts to manage relationship/connection and communication/expression strategies. Children may attempt to restrict relationship, approach it haphazardly or ineffectively, or try to maximize it out of a desperate need to connect. Influencing this area of response are strategies that may be constricted, ineffective, or unboundaried. Common patterns include the following:

■ In the face of shame and a need for secrecy, children may *restrict relationships and fail to share internal experiences* with others—they may:
  ◆ Put on a "false front" (e.g., "Everything's fine").
  ◆ Isolate themselves.
  ◆ Substitute acceptable emotions for unacceptable ones, or powerful emotions for less powerful ones.
  ◆ Minimize emotional experience.
  ◆ Deny or appear unaware of emotional, physiological, and relational needs.
■ Emotions and needs that are not expressed in healthy ways may emerge in other forms, such as:
  ◆ *Somatic expression:* for example, headaches, stomachaches, fatigue
  ◆ *Behavioral expression:* for example, disorganization, agitation, withdrawal
  ◆ *Need substitution:* for example, overeating or hoarding food to replace need for connection and relationship
■ Children may also *attempt to form relationships and communicate their needs and emotions in ineffective ways*. For instance, they may:
  ◆ Substitute actions for verbal communication (e.g., punching instead of telling someone they are angry).
  ◆ Externalize emotions by projecting them onto others (e.g., "I think my mom is really sad about this").
  ◆ Attempt to engage others through ineffective strategies (e.g., act silly or talk too much in an attempt to relate, but fail to read others' annoyance).

■ Some children ***overcommunicate***—that is, they share information indiscriminately, without awareness of appropriate boundaries. This response may occur for different reasons:

 ◆ **Inability to contain intrusive traumatic material.** Children may experience recurrent, intrusive memories that are triggered by thoughts, feelings, or interactions. In the face of this ***reexperiencing,*** indiscriminate sharing (i.e., detailed retelling of traumatic experiences) may be an attempt to gain mastery over devastating internal material. However, in the absence of modulation strategies, this attempt at mastery may actually be retraumatizing. Furthermore, an inability to discriminate appropriate contexts for sharing this material may have negative social and emotional consequences.

 ◆ **Poor relational awareness.** Children may also overcommunicate about nontraumatic material. In an attempt to connect, form relationships, or meet emotional needs, children may share overly personal information with individuals with whom they have not yet developed relational intimacy. This ineffective attempt to share emotional experience often ends up backfiring, as others may distance themselves in an attempt to regain appropriate boundaries.

 ◆ **Desperate attempts to get needs met.** Children who have learned that responsiveness from others is unpredictable or unavailable may have learned to maximize opportunities for connection by flagging their emotions, needs, and experiences. These children may dramatically express emotion, may present as highly demanding of others' attention, or may behaviorally act out or engage in high-risk or sensational behaviors in order to be noticed or to connect. This strategy, although developed to increase opportunities for connection and support, may lead to further experiences of rejection, as others feel intruded upon or frustrated by the child's actions.

Therapist Toolbox
What's the Stake?

■ The very factors that interfere with children's ability to connect with others are those factors that make this treatment target particularly challenging. For children who have been explicitly harmed, rejected, and betrayed in relationship, survival has mandated that they develop careful and often rigid strategies to manage connection. Challenging or changing those strategies is experienced, in many ways, as a threat to safety or survival.

■ Because children who struggle with connection may present with a range of relational patterns, understanding their current organization around relationships is crucial for engaging them in therapeutic work focused on shifting how they approach relationship. For instance, consider the following:

 ◆ For the child who has managed relationship by **disconnection,** isolation, and constriction, it may be important to focus on the concrete outcomes of connection: When we connect with others and communicate our needs, it may help us to get those needs met. For these children, it is likely going to be important to acknowledge and explore the ways that relationships have been painful, threatening, or unavailable over time, and why it has been important or helpful for the youth to minimize connection. An early emphasis on concrete needs (vs. relational or emotional ones) may be the most tolerable for these children.

◆ For the child who has managed relationship by **overconnection** and intrusive communication, attempts to shut down communication and connection ("You need to back up, you're all over me, stop talking so much") may well backfire, as they are experienced as a threat to the child's relational needs. For this child, it will be important to witness, validate, and offer opportunities to meet the need, often repeatedly, while gently exploring the ways the expression of the need is interfering with the outcome. For instance: "It sounds like it was so important to you that your mom understand that you were upset, that you yelled and screamed so she would notice you. It's so important to feel taken care of when we're upset. Let's think together about how to make sure that happens, instead of everyone getting angrier and not wanting to be with each other. Maybe we can bring your mom in to help us think that through."

■ Although it would be impossible to characterize fully every child's approach to connection and communication, the likelihood is that children who struggle in this area are doing something to manage relationships and to attempt—or withhold—communication. Before working to change the child's patterns or to build skill, providers and caregivers must attune to current strategies and validate the ways they have served the child over time.

Behind the Scenes

■ A primary goal of this work is to support children in learning to effectively share internal experience with others, in order to meet emotional or practical needs.

■ Because communication and relational connection may be impacted in a number of ways, different skills and capacities may need to be targeted. Consider the range of possible factors that may interfere with connection; these include internal experiences (e.g., feelings of vulnerability in relationship, motivation to connect), availability of relational resources, and concrete skills for accessing and maintaining relationship. The provider's attunement will serve as a crucial foundation to this work. Because the goal is *effective* communication and connection, it is often important to pair modulation skills with this work. For instance, a child who is in a calm state will be more effective in communicating frustration to a teacher or caregiver than one who is angry or hyperaroused.

■ Effective communication is largely governed by context. What is effective and appropriate in one setting (e.g., with peers) may be ineffective in another (e.g., with grandparents). Clinicians should explore the nuances of effective communication, including issues such as language choice, boundaries, and style of interacting, in building communication skills. An additional consideration here is the caregiving/attachment system and its capacity to effectively respond to child communication strategies. Consideration should be given to how well caregiver(s) are responding to work in the attachment domain.

■ The ways in which humans express emotions are strongly influenced by culture. The use of language (or not), the role of nonverbal cues, the nuances of interaction, and even choosing with whom to share are all impacted by culture. Consider the following example.

> In certain Native Alaskan tribal cultures, direct eye contact by a child toward an adult may be considered disrespectful. Facial expressions, to an outside observer, may appear constricted and flat. A clinician began treatment with a 12-year-old boy of Native Alaskan background who had been terminated from three prior therapies due to the therapists' belief that he could not "do the work." In building a forum for therapeutic

communication with this child, the clinician learned that the most comfortable expression for him occurred when he was engaged in parallel, nonverbal activities.

In this example, had the clinician failed to take into account the role of culture in this child's interaction, he might have misinterpreted the child's behaviors as avoidant or resistant. In working with this child, pushing him to make eye contact (as described later in this section) would have run counter to his cultural norms and would be likely to cause distress. When working with children and families, it is important to understand the role of cultural norms in typical emotional expression, as well as the ways these intersect with the dominant culture.

■ Much of this work happens in the moment. Tune in to signs or statements that reflect internal experience. Ask questions to expand children's communication. Reinforce attempts to share experience and to connect. Work with caregivers to model effective strategies, and to invite and provide opportunities for connection and communication.

Teach to Caregivers

■ *Reminder:* Teach the caregiver the Key Concepts.

■ *Reminder:* Teach the caregiver relevant Developmental Considerations.

■ *Reminder:* Review trauma response and triggers. Because children will be less able to access language when triggered, the caregiver(s) will often need to practice modulation support strategies prior to eliciting the child's expression.

■ Attunement work with caregivers will help support children's attempts to connect, as described in detail later. As appropriate, integrate caregivers into sessions or into milieu routines so that communication about internal experience can be practiced in the moment. Treatment often provides a safe forum for familial communication. Have caregivers reframe the child's somatic and behavioral expressions by linking them with possible "I" statements.

■ Teach caregivers the tools outlined in the next section and, when possible, provide experiential opportunities for learning. For example, ask the caregiver to complete the circles exercise to explore his or her own communication resources and reflect with the caregiver on strategies that he or she utilizes to meet specific needs.

■ Teach caregivers to support effective communication:

◆ In the Therapist Toolbox section, we describe concrete skills to explore and build with children. However, because this target is, at its core, about relationship *between* the child and another person, it is equally important to address these same skills with caregivers or other relational partners as well. Core targets for caregivers include the following:

1. *Integrate attunement into communication and connection plans.* Work with caregivers to understand *why* children may struggle with connection and communication, and to understand the ways that children are currently communicating. Invite caregivers to be curious and to engage their detective skills, with an emphasis on seeing and understanding child behaviors as communication strategies. For instance, if a parent is attempting to talk to her teenage daughter about school and the teen crosses her arms, looks down and shrugs, what might she be communicating?

2. *Use communication routines to invite and facilitate communication:* Help caregivers develop routine forums in the home or milieu to encourage communication. Forums can be informal or formal. For instance, informal forums include eating a meal together, bedtime rituals, or family meetings. Similar methods can be integrated into the daily routine in milieu settings (i.e., schools or residential programs). Formal strategies can also be used. With younger children, concrete methods, such as a family/unit/class feelings chart, can be helpful (e.g., a whiteboard with each member's name, on which all members draw or select a feelings face each day to show how they are feeling or how their day went). For adolescents, communication logs can be used to share experience. Set up family or programmatic expectations around how the logs will be used (e.g., each person must write one entry in the log each day, such as how he or she felt about one thing that happened that day). A primary goal is to support caregivers in becoming communication facilitators. When possible support them in generalizing "check in" routines to the home environment.

3. *Encourage children to communicate needs.* Some children who struggle with connection may need to be given concrete and repeated opportunities to connect and communicate, as noted previously. Other children, however, may already be attempting to access relational connection. One way for caregivers to establish themselves as an available resource is to explicitly explore with the child various concrete strategies for letting someone know that he or she has something to share. The caregiver might build on current strategies being used within the family or system, or develop new strategies specific to the child's or caregiver's preference. Offer some examples of the types of strategies that are generally used to initiate communication. See Initiation of Communication Table (Skill #2 in Tools Section) for examples of ways to support children in identifying preferred strategies.

> An aunt who was attending a caregiver workshop described her experiences and specific support strategies for three trauma-impacted, high-need children who had recently come into her care. She explained that when the children came into her care they had many, many needs, including the need to be connected and reassured by her often. She could not attend to every need at every moment, so she had to develop support strategies. Her emphasis was on building a communication system that ensured the children opportunities to express need and allowed her to respond as possible. She went to the store and bought each child a different colored blanket. When explaining the blankets, she told the children that they should each hang the blanket on their bedroom door hooks if they needed her. She went on to tell them that if she noticed a blanket, she would be sure to connect and check in before they fell asleep at the end of the day.

◆ In this example there is something that the aunt did that should be highlighted (and will be highlighted in work with children as well). She was clear about her response plan, which can be characterized as a delayed rather than immediate response (" . . . before you fall asleep at the end of the day"). It is important to support caregivers in developing realistic response plans for specific needs that may be communicated. These response plans may include discussion about the rationale behind the plan, specific details about timing, and the like.

4. *Support nonverbal communication.* Family norms, culture, and other contextual variables all impact acceptable nonverbal signals. For instance, in some families, a

child looking directly at his or her parents may be considered a sign of disrespect; in others, not looking directly may be considered disrespectful. Take the time to assess, with both the child and the family, their understanding of nonverbal cues as well as nonverbal strategies that each family member uses to communicate specific experiences. In addition, assess with the caregiver the specific strategies used by child(ren) to communicate needs and note the caregiver's perception of whether or not the strategies are accepted, tolerated, and effective within the familial context.

5. *Support verbal communication.* Language is the most direct means of communication, and children's words will be the first and foremost communication method that others will often pay attention to. Support caregivers in their ability to prompt verbal communication, when possible. This may begin with external language support— for instance, using a reflective statement to put words to an action ("You really want my attention, don't you?") or to offer an interpretation of behavior for a child ("I think when you pushed me away you were saying, 'I don't want to talk to you!'"). This level of support can progress to simple prompts such as "Can you use your words?" or "Let's put words to that," and then advance to more sophisticated skills such as "I statements" (which are the focus of Skill #4 in the upcoming "Therapist Toolbox" section). Involve the caregiver in skill development whenever possible.

Tools: Relational Connection

Teach to Kids: Psychoeducation and Exploration of Historical and Current Relationships

■ There are many reasons that children whose lives have been affected by trauma may resist or have challenges with relationship and connection, and skill set is only one facet. Even in the context of excellent social skills, a child who feels inherently unsafe in relationship or who believes that no one cares about his or her needs will struggle with forming connections. A crucial foundation for approaching this goal is therefore to support children in exploring both historical and current relationships. Using age-appropriate conversation and activities (e.g., through use of Me Books, family trees, timelines, drawings, and narrative), explore the following with the child.

Historical and Current Relationships

Goal	Teaching point and possible areas of exploration
Explore historical relationships.	*Teaching point:* All of the relationships that we have had in our lives teach us something about how to manage other relationships.
	Work with children to identify important relationships they have had in their lives. These relationships may include people who have been generally positive, people who have been more challenging, and people with whom the child's relationship has been mixed. Explore: ■ What was the nature of your relationship with this person? When did you know him or her? For how long? In what way? ■ What role(s) did this person play in your life? What role(s) did you play in his or her life? ■ What did you learn about relationships from this person? ■ In what ways did you and this person communicate? What did you learn about communication?

Goal	Teaching point and possible areas of exploration

- Did this person meet any of your needs? Which ones? Were there needs that were not met?
- Did you have to work to meet this person's needs? Which ones? How did that feel to you?

Explore current relationships.

Teaching point: Most of us have a mix of different people in our life who serve different roles and who help us feel more or less comfortable connecting.

In Skill #1, below, the focus is on helping the child identify a range of resources. Broadly, it is important to explore and be curious with the child about the different people in his or her life, and the ways that these people help the child feel safer or less safe, heard or not heard, comfortable or uncomfortable. This may include people who *might* be able to meet needs (e.g., those who are identified as possible resources), but may also include those who have failed to meet the child's needs, who make his or her life feel harder, or who are hurtful. Help the child to identify key people who currently play some role in his or her life and/or have some influence on them, such as caregivers, relatives, teachers, friends, providers, and others. Explore similar questions as those noted in the first point, above.

Explore the goals of expression and connection.

Teaching point: There are reasons that it is important to connect with other people and to communicate about our internal experiences.

A foundation for the work on this goal is to understand *why* it matters to connect and to communicate with other people. Our premise is that, at their simplest, connection and communication help us to get our needs met, whether these needs are concrete (e.g., getting a ride somewhere) or emotional (e.g., feeling loved). Below, we describe ways to speak with children about their current connection strategies. First, consider engaging children's curiosity about the following:
- "Why do you think people might want to have relationships with others?"
- "What are the different kinds of relationships people have?"
- "Do you think some kinds of relationships are more important than others?"
- "Do you think that relationships or people might serve different roles, or be able to meet different needs?"
- "Why do you think it might be important to share things with other people— like, what you think or feel, want or need?"

Explore barriers to expression and connection.

Teaching point: There are many different things that can make it hard to communicate with others and to be willing to connect.

It is important to acknowledge with children that communication and connection are not always easy, and that many people struggle in these areas at least sometimes. Engage children's curiosity about the topics such as the following:
- "Are there people who it is easy for you to talk to or connect with? What about people who are harder?"
- "In what situations do you find it easiest to talk to or share experience with others? In what situations do you feel like it is harder?"
- "Are relationships something that you feel comfortable with or uncomfortable with?"
- "Are there things that are important to you to get from other people when you are with them? What things [situations, reactions, etc.] make it harder for you to talk to people?"
- "Are there times you can think of when you tried to talk to other people and it felt like it didn't work or like they didn't listen? Why do you think that happened? What did that feel like?"

Identify specific needs and ways others might be able to meet those needs.

Teaching point: We all have a number of different needs, and though we can meet some of these on our own, other people can help us to get our needs met.

An important component of engagement in this skill set is children's understanding of their own needs and ways that others might be able to support those needs. In upcoming material we discuss goals and sample language for speaking with children about their needs.

Skill #1: Identifying Interpersonal Resources for Expression

Goal   Building children's awareness of safe people with whom to share emotional experience

Materials   Paper, crayons or markers, photographs of safe people (optional)

Description

■ **Teach importance of expressing feelings:** Why do people need to share emotional experience with others?
   ◆ *Point 1: "When kids keep feelings all to themselves, they may come out in lots of other ways, like stomachaches, headaches, and behavior."* Check in with child: How does he or she think feelings come out? Query about different types of feelings.
   ◆ *Point 2: "Talking to other people about feelings can sometimes help kids get what they want or need."* Give an example (e.g., if mad about something a family member is doing, the child cannot tell anyone, and things probably won't change . . . *or* the child can communicate how he or she feels and work toward a resolution).
   ◆ *Point 3: "Letting other people know how we feel can help us feel better. Sometimes, we can't change what's going on, but people who know how we're feeling can help us deal with it."* Query: Can child think of a time when other people supported him or her in a hard situation?

■ **Help the child identify safe people in his or her life.** If the child has difficulty doing this, make suggestions. Consider caregivers, teachers, friends, other relatives, therapist, etc. Note that different people may be safe for different things. Help children differentiate who can help when they are angry, sad, scared, happy, etc.

■ **Make it concrete.** Create lists (or drawings, pictures, book, etc.) of safe resources. Examples of activities follow.

■ **Circles:** On a blank piece of paper, write the child's name in the center (or draw a picture). Draw a series of circles around the child. Teach the child: *"We all have different people in our life. Some of them we're really close to, and we can tell them anything. Other people we're kind of close to, and we can tell them some things, and still other people we know just to say 'Hi,' or talk about little things like schoolwork, sports, or TV shows."* With the child's help, write names in each circle, showing increasing intimacy as the circles come closer to the child. Help the child identify different types of information he or she feels comfortable sharing with people in each circle. Explore differences in communication style with different resources and across contexts. (*Note:* A sample form appears in Appendix D, "Circles of Trust.")

■ **Circles expansion:** Expand on this or similar exercises to explore the child's interpersonal relationships further. For instance, explore *roles* that different individuals play. Have the child circle, in different colors, people to whom the child can talk about important things, people with whom the child has fun, people who comfort the child, etc. Any individual can be circled more than once. Use this technique to explore types of relationships the child has, and/or the types of relationships the child may want to build. Use arrows to indicate the child's satisfaction with level of intimacy: An arrow pointed inward may indicate someone with whom the child wants to become closer; one pointed outward may indicate someone from whom the child wants distance.

■ **Draw a house activity:** On a sheet of paper have the child draw a house that includes the following: a foundation, walls, a roof, a door, a chimney, and a billboard nearby. After the house is drawn, ask the child to add the following responses to the specified parts of their picture:
   ◆ Foundation: *"On the foundation write down your values or the things that are important to you."* Examples may be provided, such as honesty, helping, trust, etc.
   ◆ Walls: *"On the walls write down the people who support you."* (We may change language with younger children—for instance: *" . . . the people who help you at home/school. . . ."*)
   ◆ Roof: *"On the roof write down the people who protect you or who keep you safe."*
   ◆ Door: *"On the door write down, or just think about, the things about yourself that you keep hidden from others."* (In our experience this is too abstract for very young children, so you may omit this or modify the exercise to be more developmentally appropriate.)
   ◆ Chimney: *"Near the chimney write down things that you do to blow off steam or to help keep you comfortable, calm, and so on."*
   ◆ Billboard: *"On the billboard write down the things that you are most proud of."*
■ *Other modifications:* We have found that children like to add things to their pictures—for example, clouds with the names of people that children "think about"; birds with people that we can't see but who watch over us, and many other wonderful creations. When completing this activity, use your own attunement skills to individualize, as needed.

Effectively Using Resources

■ Even with awareness of social resources, children who have experienced trauma may have difficulty effectively communicating emotional experience or needs. Given a history of failed or rejected attempts at connection, and/or a lack of modeling and early "practice" in sharing experience, these children may have failed to develop key skills. Initially it is helpful for children to gain an understanding of how they are attempting to communicate needs. The intent to communicate is the foundation of effective communication. When possible, find ways to label and reinforce the desire to communicate while suggesting strategies that may be more effective.

Teach to Kids: Psychoeducation about Their Current Connection and Communication Strategies

■ Examples of how to speak with children about key teaching points are provided. As discussed in previous chapters, keep in mind, however, that psychoeducation should be provided in a developmentally appropriate way, so language will vary from client to client.

Understanding Needs and Communication Strategies

Teaching point	Important information as sample language
Everyone has tools or strategies that we use to communicate how we are doing or what we need.	"All of us—kids and adults—have a lot of different tools or strategies that we use to let other people know how we are doing or what we may need from them." "There are no 'wrong' tools or strategies, but some work better than others. For example, if you tell a teacher that you need help with math because it's a little hard, then your teacher is more likely to give you the help that you need. If you tell your teacher that math is hard using your behavior (e.g., refusing to do math or misbehaving during math), then your teacher may not know that you need help and may just think that you feel like breaking the rules."
Kids and adults have different needs that are important to their survival and overall well-being.	"It is important to think about all of the different needs that kids and adults may have at different times in their life. Here are some of the things that we have learned are important: ■ "Basic needs like food and sleep ■ Safety needs ■ Connection ■ Control." *Note:* The clinician can collaborate with the child (and/or caregiver) to provide specific examples in each category.
There are lots of strategies that kids use to tell the people around them that they need something.	*Behavior:* "Sometimes we communicate our needs in what we do, what we say, or how we act with other people, and a lot of the time people communicate in very different ways. For example, some kids ask for attention from parents or other adults by engaging in big, obvious behaviors such as misbehaving or being really, really silly. Other kids may communicate the need for attention by becoming really quiet, and still others may communicate the need for attention by being really, really good at following the rules. It usually depends on the person, why attention is needed, where you are, and who's around." *Body:* "We might tell people that we have a stomachache when we're sad or a headache to communicate that we're really angry, upset, or when we just need some extra attention."

Teaching point	Important information as sample language
	Facial expressions/body language: "Most of us use our facial expressions and body language to communicate our feelings and/or our needs to others. If we want someone to leave us alone, we may look down, turn away, move away, or roll our eyes when he or she attempts to connect with us. If we want someone to help us or to come closer, we may look at them, gesture them to come, smile, or move toward them."
	Voice/vocal tone: "Sometimes we use our voices to communicate our needs. What we need may be communicated with our tone of voice or with the words that we use."
	Other strategies: "Are there any other strategies that you can think of that people use or that you use to communicate *to others* either how you are doing or something that you need—at home, in school, with friends?"
It is important to be a "detective" about our needs and our communication strategies.	"Knowing about what we need and how to communicate that to other people is really important. Sometimes our needs are about really concrete things like knowing when we are going to eat, and sometimes our needs are about feeling comfortable, protected, and cared for. All of these things are important and, for the most part, are difficult to accomplish on your own. This is especially true for kids!"
	"One of the things we are going to work on is becoming 'detectives' about your needs and your communication strategies to figure out which strategies are working, which strategies are not working, and to learn some new ways to get your needs met."

■ The activities in the following table target several areas of vulnerability that may interfere with a child's ability to effectively communicate with identified resources. These vulnerable areas include initiating communication, using effective nonverbal communication, and using effective verbal communication.

■ The overarching goal of these activities is to support children in effectively communicating their feelings and needs to identified interpersonal resources in service of building safe relationships. However, be aware that failure to share experience is often due only in part to skills deficits; difficulty with trust and lack of perceived safety in relationships also play a key role. It is therefore important to pair this work with work around identifying safe resources, as described in the first table in this section (p. 245), as well as with foundational psychoeducation and exploration of the child's historical experience with relationships.

Skill #2: Initiating Communication

Picking your moment	*Rationale:* It is important for children with trauma histories to successfully share their emotional experiences with others, because past communication has often been met with rejection, punishment, or indifference. Teaching children how to identify appropriate moments to initiate support can help with successful interaction.
	Steps: Consider the following steps:
	■ Teach children that communication is more effective if the other person is ready to hear them. Ask children to consider when they might not want to listen to someone else. (If a child has a hard time, give examples: when busy, when in a hurry, when talking to someone else, when mad or grumpy, etc.)
	■ Help children identify "good times" and "not-so-good times" to share their feelings with people in general.

- Select the safest (most talked to, most liked, etc.) people on the child's list of identified interpersonal resources. Help the child identify specific "good" and "not-so-good" times for each of those people. Help the child describe specific cues (e.g., "How do you know when your mother is busy?").
- Ask the child, "Have there ever been times when you tried to communicate with one of those safe people, and it didn't work?" Problem-solve together about why the interaction might not have gone well.
- If appropriate, invite the child's caregiver(s) or other safe person to do a portion of this work dyadically. Have the child and the caregiver problem-solve together about good ways to initiate communication.
- For younger children it can be helpful to include visual aids in this discussion (e.g., picture of a grumpy person/character vs. a calm and approachable person/character).

Initiating conversation	*Rationale:* Often, children who have experienced trauma have historically attempted to communicate through indirect means. The goal of this skill is to teach them to directly communicate a need to share experience.

Steps: Consider the following steps:
- Teach children that the first step in effective communication is letting someone know you want to communicate. Ask the child, "How do you know when different people in your life want to talk to you?"
- Teach children how to let other people know they want to talk. Consider multiple modalities:
  - *Verbal:* "I'd like to talk to you."
  - *Gestural:* Secret hand signal (that both parties know in advance).
  - *Written:* Leaving a note for caregiver.
  - *Symbolic:* Door sign or other symbol requesting communication.
- Differentiate *immediate* versus *delayed* responses to communication bids. Sometimes a caregiver will be able to respond immediately to a child's request for communication, but other times this response will necessarily be delayed.
  - Discuss reasons why it may sometimes be necessary to delay communication.
  - Set up rules or expectations with the person identified as the child's communication resource. For instance, if the child leaves the caregiver a note or hangs a door sign, by when will the caregiver respond (e.g., before bedtime? by dinner?).
  - Help children identify modulation strategies to equip with tools for tolerating delays in communication.

Skill #3: Building Nonverbal Communication Skills

- When working with children on nonverbal communication skills, keep in mind that there is significant variation in what is considered normative and appropriate. A key aspect of working to build and support nonverbal communication skills is engaging *curiosity* and *interpersonal awareness*. Concretely, this means approaching this work in a manner that does not assume there is a single appropriate set of nonverbal signals that support communication, but rather building the child's understanding of the ways his or her nonverbal communication signals are intended ("What do you think you're trying to tell people when you look away or fold your arms?"), and are potentially interpreted by different individuals and in different contexts ("What do you think your grandmother wants you to do when she and you are talking? How can she tell you are listening?")

Nonverbal Communication Skills

Rationale	**One of the contributors to trauma-impacted children's difficulty with effective expression and connection is difficulty using nonverbal cues to communicate effectively.**
Teaching point	▪ Teach children that communication involves more than words or language. Often, nonverbal cues (eye contact, tone of voice, etc.) are important clues that help other people read or understand what we are trying to communicate.

■ *Ask: "Have you ever thought someone was angry at you, even if he or she didn't say anything? How could you tell? If someone is yelling at you, does that make it easier or harder for you to talk to them? Learning about nonverbal cues—what we do with our voice and body—helps us communicate more effectively."*

Target the following specific skills:

Tone of-voice

Goal: Teach children about the ways that vocal tone (loudness, softness, inflection) contributes to our interpretation of what someone says, as well as our ability and willingness to listen. Explore the ways this may vary by relationship, context, or situation.

Possible activities:

■ Select an emotion and a situation. Role-play a conversation between two people. Have one conversation in an overly loud (or overly soft) tone of voice. Repeat the role play in a different tone of voice or using different inflection.
  ◆ Afterward discuss what the conversation felt like to the child. Was it different, using different tones of voice?
  ◆ Play out different possible endings. Be realistic—how might someone respond if the other person is yelling? Speaking calmly? Speaking sarcastically? Whispering?
■ Refer back to feelings detective work (in Chapter 10, "Identification"). Have children create a list of their own "emotion clues."
■ Work with both child and caregiver to develop a list of nonverbal clues (one for caregiver, one for child) connected to different emotions.
■ Work with both child and caregiver to pick a topic and practice communicating in a calm tone. Start with a neutral topic and work toward more difficult topics. Provide lots of reinforcement for successful communication!
■ Have caregiver and child create a list together of "communication rules" describing how they can communicate respectfully with one another. Pay attention to respectful communication by the caregiver as well as the child.

Physical space

Goal: Teach children how to maintain comfortable/appropriate physical boundaries when communicating, and how to read other people's "physical space" cues.

Possible activities:
■ **Teach child:**
  ◆ "We all have a 'personal bubble': an invisible area around our bodies that is ours alone, and other people should not enter that space without permission."
  ◆ "Our personal bubble can grow bigger or smaller, depending on who the other person is, what kind of mood we're in, what kind of mood the other person is in, etc."
  ◆ "Our personal bubble helps us to feel safe."
  ◆ "When we're talking to other people, we have to pay attention to their personal bubble, too. If we're too close or too far, it's hard for them to listen to us, because their brain will be too focused on not having enough space or having too much."
■ **Own your zone:** The child stands still, and the therapist (or caregiver, other child) should stand across the room. When the child gives permission, the second person should begin walking toward the child. When the child decides the other person is "comfortably close," the child says, "Stop." Once the second person stops, the child can make adjustments, as needed (e.g., take a small step back) until comfortable. Possible additions:
  ◆ Use a measuring tape to measure child's preferred space, or mark the distance with tape on the floor.
  ◆ Pretend that the second person represents different people (e.g., child's mother, teacher, best friend, biggest enemy). Repeat the exercise and make note of different space requirements.
  ◆ Have second person convey different emotional states while walking toward child (e.g., very angry, very excited). Make note of different space requirements.
  ◆ With child's permission, enter his or her personal bubble. Have child (1) notice what she feels and (2) notice what she does (e.g., leans back, steps back). Teach child that these are cues others may give if she enters their personal bubble.
  ◆ Reverse roles. Have the child walk toward second person; repeat exercise and/or variations.
■ **Personal bubble homework:** Ask child to observe two different people during the week (e.g., the child's mother and a person in his or her class at school). Ask the child to notice how big or small these individuals' personal space zones are in different situations, and how they communicate their personal space needs. Talk about what kinds of things seemed to affect the observed personal space needs (e.g., time of day, mood, with whom the person was interacting).

- **Create an actual personal bubble:** Have the child create a circle with his or her arms, or use a piece of string to create a circle around the child. Teach the child that everything enclosed by the circle is his or her personal space, and that other people have the same amount of space. Practice (and model) asking permission to enter the other person's space.
- **Coping with space violations:** Although it is important to know our spatial needs, sometimes we are unable to control our boundaries as much as we would like (e.g., on a crowded train, in a busy line in the school cafeteria). Work with children to identify strategies for coping with inadvertent spatial violations.

Eye
contact

Goal: Teach children that eye contact is one way we communicate with others that goes beyond talking. Eye contact and/or averted gaze can be ways to show that we are listening and paying attention to what others are saying, that we are interested in the conversation, and that what they (or we) are saying is important. Use of gaze aversion or eye contact might—in varying situations and relationships—communicate respect or disrespect, might help increase or decrease arousal and intrusiveness or engagement, and might communicate threat or safety, depending on the situation, context, and cultural meaning ascribed to it.

Possible activities:

- **Messages we send:** Pick a scenario that involves interaction between two people. Consider scenarios such as asking to have a need met, asking for support, giving advice or support, etc. Act out the scenario two times (at least). The first time, do not make eye contact; the second time, do. Play out possible different interpretations the individuals might make: How interested is the second person? How available is he or she to the conversation or to the request? Discuss afterward.
- **Active listener:** Have the child tell a story to you (or to caregiver, other child, etc.). The second person may *not* speak. For the first minute, have the second person sit with face turned away; for the second minute, allow the second person to make eye contact while listening. Explore what it feels like when someone is looking, versus not, while listening. Be curious about what might affect how eye contact feels. For instance, does eye contact feel better or worse if someone is talking to you about very personal content? How might it feel different if you felt like the person talking liked you or didn't like you? If you or the other person felt angry or happy? Explore the nuances of how eye contact might contribute to felt experience in relationship. Reverse roles.
- **Ball toss (group activity):** Have group members sit in a circle. Toss a ball around. Each child must throw to the same person each time, and everyone must be thrown to within the pattern. Before tossing the ball, the child must say the person's name and make eye contact. Tell children, "See how fast you can get!" Discuss tuning into how eye contact helps make throwing more accurate.

Listening
skills

Goal: To teach kids that an important part of learning to communicate with another person is learning to be an active listener. Learning to listen requires attention and focus.

Possible Activities:
- **Children:**
  - **Sound hunt:** Children who are in your office can "hunt" for sounds (e.g., "Name four different things you hear right now") or, if possible, you and the child can walk around inside the building on a sound hunt to find "all of the different sounds in the building."
  - **Guess the sound:** Fill containers up with different items (e.g., rice, M&M'S, beads), shake the containers, and tell the child to try to guess what is inside.
  - **Tongue twisters:** Read a couple of sentences from a tongue twister (Dr. Seuss books are a good resource for this). Have the child listen and repeat back what he or she heard.
- **Teens:**
  - **Interviews:** Have teen interview someone (may be the provider) and share three things that he or she learned.
  - **Telephone games (for group format):** Create a telephone game by having the teens sit in a circle. Whisper a sentence into the ear of one teen, such as, "Active listening games help teens build an important life skill." Each teen must whisper the sentence into the ear of the player next to him or her. However, they can only take one try to whisper it correctly. The object of the game is to try to pass the sentence, word for word, all the way around the circle. For a challenge, divide the players into two teams. Whisper the same sentence into the ear of one player from each team. The first team to get the correct sentence all the way around the circle wins the game.
  - **What changed (individual format)?** Read a story one time. Ask the teen to actively listen to your narrative. Read it back a second time, changing one or two details in the story, and see if he or she can identify the changes.

Skill #4: Building Verbal Communication Skills

Verbal Communication

Rationale	Language is the most direct means of communication: Before anything else, people listen to the words we say. Using appropriate, direct language is often the best way for children to get their emotional needs met and to share experience.
Verbal communication routines in therapy	Build on check-in routines to incorporate an emphasis on verbal communication about experiences, preferences, interests, etc. Some of this work overlaps with self-development and identity work, which is discussed in Chapter 14. **Examples** of sentence stems to elicit use as part of check-in routines may include: ■ "One good thing that happened this week was. . . ." ■ "Something that made me feel happy today is. . . ." ■ "One hard thing that happened this week was. . . ." ■ "Something that I like to do when I'm mad is. . . ."
Reflection	Engage children in reflecting on their experience both in clinical interactions as well as in daily/weekly life. **Example:** *Reflecting on therapeutic activities.* For instance, following a game of "Simon Says," ask the child to complete an evaluation of the activity and to share their thoughts with you. Sample questions may include: ■ "On a scale of 1–10, with 1 being the worst activity ever and 10 being the best activity ever, what rating would you give this activity?" ■ "Are there any changes that you would make to the activity to improve it?" ■ "Would you like to do this activity again?" ■ "Would you recommend this activity to a friend?" **Example:** *Reflecting on daily life.* As part of a routine check-in, ask the child to share one thing that happened during the week that was interesting. Engage the child in describing the activity, describing what made it interesting, the best/worst part of doing the activity, the ways in which the child was involved, what the activity led the child to be curious about, etc. When appropriate, write down the child's words.
"I statements"	**Possible activities:** ■ Teach child that "I" statements are ways to let other people know how we feel. There are a lot of different ways we can start a sentence: ■ I feel _____ (or, When _____ happened, I felt _____). ■ I want _____. ■ I would like _____. ■ I need _____ etc. ■ It makes me feel _____ when you _____. ■ Have children practice using above statements to describe past and/or current experiences. **What I Need:** Help children develop a list of what helps when they are trying to share emotional experience (e.g., a hug, silence, brainstorming, help thinking of ways to feel better). Keep in mind that the list may differ when communicating with different people or for different feelings. Help the child practice using "I statements" to ask for those communication helpers. If possible, bring caregiver into session and do this exercise interactively. Use this technique in the moment and connect it with affect identification skills. When a child describes an experience that involves emotions, prompt him or her to use "I statements" to describe the emotional experience (e.g., "When your aunt got frustrated with you, how did that make you feel?").
Individualized verbal communication strategies	Some children and youth find their own unique language for communicating experiences, needs and wants. Allow children the opportunity to develop and share their own unique strategies for communication; work to help label observed communication strategies as such. Consider the following case examples: ■ Colors: An adolescent male communicated with staff by identifying the "color of the day." For him, a good day was coded as sea-foam green, whereas a tough day was dark purple. ■ Weather: An adolescent female communicated about her day using the weather. Clouds, sun, wind and rain all communicated something different and unique about her daily experience.

Children who have experienced trauma may also benefit from alternative or augmented communication strategies. Alternatives may be particularly important for children and youth who present with additional developmental vulnerabilities that impact expressive and receptive language skills. Consider the following strategies.

Skill #5: Alternative or Augmented Communication Strategies

Sign language	In work with very young children, children with developmental delays in communication, and hearing-impaired or deaf children, we have used basic sign language for elements of our therapeutic structure and teaching. Here are some examples of how sign language may be incorporated into the work: ■ Emotion check-in's: Showing and/or giving signs for basic emotions (media support is often used: e.g., "Signing Time"). ■ Pause or stop cues: Can offer the basic sign for "stop" and "go." ■ Modulation language: Offer basic signs for high, medium, low; fast and slow; big and small, more, etc. ■ Reciprocity: Offer basic sign for "my turn" or "your turn."
Pictures	Similar to what we described about the use of base sign language, pictures may be used to facilitate communication of experience. Suggestions about visuals were incorporated into Chapters 10 and 11. Consider the following suggestions: ■ Feelings face visuals (e.g., emojis) ■ Energy visuals (e.g., a rabbit and a turtle, or one child running and one child sleeping) ■ Activity visuals (preferred/nonpreferred selections by child; e.g., pictures of a board game, art materials, and a trampoline) ■ Coping/modulation skill visuals (e.g., blankets, a quiet space, a preferred staff member) ■ Visuals of relational resources (e.g., photos of family members, friends, staff members available each shift) ■ Visuals related to rules and expectations (e.g., "safe hands," talking to an adult, asking for help) ■ Visual showing schedules/routines (e.g., activity order for the day, daily classroom schedule, nighttime routine) The type of picture in each category should be determined based on individual needs. For instance, some children may prefer real-life pictures, whereas others may respond to symbols.

Special Consideration: Self-Expression as a Form of Communication and Connection

■ Expression of internal experience may include creative or symbolic communication that moves beyond the concrete. Creative self-expression forums offer children and adolescents an opportunity for connection and communication, as well as a way to symbolize, express, and share internal experience.

■ Keep in mind that many expressive strategies may lead to an increase in children's arousal; conversely, many of these strategies may themselves offer opportunities and sources of regulation. Support children in pairing creative expression with previously learned modulation strategies, as needed.

■ Possibilities here are almost endless. Various modalities for self-expression are suggested in the following table. Help children identify and refine their own preferred means of self-expression.

Self-Expression

Play	As one of the most important ways young children share their experience, play in any form—with puppets, dollhouse characters, animals, and other figures—can be used to help children express and communicate experience in a displaced manner. Clinicians (and caregivers) can introduce effective communication strategies, emotional support, and possible resolutions into the play when necessary. *Example:* ■ The child has previously witnessed domestic violence. In the child's play, the child character is hitting the mother character. The therapist might: ◆ *Observe:* "Wow, that boy looks really angry." ◆ *Query about communication:* "It looks like that boy is hitting to show how mad he is right now. I wonder if there are other things he's doing because he's mad." ◆ *Take on a role in the play:* [Therapist enters as "neighbor."] "I heard lots of yelling. Is everyone okay? Can I help?" ◆ *Suggest communication:* "What if that boy tried telling his mom that he needed to talk? What do you think might happen?"
Art	Use drawing, painting, clay, etc., to help children express themselves. With young children, structure is often helpful; however, create a balance between structured and unstructured time to allow for children's creativity. ■ In addition to general activities, consider incorporating art into familial (or other) communication. For instance, use strategies such as "picture of the day" to allow children to draw as a way to communicate experience with their families. ■ *Collages* are a wonderful group project for self-expression, but also useful one on one. ■ *Outside–Inside:* Masks, boxes, two-sided faces, etc., can be used to help children express what they think people see on the *outside* (labels, masks, "fake fronts," etc.), and how they feel on the *inside.*
Writing	Support children in the use of writing for self-expression. Forms of writing might include poetry, journaling, fictional/nonfictional stories, lyrics/raps, etc. Consider providing a journal for each child (and/or creating one in session through the use of construction paper, blank paper, etc.). Invite children to share some of their writing, if comfortable, with one of the safe interpersonal resources discussed in Skill #1, this chapter, p. 245).
Movement	Movement includes dance as well as more focused expressive movements. For instance, a child who wishes to express pride can embody what it feels like to "stand tall"; a child who expresses a wish to have fought against an aggressor or victimizer can push against a wall or another object; a child who is naming unexpressed anger can build with and push down clay. Keep in mind that these types of activity may increase arousal and should be paired with modulation strategies.
Drama	Acting is a way for children to express feelings, experiences, etc., in a displaced way. Acting techniques can be incorporated into sessions, and/or children can be encouraged to take part in adjunctive, theatre-based programs.
Music	Music provides a powerful nonverbal expression strategy. Even children who do not have an immediate interest in, or talent for, a musical instrument can effectively express themselves on drums or other simple musical instruments. In addition, the process of sharing music (e.g., having a child bring a favorite song or playlist to the therapy session) can act as a vehicle for communication of internal experience.

ﾟ Developmental Considerations

Developmental stage	Relational connection considerations
Early childhood	Caregivers are generally the primary resource for shared communication for young children. It is particularly important to include caregivers in sessions for this age group.
	Young children's communication is generally more concrete and less sophisticated than that of older children or adolescents. Often, their sharing of experience will simply let important adults know how they feel. It is important that adults take greater responsibility for noticing and eliciting communication and identifying child needs.
	Because early childhood is an egocentric stage, young children will have greater difficulty considering others' perspectives, reading cues, etc., and expectations for these skills should be limited.
Middle childhood	Peers, teachers, and other adults may become important resources for communication in addition to primary caregivers.
	Because children's social worlds are expanding during this time period, understanding of appropriate boundaries and social resources becomes particularly important. Help children learn to differentiate with whom they can safely share different kinds of experience.
Adolescence	The peer group becomes a primary resource for communication during adolescence, and a desire for increased privacy from caregivers is a normative developmental shift.
	Work with caregivers to tolerate decreased detailed communication and to tolerate the adolescent's increased need for independence. However, help caregivers and adolescents strike a balance. For instance, it may be important for an adolescent to communicate to a caregiver, "I'm angry and need some space," but the details of the emotion or precipitating events may not necessarily need to be shared immediately.
	Avoid all-or-nothing interactions. It is important that (1) caregivers remain available for communication, (2) adolescents continue to view them as a resource, and (3) certain lines of communication remain open. Help adolescents define material that may be important to share with caregivers.

Applications
Individual/Dyadic

Work with the child on the skills identified in the section titled "Therapist Toolbox." Because therapeutic work on relational connection generally involves expression of experience *to* someone, integrate caregivers or other appropriate adults directly into this work whenever possible. It is particularly important to work with caregivers when building communication strategies. Help caregivers and children develop communication routines together. Consider the following example.

> The grandmother of an 8-year-old boy expressed concerns that her grandson didn't talk to her about his day. When he returned home from school each day, she would ask him how the day went and he would reply "Fine." Follow-up questions were met with a shrug, accompanied by an "I don't know." Although she did receive reports from the school about the basics, she was concerned about how he was experiencing a recent transition into her care and adjusting to a new school. The provider inquired more about the after-school routine and learned that his client loved to get the mail on his route from the bus to the home and that he took pride in bringing his grandmother a "special delivery." Together the

grandmother, her grandson, and the provider developed a "daily postcard" that had a picture of a thumbs up, thumbs in the middle, and thumbs down to describe his day at school.
The words "good," "okay" and "not so good" were paired with the thumbs. The postcard and
a pencil were placed on a table by the front door. It was agreed that the postcard would be
filled out upon entry into the home and would be included in the daily "special delivery."
In this example, the little boy appeared to need support with developing a language for
communicating his experience. The grandmother was able to develop a system around an
existing connection strategy and her grandson's positive identity as the family's "mailman."

Beyond primary caregivers, work with the child and the surrounding systems (e.g.,
school, day care) to develop communication plans and resources for when the child is not at
home. Develop concrete plans for how a child could access safe communication resources
when needed (e.g., at school, while at friends' homes). Consider working with collaterals on
appropriate ways to invite communication from the child and/or cue the child to use identified resources, when needed.

In addition to the specific skills listed, this target involves an exploration of the meaning and understanding of interpersonal relationships, both present and historical, and the
impact of making oneself vulnerable in relationship. For older children and adolescents, in
particular, it will be important to take the time to explore these ideas and to process any
thoughts and feelings that may emerge.

Group

Many relational connection exercises lend themselves well to a group format. Consider
using role play or other improvisational theatre techniques as a way to have group members practice appropriate communication or identify inappropriate communication (often,
a more fun exercise for kids!). "Own your zone" (boundaries) and the ball toss exercises
(eye contact) are great group activities and good forums for eliciting discussion of individual
differences and similarities in nonverbal communication cues. Exercises targeting identification of resources also translate easily to group format, but be cautious about the need for
privacy, particularly with adolescent clients; allow clients to use initials or other symbolic
markings to keep their information private. Film or television clips provide a good context
for group discussion of both verbal communication skills as well as the ways nonverbal cues
influence communication and connection.

Milieu

Integrate group activities described above into milieu clinical programs. Within the milieu,
work with individual clients to identify communication resources. Troubleshoot communication plans: for instance, a child might identify a particular staff member as his or her
"safest" resource, but what will the child do on a day when that staff member is unavailable?
Build strategies that allow all residents to communicate feelings, needs, and thoughts both
verbally and nonverbally. For example, in residential programs, we have found door signs
and door magnets to be useful communication techniques. Door signs can be decorated by
the resident so that one side reflects a positive mood, or a desire for interaction, whereas the
other side reflects harder feelings, a desire for comfort, or a desire to be left alone. A magnet

on the door can be used to request one-on-one time with a staff member. It is crucial that all staff members receive training about the rationale behind the use of these strategies and the importance of consistent follow-through with the established response.

When working with staff members to support youth expression, it is important to differentiate the *goal* of expression from the *method* and the *message*. In other words, support staff in reinforcing youth attempts to communicate, even if the communication itself is less than ideal. Consider the following example:

> A 15-year-old girl in a residential program walks out of a group session. When a staff member follows her and asks her what is going on, she yells, "This group sucks—I'm sick of it. You all must think I'm some kind of *** to sit and talk about this stuff."

In her own way, this adolescent is attempting to communicate. What are the possible responses? One possibility is to respond to her *method* of communicating: "You're being really inappropriate, and you've just lost 5 points for swearing." A second possibility is to respond to her *message:* "It seems like everyone else is getting something from this group, so you just need to try harder." A third possibility is to respond to her *attempt at communication:* "I can see that you have pretty strong feelings about this group, and I'd really like to hear them. It's hard for me to do that when you're this upset. Can we try to find a way to calm down first and then talk about this?" *Note:* Although the third option is, from our perspective, a more therapeutic response to the adolescent's attempt to communicate, we do not negate that within a program, the first two options may be equally valid responses. In selecting a response, we urge staff to consider timing: First support expression, along with appropriate modulation, before addressing limits or other consequences for behavior.

◯ Trauma Experience Integration: State-Based Skills Application

More than perhaps any other target described in this book, capacity for relational connection hinges upon the present state of both the child and the connection resource—which may or may not be the primary caregiver in a given moment. When considering approaches to supporting this treatment target, it is important to take into account the state and needs of the child, as well as the state and needs of the adult or other resource.

Distress Tolerance and Regulation

Youth and caregivers who have experienced trauma and who are experiencing current significant overwhelm and distress often handle that distress by managing relationships. Both youth and caregivers may swing between disconnection and intrusiveness, and relationships and connections are likely to be one of the primary triggers for trauma-related affect and arousal. Ironically, it is during this state that youth may most need to make effective use of relationships, as their ability to meet needs independently is likely to be constrained. When youth are working on present-oriented distress tolerance, interventions focused on relational connection are likely to emphasize a few targets:

1. A primary emphasis is likely to be on engaging relational resources who are able to initiate connection and communication, rather than relying on the youth to reach out. For example, rather than having the child to speak to a teacher when upset as the plan, a better plan is likely to be engaging a teacher in proactively checking in with the child several times per day, as feasible. This is because intense affect in the absence of (still forming) effective internal resources is likely to interfere with any child-directed plan developed during a calm state.

2. When youth are particularly protective of themselves in relationship or struggle to maintain good boundaries, an emphasis on specific concrete needs and ways to address these may be more useful than a focus on the more intimate aspects of relationship. For instance, "What are the ways you might let your mom know you need a ride?" might be easier early in the work than, "How can you talk to your mom about having a super hard day at school?" Keep in mind that what is easier for one child may be harder for another; the bottom line is that the most vulnerable relational needs are likely not the best direction in the beginning.

3. Acknowledgment of the inherent challenges of relationships and of the ways the youth has learned to keep him- or herself safe in relationship up to this point is essential, including validation that, at times, relationships may continue to feel unsafe, unresponsive, and/or unrewarding. An important goal early on is to identify ways that relationships might be able to meet some needs and to build some connections, while acknowledging the ways that many needs have been, and may continue to feel, unmet.

Curiosity and Reflection

As youth are increasingly able to reflect upon their experience and to harness or make use of supported modulation resources when distressed, much of the reflective work that is the foundation for building or expanding healthy relationships becomes possible. This work includes:

- Reflecting upon the range of relationships the child has had in his or her life, the roles they have played, and ways they met or did not meet the child's needs or wants
- Exploring current relationships across roles and settings
- Exploring and concretely addressing current skills challenges
- Addressing and problem-solving identified trouble spots in relationship and connection

Engaging Purposeful Action

Over time, working with a trauma-impacted child on building safe relationships will necessarily require exploration of the most challenging relationships in the child's life: those relationships that have been involved in traumatic experiences, and/or have failed to protect children from those experiences. Direct exploration of the ways these connections have influenced the child's sense of self, capacity to negotiate in relationship, and ability to trust or reach out to others will provide a foundation for (1) child processing of historical experience, (2) initiation of repair if/when possible in current relationship, and (3) building increasingly safe future connections. To the degree possible, and as caregivers are able to tolerate this work themselves, direct incorporation of the caregiving system into these conversations can provide a rich forum for perspective taking and relational repair.

Real-World Therapy

Practice, practice, practice. Tolerating connection and communicating vulnerable experience to others are difficult, particularly for children and adults who are not used to doing either. The ability to do so in session does not always translate to an ability to do so in the midst of a crisis. However, the more practice there has been, the more likely that effective communication will eventually occur (particularly if practice takes place in a dyadic and/or familial context).

Be realistic, patient, and respectful. Sharing internal experience brings vulnerability. Children, like adults, will be better at (and more open to) sharing certain emotions and experiences than others. Praise any attempts at communicating internal experience, and *slooooooooowly* support expanded risk in communication.

13

Strengthening Executive Functions

🔑 THE MAIN IDEA AND KEY SUBSKILLS

Work with children to act, instead of react, by using higher-order cognitive processes to solve problems and make active choices in the service of reaching identified goals.

★ Support active recognition of capacity to make choices.
★ Build age-appropriate active evaluation of situations.
★ Build child capacity to inhibit response.
★ Build and support ability to generate and evaluate potential solutions.

★ Key Concepts

★ What Are "Executive Functions"?

■ *Executive functions,* as a unit, can be thought of as the "captain of the cognitive ship." They help human beings navigate through the world in a goal-directed, thoughtful way.

■ Many skills are classified as executive functions. Among them are the following:

   ◆ Delaying or inhibiting response

   ◆ Active decision making

   ◆ Anticipating consequences

   ◆ Evaluating outcomes

   ◆ Generating alternative solutions

★ Why Build Executive Function Skills?

How Does Trauma Impact Executive Functions?

■ Development of executive functions parallels development of the **prefrontal cortex**. Normatively, executive functions develop over the course of childhood and adolescence, allowing children to become increasingly sophisticated in their cognitive meaning making and problem solving. Goal-directed human behavior is guided by this part of the brain much of the time.

■ Along with many other brain systems, the prefrontal cortex is implicated in the traumatic stress response. When stress overwhelms normal coping mechanisms and the danger response is activated, key survival systems (e.g., the **limbic system**) take charge, and "nonessential" systems are deactivated. In the moment of significant danger, higher cognitive processes are considered nonessential! (Think about it—if you are in the middle of the jungle and a lion is speeding toward you, do you want to be thinking, or do you want to be running?)

■ The limbic system and the prefrontal cortex are mutually inhibitory: As one increases in activation, the other decreases, and vice versa. Consider the way in which frustration, for instance, interferes with your ability to remain focused on a difficult task and continue to work toward a solution: As arousal goes up, cognitive processes begin to fragment. Conversely, consider the ways in which using your "thinking brain" (e.g., focusing on logic, breaking tasks into step-by-step solutions) can help decrease feelings of being overwhelmed: That is, the act of harnessing higher-order cognition can serve to regulate arousal levels.

■ For children who experience chronic trauma, the ongoing exposure to danger (both real and perceived) takes a toll on the development of higher cognitive abilities. With increased sensitization to danger signals, the brains of chronically traumatized youth are frequently readying the body to run from the lion, and therefore prioritizing limbic over prefrontal activation. Because there are many potential triggers of danger, these children may be as likely to be under limbic control in the midst of math class as they would be in the midst of the jungle.

■ Research indicates that children who have experienced trauma lag behind their peers over time in development of age-appropriate executive function skills. They do less well on tasks requiring several distinct abilities: to inhibit responses, to plan and make active choices, and to sustain attention.

Why Target Executive Functions?

■ Executive functions allow us to participate actively in our own lives. They provide a sense of control and agency. In the absence of higher cognitive control, we are caught in stimulus–response mode: Life throws something at us, and we react. Executive functions bring *conscious thought* to our actions; rather than simply reacting, we consider our actions in context.

■ Research on resilience highlights the importance of these executive abilities. In study after study, the ability to problem-solve, make active choices, and function independently predicts resilient outcome among high-risk youth.

🧰 Therapist Toolbox
🐾 What's the Stake?

■ Taking the time to delay behavior and consider alternatives may feel very foreign to children who have experienced chronic trauma. For these children, the surges of emotion or arousal they experience in response to often misunderstood or misinterpreted environmental cues feel like a call to action, and any suggestion that they stop and think is unsettling and potentially threatening.

■ Clinical work and day-to-day adult supports for these skills may feel like blame to the child: "What choices should you make? Why didn't you make this choice?" At heart, though, this skill set is based on the goal of increasing, not decreasing, the child's felt and actual power. When we are able to pause, slow down our responses, consider our options, and make a choice that works for us, we are increasingly able to be powerful in our world.

■ Engagement in this skill set requires patient support by adult caregivers. In the best of circumstances, it is hard for any of us to slow down our reactions and make good choices when we are frustrated; for a child who has limited internal resources, unreliable external resources, and a highly active arousal system, this skill may feel almost impossible. Adult scaffolding is required to help children be successful in approaching their challenges actively and tolerating the frustration inherent to this work.

■ Engagement in this work may be increased by:

   ◆ Paying attention to timing. When a child is in a strongly hyper- or hypoaroused state, providing support for regulation is a priority over support for engaging executive functions.

   ◆ Observing and validating the choices a child is already making before trying to change them. For example: "I think I understand why you walked out on your mom in the middle of that conversation. It sounds like you were feeling really angry and frustrated, and I'm guessing you needed to take some space."

   ◆ Validating the many reasons it feels hard to slow down. For example: "Most of us have a hard time using our thinking brains when we're really frustrated or upset and that arousal takes over. I doubt there's anyone who hasn't acted too quickly sometimes, and done things he or she might not have done if there had been time to think about it."

   ◆ Engaging the child's own curiosity about why they make the choices they do. An important message here is the belief that all of us engage in behavior for a reason: Our behavior serves a function and gives us important information about our goals. "I wonder what you might have been trying to communicate when you walked out of class."

   ◆ Engaging the child's curiosity about goals, both immediate and longer-term (as developmentally appropriate). "I know that you've been getting really upset at school and taking off before the end of the day. I get why that's working right now as a way to manage your feelings, but let's talk about where you go from here. I'm curious what you see yourself doing when this year is up. Do you have plans that you need a high school degree for?"

■ In the sections that follow, psychoeducation is woven in to descriptions of work with caregivers as well as with children and adolescents. For children who feel as if they have no choices, and for adult caregivers who are frustrated and overwhelmed by child behaviors, transparency about the goals, timing, and skills involved in engaging executive functions, and psychoeducation about the role of the brain in reacting versus acting, are crucial to depathologizing child behaviors and increasing felt power.

📋 Teach to Caregivers

- *Reminder:* Teach caregivers the Key Concepts. It may be helpful to use visual tools or media to support your teaching about executive functions.
- *Reminder:* Teach caregivers relevant Developmental Considerations.
- Teach caregivers to support and facilitate executive function skills, including:
    - Helping empower youth to make choices and giving them ample opportunity to do so
    - Supporting inhibition of immediate response through external support for youth modulation
    - Engaging youth in evaluating situations ("What's the problem we're dealing with here?") and identifying goals ("What do you/we/others want to happen?").
    - Learning and actively supporting problem solving, including the generation and evaluation of ideas and active experimentation
- Ways that caregivers can engage in each of these areas is detailed later in this chapter.

Caregiver goal #1: Empower and provide opportunities for youth to make choices.

- One of the most important foundations of the skill set for making choices is the *belief that you can* make choices. Many children and adolescents have had limited opportunity to be active participants in their lives, and in fact as part of their traumatic experiences too often had choices taken away. A key role of caregivers, therefore, is to support awareness of choices that children are making, and to provide additional opportunities for youth to be active in making choices.
- Work with caregivers to notice and name choices, even minor ones, and related or anticipated outcomes ("It sounds like you want to make the choice to walk today, instead of taking the bus? That's fine, but I'm guessing you'll want to leave a bit earlier, right?").

It is important to support caregivers in their attunement to their child's (and their own) ability to engage these skills every day and particularly during daily routines. There are many opportunities to exercise executive function skills every day. For example, when an older child or adolescent wakes up in the morning they make choices about when they will get out of bed, what they will eat for breakfast, wear, and so forth. It is important to encourage caregivers to reflect on these opportunities and to incorporate the language of choice and outcome (if–then or because–then statements; for instance: "If you do X, then Y might happen"; "Because you did X, then Y happened later") into these daily routines.

- Prior to asking caregivers and children to apply these skills in more challenging situations, it is often helpful for caregivers to actively tune in to and reinforce positive choices and to focus on strengths *or* successes in decision making, rather than on "poor choices," as an opportunity to build mastery of this skill. However, it can be equally important to work with caregivers to engage attunement skills to validate the possible reasons for less positive choices.
    - For instance, a caregiver might notice a positive choice such as this one: "You know, I saw you trying to keep your temper when your sister was yelling at you, and even though she didn't like your walking away from her, I know that it was a really good

choice for you that kept you from getting caught up in the drama with her. I'm guessing things didn't heat up as much as they could have because you were able to walk away."

♦ In the same situation, with a different set of behaviors, the caregiver might also validate less positive choices: "We've talked about how important it is for you to try to walk away when you're getting really angry, so that you don't lose your temper and lash out like you did earlier. But I get why you felt the need to say those things to your sister. I'm guessing it felt really important to let her know how you felt, even if you spoke to her in a way that I know felt hurtful to her."

♦ When providing a mirror for less positive choices using attunement skills, it is important that caregivers understand the distinction between validating the *reason* behind the choice (why does the child's behavior make sense?) and validating the *choice itself* (why might you still set limits on or disapprove of a choice, even if you understand the reason for it?) The more that caregivers can communicate both facets, the more their attunement skills will support child awareness of choices in a way that the child can hear them.

♦ Opportunities to make or contribute to choices can be built into a wide range of activities and experiences, from the more mundane ("Which show should we watch tonight?") to the more significant ("I'm trying to decide whether it's better for you to stay in the class you're in now or to switch to that new one we talked about. Let's you and I talk through which choice makes more sense for you"). When the child is unable to be part of making a choice that strongly affects him or her (e.g., decisions that lead to a child switching therapies, leaving a foster home, not being able to reunify with a parent, remaining in a disliked school), transparency by those in power about why the choice was made can be vital for minimizing the child's feeling that decisions were made randomly and without considering the child's wants or needs.

Caregiver goal #2: Support inhibition of immediate response through external support for youth modulation.

■ To engage executive function skills successfully, a person must be in a reasonably regulated state. Delaying impulsive reactions depends on first calming down a heightened arousal system. As described in depth in Part V on regulation, many children are unable to do this independently, particularly early in treatment. One of the most important ways that caregivers can support children in being *ready* to consider options and to make decisions is by supporting them in (co)regulating experience in the moment.

■ In the "Teach to Caregivers" section of Chapter 11, we provided important psychoeducation and steps that caregivers can take to externally support child modulation in the moment. As a reminder, these steps include:

1. Develop a "modulation support plan": Work with children and caregivers to proactively identify situations that might lead to dysregulation and common dysregulation patterns. Engage the caregiver's problem-solving capacities to brainstorm potential responses. Be sure to include the caregiver's own in-the-moment self-care plan.

2. Identify early signs of dysregulation and use simple reflection skills to mirror the child's experience.

3. Cue, support, and reinforce the use of previously identified and practiced skills.

4. Offer simple opportunities for control and choice in the moment, to increase the child's felt safety.

5. Delay more cognitively involved problem solving until the child is in a more regulated space. *However,* it may be important to signal to the child the adult's awareness that there is a problem, and a willingness to support the child in solving it.

■ Example of putting the above steps into action: A caregiver might recognize that a child is getting agitated and frustrated while doing homework. Knowing that this situation has led to intense angry outbursts in the past, the adult might state: "You know what, I can see that you're getting super-frustrated with that homework [*simple reflection*]. I really want to help you figure out what you need to do [*communicate desire to help*], but I think we'll do a better job of it if we can calm down your energy a bit [*support regulation*]. Do you want to take some space and take a walk, or do you want to just sit here with me for a bit and relax [*offer choice and control*]?"

■ The more the child is in a state of physiological readiness, the more successfully he will be able to use higher cognitive capacities.

Caregiver goal #3: Engage youth in evaluating situations ("What's the problem we're dealing with here?") and identifying goals ("What do you/we/others want to happen?").

■ To solve a problem, a person must first be able to identify both what the *problem* is and what the *goal* is. In the Therapist Toolbox section later in this chapter, we provide examples of psychoeducation and strategies for supporting children in recognizing difficult situations and identifying goals. This psychoeducation is equally important for caregivers, because a key part of their role is to help the (regulated) child engage curiosity about her own experience, about the reactions of others around her, and about her wants and needs. "Problem identification" is, in many ways, simply an outgrowth of identification skills, described in Chapter 10: A situation is a "problem" if the child is feeling distressed, or if people around the child seem to be feeling distressed.

■ Both primary and milieu caregivers may use the steps described in the table beginning on page 268, particularly Step 1 ("Notice there is a problem") and Step 3 ("Identify and understand the problem") to support children in recognizing and defining opportunities to solve problems.

Caregiver goal #4: Learn and actively support problem-solving, including generation and evaluation of ideas and active experimentation

It is important for caregivers to think of themselves as facilitators of problem solving—as teachers and supporters of this skill set rather than as the "problem solver" for a child or teen. If adults simply provide solutions for the child, then the child will not learn the numerous skills involved in the process. For example, it is very common for providers or caregivers, having just heard a child present a potential problem, such as "I'm going to punch her in the face," to react by discussing all of the reasons why the child should *not* make that choice rather than supporting the child through the process of evaluating the consequences (positive and negative) of this choice. When possible, caregivers should allow children to come to their own conclusions. They may make the "wrong" choice sometimes or the choice that is least effective for them in the long term. However, these "failures" or lack of success are a very important part of the learning process. This point relates to the importance of framing much of our work with children and teens as an experiment with many possible outcomes. The language of experimentation supports executive function skills because it implies the possibility of multiple outcomes and it normalizes the idea that some outcomes will not feel successful—and that's okay. Learning through trial and error is an effective way to learn; in fact, it is inherent in the learning process itself.

There are a number of ways for caregivers to support and facilitate children's ability to make decisions and engage executive functions—in daily routine, in play and other normative activities, in response to challenging behaviors, and by "catching the moment" and supporting children in considering alternatives.

- There are a large number of normative activities that support executive functioning in our children and youth. In the table on page 267 we provide examples of activities by developmental stage. Support the caregiver in his or her ability to facilitate suggested activities as part of daily routines and family engagement. Many of these activities can be built into therapy sessions or milieu routines.

- In Part IV on attachment, one of the targets for intervention is to support the caregiver in developing increasingly effective responses to child behaviors. It is important to remind caregivers that one of the goals of learning effective responses is to create behavioral response plans that help children to anticipate outcomes (reinforcement, limits/consequences, having to take breaks from activities, etc.) and over time to make active choices in service of achieving a desired outcome, whether it be connection, a reward or the removal of something aversive.

- In the "Tools" section later in this chapter, we outline a number of opportunities to "catch" problem solving in the moment. Work with caregivers to recognize and support these opportunities through analysis of situations after the fact; through modeling, practice, and coaching in session; or, for milieu caregivers, in staff supervision, and by actively teaching and role-playing problem-solving opportunities.

Behind the Scenes

- Although executive functions encompass many different areas, this section specifically targets three key skills: active evaluation of situations, inhibition of response, and decision making. These skills all contribute to and are encompassed in problem-solving skills. As originally outlined by D'Zurilla and Goldfried (1971), problem-solving skills have been integrated into a wide array of cognitive-behavioral and social skills treatments for both children and adults (e.g., D'Zurilla & Nezu, 2007; Greene & Ablon, 2006; Kazdin, 1985; Kazdin, Esveldt-Dawson, French, & Unis, 1987; Kazdin, Siegel, & Bass, 1992; Matthews, 1999). We describe a variation on these steps that incorporates a recognition of the impact of the danger response on the problem-solving capacities of children and adolescents who have experienced traumatic stress.

- For children to engage in and practice these skills effectively, they must be in a regulated state of arousal. Engage caregivers in supporting child regulation, and teach children to pair the use of learned modulation strategies with these skills.

- A primary goal of this work is to increase children's recognition of their ability to actively make *choices*. Understanding the concept of choice increases children's sense of empowerment and fosters several key competencies: **agency,** or the self-knowledge that their actions can impact their world; **personal responsibility,** or ownership of decision making and the consequences; and **mastery,** or the ability to implement, evaluate, practice, and own personal actions and decisions.

- Often, children (and adults) are presented with two less-than-ideal choices, rather than a clearly positive and clearly negative one. At times, our choice may be between doing *something* and doing *nothing*. The process of reflecting and actively choosing remains important: There is a clear difference in internal experience between *choosing* to do nothing (when acting will invariably bring negative consequences) and *feeling or thinking that we can't do anything*. It is the difference between agency and helplessness. It is important to teach children that problem solving will sometimes involve choosing among solutions that don't necessarily feel good, but that ultimately remain the best options toward meeting their goals.

- Although the problem-solving steps are taught in sequence later in this chapter, we can apply them in any order. For instance, in some situations, we might start at Step #3 (identifying the problem) and work our way through understanding our goals, generating possible solutions, and anticipating outcomes. In other situations, we might start at the end: that is, what outcome are we seeking? Given that outcome, we can work our way back to possible actions, behaviors, coping strategies, and the situations or problems that may interfere. Or, we can work with an outcome (whether positive or negative) that has already occurred and track back to identify the precipitating factors, behaviors, and coping strategies that led to the given outcome. In the instance of a negative outcome, we might also work to identify the desired outcome and alternatives that would help clients succeed.

- It is crucial to notice and name choices when they occur, particularly with children who struggle with them. Consider the following example.

  > An adolescent girl who recently started a part-time job is talking about her frustration with the assistant manager at the store. "She keeps getting in my face, telling me what to do and how to do it, and how I need to be working faster." When the therapist asks how the teen is handling this style of interaction, she says, "What am I supposed to do? I just keep my mouth shut and do what she says." When the therapist comments that the adolescent has sometimes struggled with managing her temper in the past, the teen states, "Well, I don't want to lose this job—I need the money." The therapist responds, "I'm so impressed. You know that you want to keep this job, and it's helping you make a choice to manage your feelings and not jump into arguing or yelling back, even though you're feeling frustrated and upset."

  In this situation, it is important that the therapist notice, name, and reinforce the active choice the adolescent is making (to control her behavior, because of her goal of keeping the job). It is equally important that the therapist then work with the adolescent on possible solutions for addressing any resulting problems (e.g., how to manage the challenging feelings and arousal resulting from these interactions).

- Later in this chapter we list the key steps involved in making active choices. Following these, we highlight strategies for "catching" and applying these skills in the moment.

Tools: Building Executive Functions

Building Executive Function Skills through Play

As with the other skills taught in this framework, the most natural forum for enhancing executive functioning, particularly for younger children, is play. There are a myriad of activities (interactive games, board games, video games, cooperative activities, etc.) that present opportunities to build this skill set. The following table provides examples of strategies by developmental stage.

Activities That Enhance Executive Function Skills

Developmental stage	Examples of activities
Early childhood	For infants, consider games that challenge working memory and support a basic understanding of sequencing and cause and effect. Some example include: ▪ Peekaboo and other hiding games ▪ Pat a Cake, Finger Play ▪ Activation toys ▪ Social engagement, conversation, and basic imitation. For toddlers, the process entails building increased ability to delay impulse and an expanded understanding of cause and effect. Some fun ways to enhance these skills include: ▪ Sorting games and puzzles ▪ Any new motor challenge, such as throwing and catching, and moving through an obstacle course or jumping are fun ways to support executive skills ▪ Imitation or simple follow-the-leader activities ▪ Songs with movement such as the Hokey Pokey or Head, Shoulders, Knees, and Toes ▪ Imaginary play and/or role play For children ages 3–5 (consider developmental stage) some suggested activities may include: ▪ Imaginary play, which becomes more sophisticated as the child role-plays some of his or own early experiences (e.g., playing doctor, teacher, parent) ▪ Reading stories and/or telling stories ▪ Increasingly complex motor tasks (e.g., riding bikes, jumping rope, climbing large play sets, attempting balance beams) ▪ Increasingly complex puzzles and/or sorting challenges ▪ Educational tasks such as learning letters, letter sounds, and numbers. ▪ Cooperative board games, in which children must work together as a team toward a mutual goal, can support decision making and collaboration, while minimizing the frustration of more competitive board games
Middle childhood	At this stage children are becoming more interested in interactive game play and have a growing understanding of rules/boundaries and strategy, so games that support growth in both these areas can be helpful. Here are some suggested activities that target executive function skills: ▪ Board games that require strategy, such as Battleship, checkers, chess, etc. ▪ Memory games (e.g., Go Fish) ▪ Logic and reasoning games (e.g., Brain Teasers) ▪ Movement games that require attention (e.g., Red Light, Green Light, Mother, May I). ▪ Singing, dance, playing a musical instrument
Adolescence	During adolescence executive function skills are critically important due to growing demands in the area of educational/vocational training. Some suggested areas of focus include: ▪ Enhancing self-monitoring skills (see Chapter 10) ▪ Supporting (realistic short-term) goal-setting, organizational, and planning practices ▪ Supporting age-appropriate socialization skills ▪ Supporting organized activities such as sports, drama, art, etc.

Problem-Solving Skills

- Problem-solving skills can be used formally or informally, in conversation or in structured writing or drawing tasks, and they can be used to think about an upcoming challenge or to explore a situation that has already occurred.

- For many people, the problem-solving steps are an unconscious, rapid process used to assess situations and make various choices. For children exposed to trauma, however, these steps are skipped as they move straight to reaction. The goal of this work, then, is to build children's awareness of and capacity to consciously engage in this process.

- The steps in the following table address each of the primary skills identified in this chapter. Each step can be targeted in isolation and should be practiced separately until some level of comfort is achieved. Over time, however, the goal is to build children's ability to apply all of the relevant steps in a given situation.

Step	Description
Step 1: Notice there is a problem.	**Teach to Kids:** ■ **Connect to previous skill building.** "Lots of situations can bring up feelings. We've talked a lot about ways to recognize feelings and how to deal with them." ■ **Feelings provide useful information.** "Sometimes feelings are hard, and we want to get rid of them. But—feelings give us important information. They let us know that something is going on that we like, or don't like, or are worried about, etc." ■ **Use "feelings detective" work to recognize problems.** "We've talked about recognizing feelings so that you can cope with them, share them with other people, and understand them. Now we're going to talk about how to use feelings to help you make good choices." ■ **Emphasize building child control.** "We're going to work on using all the skills you've learned to recognize feelings and then to stop and think before you act. This helps *you, not your feelings*, be in charge of what you do." **Goal**: For children to be able to *recognize* "problem situations" (e.g., moments in which they are upset or triggered). **How to**: ■ Build children's ability to notice *internal* cues and link these cues to **Identification** work. As feelings detectives, children learn cues that indicate when they are sad, mad, worried, etc. Identify the most prominent cues, such as energy level, body sensations, thoughts, behaviors, etc., and help children practice noticing when they happen. Include caregivers, as appropriate, to help. ■ Help children tune in to *external* cues indicating that other people think there is a problem. Review signs of affects in *others* learned during identification exercises. Help children tune in to key cues, such as tone of voice, facial expressions, body language, etc. How do children know when other people are upset, angry, worried, etc.?
Step 2: Establish basic safety and inhibit instinctive danger response.	**Teach to Kids:** ■ **Teach about the brain and normalize the rapid danger response.** "One of the things feelings do is send a message to our brains that there's something going on. Different parts of our brains control different things. One part of the brain is really good at *doing stuff*, or taking *action*—like, if we touch a stove, pain is a message to the action part of the brain that we need to move our hand away quickly. Another part of the brain is really good at *thinking*, but sometimes we don't want that part to be in charge—like, if you're touching a hot stove, do you really want to spend time *thinking* before you move your hand?" ■ **Provide rationale for skill.** ◆ "Sometimes, though, it is important for the *thinking brain* to be involved. When we have physical sensations, like pain, it can be important to react quickly. But certain types of feelings, like being afraid, angry, excited, or frustrated, can make us act *too* quickly. This is good when we're really in danger, but not so good if we're not." ◆ "Kids who have been in danger before get really good at reacting quickly when situations, thoughts, or feelings come up that seem to signal danger. Most of the time, though, it's important to know what is going on before we react."

Step	Description

(Query: "Has there ever been a time when feelings made you react too quickly? Give examples—for example, yelling at a teacher or punching a sibling. What was the consequence of reacting too quickly?")

■ **Engage children in assessing real versus perceived danger.** "When you have strong feelings, the first thing that is important to do is to figure out if you're safe or in danger. We've already talked about how our brains learn to pay attention to clues that tell us that something *might* be dangerous. Sometimes there is real danger, but other times, the clues are things that remind us of something that *was* dangerous in the past. Do you remember what those are called? [Reteach concept of triggers, if needed.] Triggers activate the body's alarm system. What we're going to work on is figuring out when it's a real alarm and when it's a false alarm—like a fire drill at school."

Goal: For children to establish a basic sense of safety and then to *inhibit* initial survival reactions until children are able to make an active choice about how to respond.

How to:
■ *Step 2.1:* Before anything else happens, the child must establish a basic sense of safety. Pair a child's ability to recognize that he or she is upset with the ability to scan the environment immediately and assess: **"Am I actually in danger?"**
  ◆ *Assess for physical danger:* "Is there something in my environment that could hurt me? Is there someone *physically* threatening me? If not . . . "
  ◆ *Assess for triggers:* If not previously taught, work with children to identify their own triggers. What things elicit strong emotions or make them feel unsafe? Help children find their own words to describe situations (e.g., "People giving me a hard time" vs. "Injustice"). Pay attention to multiple types of triggers:
    ● Internal (e.g., feeling lonely or vulnerable/powerless)
    ● Relational (e.g., exertion of authority, intimacy)
    ● Sensory (e.g., smells, sounds, facial expressions, touch)
■ Help children identify cues that go along with being triggered. Link fight–flight–freeze response to triggers. What have they identified as their own behaviors or feelings when they are in the fight response? Flight response? Freeze response? Keep in mind that different reactions may go with different types of triggers.
■ **The goal here is for children to become proficient at recognizing when they are triggered (vs. actually in danger) and delaying their response until they can make an active choice.**
■ *Step 2.2:* Inhibition of response
  ◆ Help children build tools to delay immediate response. Once children recognize that a situation is "a problem," it is important that they be able to delay further response until they have had time to manage their affect and actively make choices.
  ◆ This is an incredibly hard step for many children, and significant practice is often needed.
  ◆ Consider multiple possible tools (including many of those discussed in Chapter 11, "**Modulation**"). For example:
    ● Focused breathing
    ● Cognitive tools (e.g., self-statement: "Stop and think")
    ● Visual tools (e.g., small stop sign or stop light)
    ● Social resources (e.g., caregiver or teacher cue)
    ● Grounding tools (e.g., teach child to focus on hand-held manipulatives)
■ As in affect modulation, pair regulatory skill with state of arousal.
■ Work with caregivers and other adults to support and reinforce this skill.

Step 3: Identify and understand the problem.

Teach to Kids:
■ **Getting to the root of the problem.** "Once you know you're not really in danger, you can take the time to figure out what is *really* going on. Emotions come from somewhere."

Goal: For a child to *consciously evaluate a situation* to understand the origins of his or her own and others' emotions.

How to (*or* **learn to be a problem detective**): Take the time to understand what *is* going on.
■ Once children can recognize that they are feeling something, teach them to *concretely* identify what, exactly, the problem is.
■ A situation is generally "a problem" because the *child* is unhappy about something, because someone *else* is unhappy with the child, or both.

Step	Description

■ Help children with prompts. Use the *wh-* questions to **backtrack**, as described in the next section, "Recognizing Opportunities to Apply Problem-Solving Skills in the Moment":
  ◆ "When did you start noticing that funny feeling in your stomach?"
  ◆ "Who were you with?"
  ◆ "What were you doing?"
  ◆ "Where were you doing it?"
  or
  ◆ "What made you think your dad was upset?"
  ◆ "What were you doing?"
  ◆ "What was he doing?"
■ It is important that children, to the degree possible, are the ones who identify the problem (as well as possible solutions). Help them with cues, but let them figure out what they can.

Step 4:
Brainstorm:
Identify
possible
solutions.
Don't throw
out anything
yet!

Teach to Kids:
■ **The point of knowing that there is a problem is to be able to actively deal with it.** "Once you know something is a problem, you can make an active choice, instead of just reacting."
■ **There is *always* more than one choice.** "A lot of times, kids feel like they don't have a choice when things feel hard. But—almost all the time, there *are* choices, even if the choice is to not do anything."
■ **Sometimes, the choice is about what happens inside of us, instead of about action.** "There may be times when the choice we make is to work on how we feel and think about something, rather than about taking action to address a situation. For instance, if we are in a situation we cannot change, our choices may be (a) to feel angry and resentful, or (b) to work on accepting the situation, to think about something that makes us happy, to think forward to a time when the situation will be over."

Goal: To help children identify many possible solutions, so that they can make an active choice.

How to:
■ *Step 4.1:* Name and validate current choice.
  ◆ If a choice has already been made (i.e., work is being done in the aftermath of a situation), it is important to first *name* the choice the child has already made and *validate* it.
■ *Step 4.2:* Identify the goal.
  ◆ Every situation has many possible goals. The choices we make in a hard situation will depend on what our goal is (e.g., if a child is in trouble at school for fighting, the goal may be to teach the child how to calm down from being mad, to think of ways to resolve the problem, or to think of a different solution for next time).
  ◆ Help child concretely identify what he or she is trying to accomplish. Consider expressing feelings, seeking support, avoiding a consequence, gaining a reward or privilege, fixing a difficult situation, etc.
  ◆ If the goal the child picks is not a realistic one, help him or her to examine that, and, when necessary, to identify an alternative goal. For instance, consider a child who is having difficult visits with a biological parent due to conflict with a sibling; the child's goal may be, "To make my brother disappear." Although understandable (and important to validate), help the child consider alternative goals (e.g., "How to deal with my brother so I can still see Mom").
■ *Step 4.3:* Generate ideas about possible choices.
  ◆ Help children generate as many ideas as possible. It is crucial at this point to refrain from commenting on any of the potential choices. For instance, if you ask a child all the different ways he or she could handle a confrontation at school, and the child lists punching someone, throwing a brick through a window, running off, etc., then all of these go on the list.
  ◆ Keep in mind at this stage, you're not trying to get to the *best* solution. You're trying to highlight that there *are* solutions, and that—even when it doesn't seem like it—children are making choices. For instance, choosing to punch someone is a solution, but there are almost always alternatives.
  ◆ If a child is unable to generate any positive solutions, the clinician has two choices: Continue with the steps below, evaluating consequences, and then come back and look for alternatives, *or* try to generate a few more with the child in the moment (e.g., "I wonder if we can think of a few ideas that don't involve hitting someone").

Step	Description
Step 5: Evaluate all the possible consequences (good and bad) of each solution, and then make a choice.	**Teach to Kids:** ■ **All choices have consequences, good and bad.** "Every choice we make has consequences—sometimes they're good, sometimes they're not so good, and sometimes they're both. Like—if you help out your mom, it might make you (and her) feel good, but you might not have time to watch your favorite show that day. Or—if you decide to hit someone, it might make you feel better, but you'd probably get in trouble." ■ **Make a choice.** "Sometimes there's no perfect choice. Usually, though, we can figure out what some *good* choices are, based on what you want to happen, or what you don't want to happen." **Goal**: To support children in evaluating outcomes so that they are able to select solutions in service of meeting goals. **How to:** ■ *Step 5.1:* Evaluate possible consequences for each idea generated. ◆ Work with the child to evaluate each idea on the list. It is important to acknowledge that most choices potentially have both positive and negative outcomes. ◆ Pay attention to immediate and delayed outcomes. Help the child to think through not just what will happen in the moment, but what may happen later on as a result of the choice. ◆ Go through this process for every solution the child has generated. ■ *Step 5.2:* Based on potential consequences, help the child make a choice. ◆ *Help the child actively examine all choices.* "Given the situation, the goal, the possible rewards, and the possible consequences, what seems like the best choice for you now?" ◆ *Help child to examine combinations:* "Sometimes the best choice involves doing a few different things. For instance, one of the goals may be to express your feelings, and another is to seek support. Does it make more sense to pick choices that help you do both, or does one need to have priority over the other?" ◆ *Name consequences of negative choices, but don't engage in a power struggle.* Be aware that children may select a negative choice, even after having gone through this process. Acknowledge that this may be the choice they would really like to make, but highlight that making the choice will mean that they need to accept the consequences. Emphasizing consequences increases awareness of responsibility and personal control. ◆ *Help children be realistic in their assessment.* Some choices sound good but will be difficult to implement. For instance, in choosing a solution for dealing with peer conflict, a child decides that the best choice is to "Just not get mad." The clinician may: • *Normalize emotion:* "Well, I think it would be really hard to have someone yell at you and not feel a little bit mad. Remember how we've talked about that it's okay to have all feelings, it's just important to make safe choices? And trying to turn off your feelings isn't really good for you, because your feelings will come out in other ways." • *Identify a safe way to cope with the emotion and still reach the goal.* For situations involving difficult affect, integrate self-regulation strategies into potential choices. For instance, a child might choose to calm down by squeezing a stress ball and then try talking to an adult.
Step 6: Implement and evaluate solutions and revise as needed.	**Teach to Kids:** ■ **Try it out.** "We don't always know what the best choice is, and we don't always know what is going to happen when we make a choice. Sometimes we have to experiment—that means picking what we *think* is the best solution and trying it out." ■ **Evaluate outcomes.** "Once we've tried out something, we can decide if we made the right choice. We can always go back and try something else or choose a different solution the next time." **Goal**: To support children in actively engaging in choices, and then reflecting upon them. **How to:** ■ *Step 6.1:* Act on the choice. ◆ The goal here is for children to implement the choice they have made. This is, in many ways, the hardest step. It can be difficult for children to generalize from the therapy room to their daily lives. ◆ *Anticipate:* Work with the child to identify factors that will increase the possibility of success, as well as any possible barriers. Help the child think of ways to increase positive factors and decrease or cope with barriers.

Step	Description

◆ *Role-play:* Help the child practice carrying out the chosen solution. Use role play to act out different scenarios and outcomes.
◆ *Build a team:* Help the child achieve success by drawing in other resources. Elicit suggestions from the child: "Who will it be okay to talk to about helping you with this?" To the degree possible, involve caregivers, teachers, etc., in supporting implementation. Teach the child's team to cue the child in using target skills.
◆ *Experiment:* Frame the attempt at implementation as an experiment. Teach the child that no one can completely predict the results of a new action or behavior. Have the child actively observe outcomes, and report back.
■ *Step 6.2:* Evaluate outcomes and revise as needed.
◆ In situations where the child is going to attempt a new solution, it is important to take a look at what happened. Celebrate successes.
◆ Even if the solution did not work, reinforce any *attempt* the child has made to implement a positive solution.
◆ If the implemented choice was not successful, work with the child to critically identify and evaluate possible barriers. Was it that the solution wasn't the right one? Was it the timing? Was it the other person? Was it that other feelings got so strong that the child couldn't remember the choice in the moment? Help find solutions that address the barriers to implementation, going back through the preceding steps.

Recognizing Opportunities to Apply Problem-Solving Skills in the Moment

■ Often, the best place to apply problem-solving skills is in the moment in response to child statements, or in situations in which a choice should be—or has been—made. In the preceding table, each step of the problem-solving process is detailed, with key teaching points and goals. Here, suggestions are given for ways to recognize opportunities to use and apply this skill.

"I DON'T KNOW WHY EVERYONE'S SO MAD."

■ *Entry point:* Listen for moments when children are confused about why a situation happened or show a lack of awareness that something was a problem.

■ *Goal:* To increase children's awareness of internal and external cues that signify a "problem situation" and to help them evaluate and understand what the problem was/is **(Steps 1–3)**.

■ *Note:* When applied in the aftermath of a situation, *backtracking* can be used to help children learn to track and tune in to subtle cues in their bodies and in the environment:
◆ Help children **concretely define the situation** about which they are confused (e.g., "Suddenly everyone was mad").
◆ **Track backward.** What was happening 5 minutes before "everyone was mad"? Assess the situation, the child's body state, feelings, and thoughts.
◆ **Continue to move backward to the earliest cues available.** Help children notice clues that there is "a problem"—for example, that their feelings were getting out of control, or that other people were upset. Tie in to affect identification skills.

Example:
(The child comes into session appearing sad and shut down.)
THERAPIST: You look kind of down today. What's going on?

CHILD: Everyone hates me, and I don't know why. [Language of confusion about situation]

THERAPIST: Everyone hates you? What makes you think that?

CHILD: I don't know, I was just trying to play and everyone told me to go away. [Defining the situation]

THERAPIST: Wow—I can see why you're down. Let's try to figure out what was happening. What happened right before everyone told you to go away? [Backtrack]

CHILD: I don't know. It was recess, and some kids were playing, and I wanted to play, and then they got mad.

THERAPIST: How did you know they were mad? [Tuning in to clues of "a problem"]

CHILD: 'Cause they were yelling, and they said I was stupid.

THERAPIST: Okay, sounds like they were mad. What happened right before they yelled? [Backtrack]

■ *Note:* This process can continue until child and therapist have identified early clues indicating that there was "a problem," defined/understood the situation, and then continued through the problem-solving steps (i.e., alternatives for next time).

"BUT I HAD TO . . ."

■ *Entry point:* Listen for moments when children identify a situation, either past or future, in which they did not or do not feel as if they have a choice.

■ *Goal:* Increase awareness of choices **(Step 4).**

Example:

(The child is on program restriction for shoving another resident in their group home.)

CHILD: I don't get what the big deal is. He started it, so I *had to*. [Language of "no choice"]

MILIEU COUNSELOR: Sounds like it really felt like you didn't have a choice.

CHILD: Well, I didn't. He was getting in my face.

MILIEU COUNSELOR: Okay, Manuel was getting in your face, so you chose to shove him. [Language of choice] Because of that, you got put on restriction. [Language of consequences] Let's think of why it might have happened so quickly. [Acknowledgment of the role of triggers or dysregulated response] and whether there was anything else you could have done.

"I'M GONNA . . . [INSERT BAD CHOICE HERE]."

■ *Entry point:* Listen for moments when children name a potentially negative choice that they plan on making.

■ *Goal:* Increase understanding of consequences for actions **(Step 5).**

Example:

(The adolescent has had an argument with her parents and comes into session very angry.)

ADOLESCENT: I hate my parents. I'm sick of this, I'm taking off. [Potentially negative choice] I've got friends in New York—I can always go there.

THERAPIST: Okay, sounds like things are really heating up. I can understand why you would want to take off. Can we take a couple of minutes to think about it?

ADOLESCENT: Fine, but I'm not changing my mind.

THERAPIST: Okay, well that's your choice. **[Don't engage in a power struggle; reiterate choice.]** It sounds like you're feeling like you need a break. Can we think of some different choices you might have, including taking off [**don't leave anything out when brainstorming**], and then think about what's going to work best for you? **[Generate alternative solutions, then evaluate them.]**

Note: In a situation in which a child/adolescent continues to reiterate intent to make negative or unsafe choices, despite support in problem solving, the adult may be in the position of needing to address those actions. Continue to use the language of choice, as follows:

ADOLESCENT: This is stupid! I'm serious—I'm leaving.

THERAPIST: I can understand that you want to leave, but you know that part of my job is helping you to stay safe. If this is really the choice that you want to make, then the choice I'm going to have to make is to do something to help keep you safe, like speaking with your mom about this.

"IT'S ALL [MY MOTHER'S, MY FRIEND'S, THE TEACHER'S, MY DOG'S, ETC.] FAULT!"

■ *Entry point:* Listen for moments when children externalize responsibility for a choice they have made.

■ *Goal:* Increase understanding of consequences for actions **(Step 5)**.

> *Example:*
>
> *(The adolescent comes into session angry because his parents have taken away his Play-Station.)*

ADOLESCENT: I hate my parents! I'm sick of this, they're always taking stuff away for the stupidest little things. They do it just to piss me off. **[Externalizing responsibility]**

THERAPIST: Okay, sounds like you're pretty mad. What happened?

ADOLESCENT: I told you, they're trying to piss me off, so they took away my PS2.

THERAPIST: Wow—they just took it away out of the blue? What was going on before it happened?

ADOLESCENT: Nothing—I was just playing, and I was gonna do my homework after I finished the game, and they came in out of nowhere and started yelling.

THERAPIST: Is this something you guys had talked about before?

ADOLESCENT: Yeah, I guess so, but I was gonna do it in a minute. I don't see what the big deal is.

THERAPIST: Can I make sure I understand? So you and your folks had talked about doing homework—did they tell you that you needed to do it before playing?

ADOLESCENT: Yeah.

THERAPIST: Did they tell you you'd lose the PS2 if you didn't do your homework?

ADOLESCENT: Yeah, but I was planning on doing it—I was just gonna finish my game.

THERAPIST: Okay, this is making more sense. It sounds like your folks asked you to do something, and you made a choice to use the PS2 instead of doing your homework when they asked. [Highlight choice made by adolescent.] Do you think there's any other choices you could have made, that wouldn't have gotten the PS2 taken away? [Generate future alternative choices.]

🏃 Developmental Considerations

Developmental stage	Executive function considerations
Early childhood	Executive function skills develop over the course of childhood, into adolescence and young adulthood. Young children are not able—and should not be expected—to engage these skills independently.
	However, young children are able to learn basic if–then relationships. The goal with this age group is to establish an early understanding of choice, or action, and consequence (both good and bad).
	Agency is a key developmental task in early childhood. Work with caregivers to actively notice and name child choices and actions and link them to outcomes. For example: The child builds a tower, then knocks it down: "Look at that! You hit that tower, and it went boom! That was really neat!"
Middle childhood	Normatively, there should be a progression in children's ability to control and reflect on actions and choices. Cognitive abilities can begin to be used in the service of goal-directed activities.
	With this developmental stage, increase focus on support in anticipating, planning, and evaluating possible choices and outcomes. Involve caregivers and other adults in increasing the language of choice. For example: "You have soccer today, and I know sometimes you feel frustrated at practice. What choices do you think you could make to help with that today?"
	At this stage, mastery becomes increasingly important. Work with caregivers and other adults to actively identify how choices children made have led to successful outcomes. Keep in mind that "success" should be defined in a child-specific way, and may be about effort as much as outcome.
Adolescence	Normatively, adolescents have developed the cognitive capacity for critical thinking and independent problem solving. For trauma impacted adolescents, however, this area continues to remain a challenge. Several factors are important to consider: ▪ Because adolescents often wish to keep their inner lives private, shared problem solving may feel like an invasion. Allow adolescents some degree of autonomy in selecting problem situations to share. ▪ Foster adolescents' ability to generate solutions independently and to take responsibility for the consequences. Emphasis is often on teaching and supporting the problem-solving skills, rather than judging choices.
	Keep in mind that adolescents' interpretation of situations (and possible outcomes) are often idiosyncratic. Clinician and/or caregiver goals likely differ from those of adolescents. It is important to try to understand their perspective and individual goals.

🏠 Applications

🏠 Individual/Dyadic

It is likely that, to some degree, strengthening executive functions in the form of addressing problem-solving skills will come into most individual sessions with a child or adolescent. The problem-solving steps are often taught formally (i.e., step by step), but are most often applied less formally, by "catching the moment." Identifying difficult situations, exploring and defining "problems," exploring and defining goals, examining and generating choices, and linking actions to consequences are all an important part of ongoing therapeutic work. The more this process is made explicit, the more likely it is that a child will be able to internalize this set of skills over time.

The process of solving problems and making active choices will link, in some way, to every target encapsulated within this framework. A child will use **Identification** skills to support identification of problem situations and his or her own responses; **Modulation** skills are vital to remaining regulated enough to harness higher-order cognitive processes; and **Relational Connection** skills may be a key component of generated solutions (e.g., in expressing feelings or seeking support). **Self and Identity** work, as described in the next chapter, often intertwines with choices: A child's future goals, for instance, may help in identifying situational goals; values may help in considering the benefits and consequences of various choices. **Attachment** targets are vital to supporting child executive functions: The caregiver's capacity to stay regulated and to tune in to the child's thoughts, feelings, challenges, and strengths will help in delaying response, managing impulses, identifying the problem, and cuing and supporting the child in the use of these skills. Eliciting the child's understanding of choices can assist in the application of **Effective Response** (e.g., by proactively helping a child make positive choices, rather than relying on limits and consequences). The clinician can help the child and caregiver understand the important links among the skills and goals they have worked to develop.

Pay attention to recognizing "choice" situations, either in anticipation (e.g., an anticipated problem or upcoming challenge) or in the aftermath. Notice, name, and reinforce positive choices as well as attempts toward making choices, even when less positive. Whenever appropriate, involve caregivers (parents, teachers, other helping adults) in supporting child choices or in jointly generating potential solutions. It is particularly important to involve key adults whenever a child will be attempting to implement a new skill (e.g., making a choice to seek an adult's support instead of getting in a fight). Teach children's caregivers the problem-solving steps and actively practice and reinforce their support of these skills.

In addition to supporting the child/adolescent's own problem-solving abilities, it may be valuable to use transparency around decision-making processes, particularly as these decisions apply to the child's own life. Transparency helps both in modeling the decision-making skill and in decreasing a child's perception of the "randomness" of life decisions. For instance, consider the child who is being moved to a different classroom due to behavioral dysregulation. The clinician or caregiver might describe the decision-making process:

> "Like we had talked about, Mom, Mrs. Jones, Mr. Rivera, and I all met to talk about what would help you the most to be successful in school. We thought about different possibilities, like having someone sit with you in class, or having you leave the class for part of the day. We thought the best solution was _____. The reasons we thought might not work so well were _____. So here's what we're going to try. . . ."

Explanations should be developmentally appropriate and solution-focused.

Group

There are many ways to apply problem-solving skills in a group format. When developing activities, consider the ultimate goal: increasing child awareness of choices and the capacity to actively make them in the service of reaching a goal. In group situations the process of collaborative problem solving is often a more valuable teaching tool than simply providing explicit instruction in the steps, so long as there is a follow-up process. Consider, for instance, engaging the group in a collaborative process in which members must actively generate solutions to solve a problem (examples are provided in Appendix C). Following the activity, explore the process (e.g., "What was it like to work together? What helped you to be successful? What got in the way?"), the decisions (e.g., "What was it that made you pick x instead of y?"), and the outcomes (e.g., "How well do you think you did? Can you think of anything that would have made this turn out better? What about something that would have made this turn out worse?"). When appropriate, redo the activity, this time inviting group members to use their experiences to anticipate challenges/obstacles as well as successful solutions. In a follow-up discussion, link these processes to real-world decisions: the process of making choices, the obstacles that get in the way, the supports that can help, the ways in which our choices affect outcomes, and the ways that anticipating outcomes (and practical experience) can help in making increasingly positive choices.

Similar work can be done by engaging group members in a discussion of situations relevant to their lives through use of prompt scenarios; consider the use of appropriate movie clips, books, and current events. Most useful in this work is examining ambiguous situations—that is, those in which there is no clear "right" solution. Invite the group (1) to identify what the problematic issues are; (2) to discuss and generate possible goals, choices, and outcomes; and (3) to consider the ways in which potential obstacles and resources will intertwine with choices. It is important that group leaders not steer the group toward a "correct" choice; in this work, the process is more important than the decisions made.

Milieu

Supporting the child or adolescent in active problem solving, in combination with the use of modulation strategies, should be a key goal of milieu programs. Often, it is the demonstrated capacity to implement these skills independently that is seen as indicating the child's readiness for less restrictive levels of care.

Train staff, across levels, in the key skills described in the "Teach to Caregiver" section, including the balance between supporting regulation and facilitating decision-making skills. It is particularly important to work with staff on ways to recognize, cue, and support children in making active, healthy choices, and to provide opportunities for control and empowerment. Training should highlight the role of timing: Modulation skills are the necessary first step to successful engagement of higher-order cognitive processes. Offering choice often has the power to reduce power struggles, escalation, and the need for limits.

In milieu settings staff members have many opportunities to support children in the application of problem-solving skills. The approach will vary depending on the entry point. For example, when problem situations have been identified in advance by both staff members and children—for example, common triggers such as visits or phone calls with family, unstructured social situations, transitions, and changes in schedule—it is particularly helpful to create a "problem-solving plan." Work with each child to plan for challenging situations and to identify strategies for effectively coping and achieving a desired outcome (e.g., earning rewards or avoiding consequences, using Steps 3–6 as a guide). Involve youth in planning for these situations in advance; as with all skills, the skill of actively making positive choices is most successful when it has been practiced.

Problem-solving skills can also be applied when an outcome has already occurred. Formal processing of events that led to negative outcomes, such as restriction or therapeutic holds, can include each step outlined previously. It may be helpful, when processing, to provide visual cues of different affective states (e.g., feelings faces), energy levels (e.g., high, medium, low), so on. Additionally, if the outcome is related to peer conflict, consider formally implementing problem-solving steps in the approach to conflict resolution. Each resident involved in the conflict can have the opportunity to reflect on the situation individually, share his or her perspective, and then to jointly engage in problem solving based on a mutually agreed-upon goal/outcome. Milieus often have external structures for dealing with conflict-related problems such as boundary breaches. When possible, involve youth in the process of evaluating the situation and selecting appropriate solutions, including reparation with peers or staff, as well as potential programmatic consequences.

Problem-solving steps are most often applied in the moment with residents. In this case, use staff communication forums to develop plans for implementing problem solving in the moment. Consider a meeting structure that draws on staff attunement to each client and includes discussion of client triggers; cues indicating distress; behaviors associated with fight, flight, and freeze responses; and current modulation strategies being used by client, both positive and negative (e.g., asking for space, cutting). Use that information to develop a menu of modulation strategies from which each resident can choose when a problem situation appears to be occurring. For example, a staff member may observe that a resident is experiencing distress, as indicated by noncompliance. That staff member could reflect cues to the client and offer choices such as "Would you like a break? Would you like to blow bubbles or try something else from your toolbox?"

In summary, consider the entry point when developing programming that emphasizes this skill and incorporate both formal and informal approaches.

◯ Trauma Experience Integration: State-Based Skills Application

Distress Tolerance and Regulation

Delaying response, managing impulses, engaging higher-order cognitive capacities—all of these skills will be particularly challenging for children who are operating in a state of survival, with frequently overwhelmed affect and physiology. Similarly, caregivers who are struggling to manage their own distress are likely to have a hard time engaging attunement skills and managing their own affect in support of scaffolding youth decision making.

When youth are in an overwhelmed state, the emphasis is on supporting them in their ability to manage impulses and shift automatic responses or reactions to challenging experiences, including identified triggers. Much of the work will focus on supporting regulation in moments of distress. Ideally, regulated caregivers should be engaged and coached in the caregiver skills described previously.

When caregivers are themselves overwhelmed, providers may focus on caregiver affect management (how to keep themselves calm in the face of their children's distress) and on coregulation, emphasizing the phased process: regulate first, think later. This in itself may take some pressure off of stressed caregivers who feel the need to address and solve behaviors immediately, and who—like their children—may themselves benefit from the opportunity to slow the process down.

As challenging as this work is in early stages of treatment and in overwhelmed moments, experiencing repeated opportunities for control, choice, and empowerment may be one of the primary factors that allows children to engage reflective capacities over time. To say it differently: The more that children feel powerful in their world, the more they will believe that they can be powerful in future situations. Empowerment and agency—the foundation for this work—will build on themselves over time. Reflection and other mirroring skills can be used to support children's own awareness of their choices, and to validate and support understanding of choices that have been made. Routine attention to opportunities for choice, control, and competency will support growth of child agency.

Curiosity and Reflection

As youth and caregivers increasingly build the capacity to be reflective, the focus of the work can emphasize helping youth and caregivers to accurately identify the "problem" or challenging experiences or situations, along with the functions of current behaviors and goals. When the child can tolerate the emotions and arousal generated by talking through and reflecting on challenging situations, providers can support the child by enhancing understanding of problems ("What was going on that was upsetting you?"), of behavioral function ("I wonder what you were trying to do in that moment?"), and of choices and their associated outcomes ("It sounds like when you did that, this happened"). Over time, repeated understanding of these patterns can help shed light on key trauma-related triggers ("I'm noticing that whenever you feel like someone is picking on you or targeting you, it gets you enraged, sometimes much more than you might in other situations"), the child's survival patterns (". . . and then you lash out . . ."), the goals and functions of behavior (". . . to try to protect yourself . . ."), and ways these patterns influence current outcomes and experiences (". . . but sometimes it actually ends up getting you in more trouble and gets in the way of your getting your needs met"). As the child is increasingly attuned to his or her own experience and validated in current choices, there is a greater likelihood of engagement in trying to generate alternative solutions to identified problem areas.

Engaging Purposeful Action

One of the most important end-goals of trauma treatment is to support the child's ability to be active and agentic in his or her world. The trauma response is predicated on immediate responses to danger—a powerful self-protective reaction during experiences of true danger, but a disempowering one over time, as it places the child essentially at the mercy of perceived experience. In contrast, the ability (at developmentally appropriate levels) to be reflective, to understand internal experience, to recognize choice points, and work toward short- and long-term goals allows the developing child to be truly powerful.

As a child and/or his or her caregiving system is increasingly attuned, curious, able to recognize triggered arousal and to manage and regulate distress, in-the-moment engagement of executive function skills—whether independent or supported—becomes increasingly possible. In this phase there is a growing emphasis on supporting the child and/or his or her caregivers in anticipating and recognizing challenging experiences as they arise and on accurately evaluating a range of choice points and outcomes. The provider, caregiver, and child can work collaboratively to develop plans to both address challenging experiences in the moment and/or to work toward desired goals. Ideally this work is paired with "future self" work, which is described in the next chapter.

Real-World Therapy

Practice makes . . . well, not quite perfect. These skills are hard. Children will be much better at using them in session or when supported by caregivers than independently in the "real world," particularly in moments of emotional arousal. Expect that it will take some time for children to gain any mastery over these skills, especially with difficult problem situations. Don't throw out a skill because it doesn't work the first time, or the second time, or the tenth time. Repetition will eventually increase children's sense of control; even if they are unable to make the desired choice in the moment, over time they will be increasingly aware that they *have* choices. This, in itself, is a success.

It's not just a destination, it's part of the journey. Over the years, we have heard fairly often from clinicians and other providers that they are "working toward" being able to address executive function skills in treatment, but "we're not there yet." In response to this, we would challenge our readers to try to think of a single day in which they did not, at some point, find themselves confronted by a challenge, manage (successfully or not) an impulsive reaction, try to work out the best way to handle a problem, or think about how they wanted a situation to turn out. The reality is, we engage (or fail to engage!) our higher cognitive processes on a regular basis. These processes intertwine with and rely on our regulatory capacities, but are certainly not a completely independent skill set that we are only able to engage once fully regulated. The more practice we have at engaging and solving problems, the more we believe we can do so. The likelihood is that there are opportunities to support children's power in every single interaction. Look for the moments. We promise, you'll find them.

14

Self-Development and Identity

🔑 THE MAIN IDEA AND KEY SUBSKILLS

Support children in exploring and building an understanding of self and personal identity, including identification of unique and positive qualities, development of a sense of coherence across time and experience, and support in the capacity to imagine and work toward a range of future possibilities.

★ Help children identify personal attributes (*unique self*).

★ Build internal resources and identification of positive aspects of self (*positive self*).

★ Build a sense of self that integrates past and present experiences and incorporates multiple aspects of self (*cohesive self*).

★ Support capacity to imagine and work toward future goals/outcomes (*future self*).

★ Key Concepts

★ Why Target Self-Development and Identity?

■ A key developmental process is the growth of a sense of self, an understanding of individuality, and eventually the formation of a cohesive identity.

■ Establishment of a cohesive self advances across developmental stages.

 ◆ **In infancy and early childhood, identity formation begins as a basic awareness of self as separate from, but related to, others.** This basic self-concept grows as others—primarily immediate caregivers—respond in predictable ways to child actions, behaviors, and interactions. Children internalize the typical response of others. A child who receives frequent praise and affection, for instance, internalizes an understanding of self as positive and worthy of love. A child who is routinely rejected, in contrast, may internalize an understanding of self as unworthy. These internalized messages are incorporated into the child's burgeoning understanding of self.

 ◆ **In middle childhood, understanding of self expands to incorporate the experiences from multiple domains of a child's life.** Children focus in part on concrete attributes and outcomes: "I'm a girl [or a boy]," "I'm strong [or weak]," "I'm smart [or dumb]." Attributes are often understood in dichotomies, with shades of gray developing over the course of this stage. Interactions with caregivers continue to be important to self-concept; however, the responses of peers, teachers, and other key figures are factored in as well. Over time, a sense of self grows to encompass personal attributes, likes and dislikes, and individual values.

  ◆ **During adolescence, early understanding of self grows into a more cohesive identity encompassing abstract attributes, an integration of multiple aspects of experience, and future possibilities.** Normatively, this is an active process, as adolescents explore their own likes/dislikes, goals, values, and needs. Adolescents may "try on" different attributes in an attempt to crystallize a sense of self. Integrated into this sense of self are current and past experiences as well as future goals.

■ Growth of personal identity is an ongoing process that continues throughout our life.

★ How Does Trauma Impact Self-Development and Identity?

■ Impaired establishment of a positive, cohesive sense of self is a primary consequence of early trauma and attachment disruption. Empirical studies indicate impaired self-concept beginning in early childhood, and continuing through adolescence and adulthood.

■ For children and adolescents who have experienced trauma, elements of the past frequently continue to intrude in the form of fragmented memories and their intertwined elements, which may include language, visual images, intense affect, physiological sensation, sensory input, and systems of meaning. These elements often continue to influence and define the self in the present. For instance, a child who has experienced ongoing and pervasive moments of vulnerability does not just *remember* feeling vulnerable; he or she continues to experience the self as vulnerable in the present.

■ Particularly for older children and adolescents, the response in the present may parallel the past experience but may also expand upon and compound it. In the past, for instance, the child may have felt terror, loss, or confusion; in the present, as the past intrudes, the adolescent may feel all of those, and additionally be filled with rage or shame.

■ These experiences may intrude in the form of behavioral patterns and adaptations, but may also intrude as specific memories. Because of the intensity of traumatic memory and the fear of the present response, many trauma survivors learn to avoid, disconnect from, and shut down memory intrusions. This disconnection prevents mastery over the memory: So long as the response and experience are fully feared in the present, the power of the experience is sustained.

■ There are several reasons why trauma may impact identity and sense of self.

Internalization of Negative Experiences

Like all children, children who experience trauma internalize and incorporate their experiences into their sense of self. Children who are routinely rejected, harmed, or ignored may internalize an understanding of self as unlovable, unworthy, helpless, or damaged.

- Keep in mind that broader societal messages have the potential to play a role in development of self-concept, both positive and negative. Media and other forums send messages about such things as gender roles, body image, ethnic and culturally based expectations, and language use. Any member of a group who is marginalized in some way by media or other societal messages may be vulnerable to the impact of those messages on self-concept and identity. Children who have experienced trauma may be particularly vulnerable to internalization of negative attributions.

Fragmentation of Experience

The development of identity requires the ability to integrate experiences and aspects of self into a cohesive whole. Trauma-impacted children often rely on dissociative coping methods involving fragmentation and disconnection from their experiences. As such, they may have multiple "senses of self": for instance, the frightened self, the angry self, the invisible self, and the okay self. Often, these *state-dependent self-concepts* emerge in response to specific experiences and emotions. As such, children have difficulty integrating a cohesive sense of self across experiences and affective states.

Lack of Exploration

Normatively, secure attachments provide the safety that allows children to explore their worlds, and by extension, different aspects of themselves. Children learn whether they can accomplish goals, experiment with novelty, explore likes and dislikes. Trauma-impacted children often curtail exploration in the service of safety, instead relying on rigid control and repetition. Without exploration, children are limited to what immediately *is,* rather than the possibilities of what *could be.* This limitation on imagination cuts off potential facets of self, both in the present and in the future.

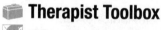 Therapist Toolbox
What Is the Stake?

- Many of the children and adolescents who present for treatment are, by very nature of their survival strategies, reluctant to explore "self." Some children have learned to disconnect from internal experience as a form of protection against overwhelming and distressing experiences of self (e.g., feeling shameful, damaged, unlovable, or other negative self-frames), and others guard and protect their internal states so as to be less vulnerable in relationship with others. These youth may have multiple experiences of others relating to them as "the problem," a "bad kid," or a series of diagnoses.

- A key premise of our intervention approach is the importance of building safe-enough relationships with children, adolescents, and families. In service of this effort, it is critically important that providers and caregivers work to be curious about, see, and accept the whole child.

- Engagement of children and adolescents in exploration of self and identity rests on a number of key components:

- ◆ Communication of interest in the whole child, and not just the negative experiences or the symptoms. For instance, a provider might say, "I can see that you like to draw when you come in here. Is that something you do other places, too?"

- ◆ Mirroring of a child's negative states, instead of minimizing or working to shift them too rapidly. So, for instance, rather than responding to a statement of "I'm so stupid!" with "No, you're not, you're a great kid," stating instead, "It's so hard to feel sometimes like we can't do anything right. I'm really sorry you're feeling like that right now."

- ◆ Accepting and validating rather than fighting a child's necessary protections, while continuing to communicate interest. When a teen shrugs and refuses to engage in a conversation about his or her likes and dislikes, for instance, rather than pushing or engaging in a power struggle, a provider might state, "You know, we don't know each other super-well, and it makes sense that you're not ready to talk to me much yet. I really do want to try to understand some of who you are and what you want, but we can go at whatever pace works for you."

- ◆ Acknowledging the aspects of self that may be discrepant from our own experience. For instance, when an adolescent states angrily, "What do you know? You have no idea what it's like on the streets near my place," it is crucial that providers respond honestly: "You're right. Our experiences are very, very different, and I can't know what it's like for you. I'll do my best to try to listen and learn from you, but it's true that I'll never completely get what it's like to be you."

🎬 Behind the Scenes

- ■ There are multiple facets involved in development of a comprehensive understanding of self and identity. These include:

  - ◆ *Unique self:* An understanding of individual characteristics, including concrete attributes, likes/dislikes, opinions, values, strengths and vulnerabilities, familial and cultural influences, and spiritual beliefs.

  - ◆ *Positive self:* Ability to tune in to, identify, and own positive attributes of self.

  - ◆ *Cohesive self:* Ability to integrate multiple aspects of self, both strengths and vulnerabilities, across experiences (i.e., past and present) and across affective states.

  - ◆ *Future self:* Ability to envision possibilities, to imagine the self in the future, and to imagine ways to become that self, incorporating both short- and long-term goals.

- ■ For all of the above, sense of identity may encompass self alone as well as **self in relation to others** and **self in context** (e.g., within the context of family, of culture, of school). It is important to explore each of these facets of self on multiple levels.

- ■ Each of these facets of self progresses over the course of development. A 5-year-old's understanding of his or her unique self will differ from an adolescent's, but the concept remains important across developmental stages. See the upcoming section, "Developmental Considerations."

- ■ A number of techniques that may be useful for exploration of self and identity are offered in this chapter. However, when working with children to build self-concept and positive identity, it is crucial to extend the work beyond the therapy room. It is important that children not just talk about who they are, but find ways to explore and express what they identify as self-attributes in their daily lives.

■ Problem-solve with the child and caregivers about potential barriers to exploring areas of interest. For instance, if a child has an interest in the theatre but is shy, can the caregiver support the child in going to the activity with a friend? Provide a safety object for the child to carry?

■ When engaging in the techniques described below, as well as in real-world applications and explorations of self-interests, it is important to include the use of modulation strategies. Many children struggle with sense of self, so activities related to self and identity may elicit a range of affective arousal.

Teach to Caregivers

■ *Reminder:* Teach caregivers the Key Concepts.

■ *Reminder:* Teach caregivers relevant Developmental Considerations.

■ Incorporate caregivers, as appropriate, into treatment. Many of the tasks described in this chapter can be completed dyadically, and, in fact, may be more powerful if done so.

■ The moments that will contribute most strongly to identity formation are likely to occur in daily life rather than in the treatment room. Work with caregivers—whether in the home, milieu, or other settings—to observe, reflect, reinforce, and support a child's exploration of self. This process may broadly involve:

 ◆ Noticing and reinforcing key concepts in the home setting (e.g., "I knew right away that this was your school book cover, because I can see all the symbols that you like decorating it").

 ◆ Using key language across settings (e.g., the language of mixed emotions: "I wonder if you might be feeling more than one thing right now—I know I'm kind of nervous and kind of excited").

 ◆ Incorporating therapeutic activities in the home setting (e.g., creating a "pride wall" at home).

 ◆ Creating unique activities specific to the home setting (e.g., a family photo album, family tree, family collage).

 Teach caregivers specific strategies for supporting each of the four identity targets.

■ Unique self:

 ◆ Provide self-expression opportunities. Let children pick their clothes, style their hair, or decorate a room in their favorite colors.

 ◆ Identify and name your child's patterns ("You pick up new ideas quickly!"). This may help him or her gain self-awareness.

 ◆ Create space for each child's or teen's unique contributions to the family or milieu environment.

 ◆ Support opportunities to identify and explore new interests.

- Pick your battles. Particularly for teens, self-expression is key. Hair, clothes, and music? Only go there if it is crucial.
- Be curious: Try to learn what influences your child/teen.
- Validate things important to the child/teen (values, religion, rituals, and holidays).
- Share and name your own unique influences and interests. Talk about family traditions, values, and historical experiences. These conversations will allow children to understand both where they fit into a larger whole, and where they are forging their own path.

■ Positive self:

- Allow children to identify and try out new interests, and reinforce effort and not just outcomes.
- Redefine success for your child/teen. What does it mean for this child/teen to have a good moment, hour, or day? Look for moments of success on the hardest days, not just the best ones.
- Find one success moment each day and praise it.
- Hang things up—like artwork or homework.
- Foster success by engaging in activities with your child/teen.
- Support more than you criticize (for every negative comment made, make sure your child/teen hears 10 positives).
- Notice small moments of success, even for behavior that is expected ("I really like how cooperative you are being"; "Thank you for being such a great helper").

■ The cohesive self:

- By definition, cohesive self strategies involve supporting the child in recognizing, accepting, and integrating multiple aspects of self across time, state, and context. Examples may include, as described next, strategies to build awareness of present self, support vulnerable aspects of self, and integrate past experiences into current-day narrative. For instance:
- The present self:
  - Capture the present in whatever way makes sense: take pictures, save schoolwork, frame artwork, keep a height chart, make a keepsake box.
- The vulnerable self:
  - Help child/teen to tolerate vulnerable aspects of self by acknowledge and normalizing challenges ("Everyone makes mistakes—I'm sorry we had such a hard day").
  - Try to tolerate children's feelings, even if you don't agree or understand them. A tolerant approach lets children or teens know that their feelings are acceptable.
  - Mirror and support before trying to shift or change a child's or teen's feelings. Even painful feelings are part of our experience of life.
  - Talk about their behavior, not them as people ("I'm frustrated by that behavior" not "You are such a pain").

- Don't label children or teens; labels will become internalized as self-definitions (the hoarder, the cutter, etc.).

- Don't limit their possibilities. Be realistic and supportive but don't assume a child's or teen's past challenges will define his or her future.

◆ The past self:

- Find ways support young people in honoring their history as part of their story. Strategies may include:

    ○ Using the trauma frame when there are opportunities to normalize responses to "hard things" that they have been through in the past.

    ○ Finding ways to reflect on past experiences by, for instance, reviewing old photos from the past, old projects, or schoolwork.

    ○ Writing down or drawing pictures to represent difficult and/or traumatic experiences from the past, if indicated (contained and supported by clinician).

■ The future self:

◆ With young children, allow and support creative and dramatic play. Exploration and imagination are the foundation of the future self. Whenever you can, engage with them.

◆ Help children and teens identify goals, both short and long term, and ways to follow through. Support success at every step.

◆ Build real-world skills in adolescence. Help teens explore vocational and academic interests. Act as a cheerleader and support team. Do not expect independence too soon.

◆ Help children and teens visualize the future. Think beyond jobs and school. Ask where they want to live, what kind of relationships they want to have, what kind of vehicle they might want to drive.

◆ Balance imagination and reality. Allow them to dream, but also identify how they can gain needed skills and develop talents and interests

In group caregiving settings (e.g., residential programs, schools) pay attention to *group* as well as *individual* identity. This may involve both a celebration of diversity (e.g., the unique characteristics of all the individuals who make up the group) and a celebration of community (e.g., those characteristics that unite group members). As with primary caregivers, milieu and other group caregiving systems can tune in to each of the primary targets of identity.

■ The unique self:

◆ *Individual:* What characteristics does *this* child contribute to the setting? In what ways does the child stand out? Use basic reflection and attunement to notice, name, and highlight unique child attributes.

◆ *Group:* What makes individuals within this (program, school, classroom) unique? What are the group values? Goals? Name and explore these. For instance, a classroom might identify and create signs to highlight class values (e.g., respect, safety) or a residential program might create bulletin boards highlighting group member "favorites" (e.g., animals, colors).

■ The positive self:

◆ *Individual:* What successes has the child had (both relative and absolute)? Work with staff to notice and name achievements. Highlight these concretely, when possible.

◆ *Group:* Establish "community pride"; work with group members toward collaborative successes. For instance, set a group goal—perhaps earning a total of *x* points across group members—and celebrate the achievement as a group success.

■ The cohesive self:

◆ *Individual:* Pay attention to ways in which a child's experience may be fragmented (e.g., across affective states, across placements, across peer groups) and name/reflect observed patterns (e.g., "It seems that you feel like you need to be a little tougher when you're hanging out with Lisa and Janice than when you're just with one of the adults"). Normalize differences in experience while working to help the child create cohesiveness (e.g., "It makes sense that the toughest part of you has to show up when you're talking with girls whom you know have been in gangs, and that you can let that part of you relax when you're with staff").

◆ *Group:* Where is there cohesiveness and/or fragmentation across group members? Tune in to the ways that group members' behavior changes when most members are excited, for instance, versus frustrated. Notice times when "factions" of group members splinter off from others and explore the group identity of this faction, while also supporting each individual in honoring unique aspects of self.

■ The future self:

◆ *Individual:* As in individual treatment or in family settings, work with children to imagine themselves in the future, to set concrete goals, and to work toward those goals, considering immediate, short-term, and long-term goals. Within programs, it is particularly important to shift the work eventually beyond the tomorrow/next-week goals and to pay attention to "life-outside-the-program" goals.

◆ *Group:* Work with group members to set programmatic, future-oriented goals. For instance, help group members identify a program-relevant goal (e.g., creating a comfortable group space in a common room, putting on a play, working as a team in a competition) and work with them to identify steps toward reaching it.

Tools: Self-Development and Identity

■ Self-development involves a number of different skills; the next table highlights key aspects of identity and sample tasks.

■ As with other skills highlighted in this framework, the best tasks are often individually targeted; use the following as a guideline, but be creative.

■ Techniques should, to the degree possible, be interactive. Use them to generate discussion between the child and clinician/caregiver.

■ Beyond specific tools and activities, for all of these areas be alert for ways to tune in to, be curious about, and explore self and identity in the moment.

Target #1: Individuality—the Unique Self

■ **Overarching goal:** *Help children identify personal attributes. These include likes and dislikes, values, talents, preferences, opinions, family and cultural influences, and spiritual beliefs.*

■ In addition to formal techniques, tune in to child statements in daily life that represent this concept. Help children expand on these.

Individuality

Sample activity	Description	
"All about Me" books	Suggested materials	Paper, construction paper (for covers), markers/crayons/writing and drawing materials, materials to decorate book, clips or ribbon to bind book, pictures of child or others, as desired
	Techniques	■ Introduce activity to children. Highlight that they will be creating a book that is all about them.
		■ "All-about-Me" books are generally created over time. Often, clinicians will choose to do one page per session with the child.
		■ Content of "All-about-Me" books varies in accordance with child needs and developmental stage.
		■ Content often shifts over time when working in a longer-term therapeutic relationship. It may be important to complete a book and then begin another as a child enters a new developmental stage or life phase, rather than continuing the same book. Creating a new book highlights the theme of change and growth.
		■ Provide structure for young children. For instance, create a page listing the child's favorite colors, names of pets, favorite foods, etc. The focus is generally on concrete attributes. Drawings can be used in lieu of words.
		■ Consider using more abstract concepts with older children. Incorporate affect. For instance, list or draw exciting or frightening experiences that the child has had.
		■ Pay attention to including *personal values*: What is important to this particular child? Keep in mind ways that developmental stage will impact these values (e.g., for a 5-year-old, "Be nice" is a value; for a 15-year-old, "It's important not to pick on people who are weaker than me" is a value).
		■ Tailor entries to child milestones, achievements, and current experiences. Listen for opportunities in the session. For instance, if a child is describing an experience that seems important, suggest writing or drawing about it, and including it in the "All-about-Me" book.
Personal collage	Suggested materials	Posterboard or sturdy construction paper, glue, magazines, pictures, drawings, stickers, letters, etc.
	Techniques	■ Collage is a way for children to represent aspects of the self without a need for words or verbal explanation.
		■ Introduce the technique to children; highlight that they will be creating a collage, using provided materials, to represent different aspects of the self.
		■ Invite children to find materials that either represent something about who they are or that appeal to them. They do not need to be able to explain *why* they are choosing the picture, material, etc.
		■ Collages can be *general* (e.g., "All about you") or they can target *specific ideas* (e.g., "the you no one else sees"; "who you are at school"; "things you enjoy").
Values jar activity	Purpose	To support individual and/or family in identifying values that are an important part of individual and/or family identity.
	Materials	A plastic container, plastic cups and spoons, a small funnel, and various colors of sand (may also use M&M'S).
	Directions	Place each of the sand colors (or M&M'S into a plastic cup. Have the child/youth/caregiver identify and assign an important value to each color (e.g., blue may indicate

Sample activity	Description	
		respect; red may indicate kindness to others; yellow, spirituality). Ask the child/youth/caregiver to determine "amount" of importance attributed to each value and to place that amount of sand into the container.
		Follow up: Develop a plan to follow up on the activity during family meeting; dinnertime go-around, etc.
Artistic self-expression	Suggested materials	Dependent on modality; may include clay, paints, drawing materials, music, pen/paper/journal, etc.
	Techniques	▪ Use array of fine and expressive arts to help children communicate aspects of identity. Consider drawing, writing, poetry, rapping, sculpture, movement, etc. ▪ Artistic self-expression can be done in a structured or informal way. For instance, the clinician may provide a prompt and have the child generate a poem or rap; *or* clinician may encourage child to engage in artistic self-expression, which child may (or may not) choose to share in the session. ▪ Consider incorporating caregivers; have caregivers work with children on artistic projects (this is particularly important with younger children). Encourage older children and adolescents to share the results of their projects with caregivers; if appropriate, invite caregivers into session.
Try it out	Suggested materials	Varies
	Techniques	Exploring identity only goes so far if it is restricted to the office. Help children identify an interest (e.g., hobby, sport, extracurricular activity) and encourage them to "try it out." Incorporate caregivers as allies.

Target #2: Esteem and Efficacy—the Positive Self

▪ **Overarching goal:** *Build internal resources and identification of positive aspects of self.*

▪ In working on self-esteem and efficacy, it is important to take note of both *absolute* strengths (e.g., a child's skill at math or athletics) and *relative successes* (e.g., working hard at a difficult task or recognizing an area of vulnerability and choosing to address it). Help children and the system reframe the concept of success.

Esteem and Efficacy

Sample activity	Description	
Power book	Suggested materials	Paper, construction paper (for covers), markers/crayons/writing and drawing materials, materials to decorate book, clips or ribbon to bind book, pictures of child or others, as desired
	Techniques	▪ Introduce activity to children. Highlight that they will be creating a book about things that make them feel powerful. ▪ Like "All-about-Me" books, power books are generally created over time. Often clinicians choose to do one page per session with a child. ▪ Help children create a cover for the power book. The only rule is that the cover must embody strength or individual power in some way; encourage children to use their imagination. ▪ The goal of a power book is to highlight children's (real and potential) strengths, successes, positive experiences, and internal and external resources. Note that resources do not need to be reality-based; encourage children to use their imaginations to picture *possibilities*. For instance, children might imagine qualities that would make them feel powerful and then picture themselves as an animal, superhero, athlete, etc., who has that quality.

Sample activity	Description	

There are two primary ways to complete power books:
- ◆ *Provide structured prompts* to elicit drawings or writing. For instance, ask children to list their five best qualities; to draw themselves as a superhero; and/or to draw themselves doing something at which they are good.
- ◆ *Include spontaneous success.* Tune in to moments when children display strength, success, or power. Note that definitions of success should include effort as well as relative successes (e.g., the child who is able to get through the day without fighting). When spontaneous successes occur, write or draw about them and include them in the power book.

(*Note* that the above two are not mutually exclusive and that most power books will contain a combination.)
- ◆ Review power books regularly; include them while reviewing treatment plans and goals with child and family. Power books provide a concrete way to track child and family successes.

Pride wall	Suggested materials	Bulletin board or blank wall; index cards or award cards; pen or marker (or other writing utensil); tape or thumbtacks
	Techniques	

- ■ A pride wall is similar to a power book in that the goal is to notice and reinforce moments of success. There are several ways to create a pride wall, depending in part on the setting. Examples are given here.
- ■ *Therapy office:*
  - ◆ Designate a wall or area of the office as a "Pride Wall" (or "Power Wall"). Create a sign or lettering to mark it as such.
  - ◆ Near the pride wall, place a basket or other container with index cards, award cards, etc., as well as pens or markers.
  - ◆ Invite children (or families) to add things of which they are proud to the wall. Children should write a statement about what they are proud of (e.g., "I cleaned my room when Mom asked") and place it on the wall. Note that children should *not* include their name (for reasons of confidentiality).
  - ◆ Invite caregivers to also add pride statements about their child to the wall.
- ■ *Home:*
  - ◆ Pride walls at home are an excellent way to help caregivers "catch their children being good." Invite a family to designate a wall or other area (e.g., large bulletin board) as the pride wall. Again, have index cards and other materials available nearby.
  - ◆ Pair the pride wall creations with attachment work. Help caregivers to notice and reinforce positive child effort and behavior as well as accomplishments.
  - ◆ For families who have difficulty providing positive forms of attention, create structure (e.g., the family must place one item on the pride wall every day).
  - ◆ A family pride wall should include not just individual successes but family successes and accomplishments.
- ■ *School or milieu:*
  - ◆ If treatment is provided in a school or milieu setting, work with staff to create a program pride wall. The wall can be classroom- or group-specific, or placed in a hallway or other public area.
  - ◆ Create rules about who may add to the pride wall, and when. It may be helpful to designate a time when people may add to the wall. Encourage self-nominations, peer nominations, staff nominations, etc.
  - ◆ Celebrate success whenever it happens.

Superhero self	Suggested materials	Drawing materials (e.g., paper, markers/crayons); writing materials; clay or other sculpture materials; other arts materials (e.g., popsicle sticks, felt, pipe cleaners)
	Techniques	

- ■ The goal of this activity is to help the child imagine him- or herself as a superhero.
- ■ Help children define qualities that make a true superhero. Note that these qualities should go beyond simple muscular strength. Have a conversation about what it means to be "strong." Consider that there are many kinds of strength. Help children think of examples of strength they have witnessed, heard about, felt, or

Sample activity	Description
	learned of via movies or books. Provide examples, if necessary (e.g., the strength to raise a child by yourself, the strength to be kind to someone when others are not, the strength to stand up to a bully, the strength to walk away from a fight).
	▪ Help children create a list of superhero qualities: What qualities do the children admire? What qualities are shared by their (real and imaginary) heroes? By people they know and like?
	▪ *Trauma note:* Many children who have been harmed at the hands of a primary caregiver may retain an idealized version of that caregiver, particularly if they have been removed/separated from that caregiver. It is not uncommon, then, for children to name that person as someone who has qualities they admire. If this happens, consider the following steps:
	◆ Validate the child's feelings. It may be important for the child to retain a positive sense of that caregiver.
	◆ Normalize the reality that all people have both positive and not-so-positive qualities.
	◆ Name the qualities (or help the child name the qualities) that the child still admires about that person and/or feelings the child has. This may be as simple as "He's my dad," or "I love him."
	◆ Reinforce for the child that it is okay to have more than one feeling about a person, and that the child can love someone (for instance) and still be angry at that person or sad about things that have happened. (*Note:* Don't push this part of the conversation; some children may not want to go there. The goal is simply to acknowledge the possibility of feeling more than one way.)
	▪ Once a list of qualities has been created, help children imagine themselves as a superhero with all of those qualities. What would they look like? What kind of powers would they have? They might make up a new superhero or choose to imagine themselves as an already existing one—either is fine.
	▪ Go beyond drawing or writing; act out with the child the role of superhero, or have doll or action figure characters take on the role. Imagine dealing with a problem situation as the superhero—how would the superhero use his or her special qualities? How might those qualities help with difficult situations? Play it all out.
	▪ Build on this project; be creative. For instance, children can create a small "secret symbol" of their superhero self and carry it with them, or they can build a model of their superhero self and place it in their room to remind them of strength.
Other tasks	Be creative in choosing tasks to build a child's sense of personal esteem and efficacy. Use drawings, writing, etc., to capture moments when the child succeeds. Make it concrete, so that over time each child has physical representations of moments of success. Incorporate caregivers and other adults into this work.

Target #3: Self across Time and Place: The Cohesive Self

▪ **Overarching goal:** *Help children build a sense of self that integrates past and present experiences and incorporates multiple aspects of self.* In many ways this target emphasizes the idea of developing a life narrative that may be inclusive of, but not exclusively about, the trauma narrative.

▪ A primary contributor to the fragmented self of trauma-impacted children is a difficulty with integrating emotional states. The tasks that follow focus on helping children incorporate an understanding and normalization of multiple affective states and reactions, including ways that feelings flow and change over time.

▪ Many children with whom we work have lived in different homes, with different caregivers, different schools, different neighborhoods, different peers, and different surrounding environments. As children move across contexts, they must enter and adjust to often vastly different cultures. They may be conscious of differences in spoken language or skin color; they may be confronted with new rules, values, food choices, customs, and rituals. These shifts involve numerous challenges. Children may feel they have to abandon the old and create a new self in each new context; they may struggle to integrate different aspects of their environment; and/or they may reject the offerings of new home environments, often leading to further placement disruption. Work with children to explore the ways in which all of their experiences have contributed to who they are and how they see themselves. In addition, work with caregivers to acknowledge, explore, and understand similarities and differences in their children's experience.

▪ Caregivers are often the bearers of children's histories: They hold the memories of "firsts" and other early experiences, of familial history, and of patterns and rhythms of the child's life over time and the ways these weave into a larger narrative. Often, caregivers are the owners of the concrete markers of children's lives, such as photographs, report cards, drawings, and writings. Work with caregivers to support their children in the development of a cohesive narrative. For children who have transitioned (and who continue to transition) among caregiving systems, it is particularly important to work with caregivers to concretely document and capture moments of the child's history, as it is developing.

▪ An understanding of cohesive self includes an awareness of the ways that experiences (emotional, behavioral, relational) relate to one another. Observe and help children tune in to patterns. Help children notice similarities and differences in their experiences over time and across contexts. A "frame" and normalizing language that may be useful for helping children, adolescents, and their caregivers explore this target is the language of parts of self. There may be other words to capture this concept so clinicians should customize language for each individual client.

Teach to Kids: Psychoeducation about Parts or Aspects of Self

▪ Examples of how to speak with children about key teaching points are provided. Keep in mind, however, that psychoeducation should be provided in a developmentally appropriate way, so language will vary from client to client.

Understanding Aspects of Self

Teaching point	Important information as sample language
Everyone has multiple aspects of who they are.	"Everyone—kids and adults—have a lot of different ideas, characteristics, and experiences that make up who we are. These ideas, characteristics, and experiences become part of us, and there are a lot of parts in all of us."
Each part of you is important because it makes you who you are.	"Every part of you is important because that's what makes you, *you*! It's important to think about all of the things that make you who you are, because it can help you understand your wants, needs, and experiences. ▪ "Sometimes our parts are about feelings. For example, there may be a part of you who is mad and a part of you that is happy, or a part of you that is really angry at your mom even though there's part of you that still loves her. ▪ "Sometimes our parts are about interests like the part of you that loves sports or music [clinician should provide specific examples related to the client], and the part of you that sometimes feels like you just don't feel like doing those things that day. ▪ "Sometimes our parts are related to talents like being a really good dancer. One part of you might know that you're great at dancing, while another part of you feels anxious every time you have to be in a show.

Teaching point	Important information as sample language
	▪ "Those parts can also be related to important qualities that we have, like the part of you that is really, really caring and honest.
	▪ "Our experience of self may also change at different times in our lives, based on what is going on or who we're living with—for instance, the way you felt when you lived with your brother and sister, and the different way you felt when you moved into your new home."
Self-protective parts of self and the trauma lens	"You know how we've talked about situations that remind you of hard stuff that's happened in your past and about some of the things that happen now that trigger a fear response—a self-protective response? Well, those protective responses that you have are a part of us as well. Here are some examples of things that may tell us something about our "protective" parts [examples should be specifically tailored to each client]:
	▪ "The part of you that needs to get away when things feel overwhelming
	▪ "The part of you that gets really, really angry when something feels unfair
	▪ "The part of you that expects something bad to happen
	▪ "The part of you that is very selective about relationships because relationships can be hard to trust
	▪ "The part of you that doesn't like to try new things out because you don't feel confident that you will do when.
	"These parts of you may not be present or prominent all the time, but kick up or rise to the surface when something feels dangerous or frightening."
Parts in context	"Different parts of us show up in different places, with different people, and at different times. For example, when you are with your friends, the part of you that likes to play/talk/listen to music may be more present. When you are with your family, because families can be hard, your angry part may come out a bit more. When you are at school. your friends and teachers see the very smart part of you who is excellent at school stuff!"
Each part or aspect of ourselves has specific patterns of thoughts, feelings, and behaviors.	"Different aspects of ourselves show up in lots of different ways. They may show up in our behavior, our bodies, our facial expressions, our thoughts, our tone of voice, and in other ways. Let's consider the part of you that loves [playing basketball]." *Note:* It can be helpful to focus on an identified competency prior to exploring more vulnerable aspects of self:
	Behavior: "When you are on the court, here are some of the behaviors, besides dribbling, shooting, passing, and defending, that come to mind: good sportsmanship, team player, and able to deal with frustration."
	Feelings: "Let's talk about some of the feelings that you experience when you play basketball: happy, proud, competitive, frustrated at times, angry when you lose, excited, and so on. There are many different emotions that you experience depending on how the game is going right?"
	Body: "We've talked about how much your energy can change during a ballgame. From very high energy when you're zooming down the court to make a lay, up to very focused and controlled energy when you are taking deep breaths before a foul shot."
	Thoughts: "Let's think about some of the thoughts that you have when playing basketball. Some may be encouraging thoughts, others not so much. All thoughts are important to put down."
	Note: When exploring vulnerable parts of self, there may be more exploration about context, including triggers as well as risk behaviors. When risk behaviors are included in this work, it is important to use your attunement skills to identify function and to reinforce modulation work.
Explore parts and patterns over time.	During this work it will be important for the clinician to use his or her attunement skills to identify parts as they present in the therapy room and work in collaboration with the client to determine which aspects of client identity are in need of attention at a given point in time during the therapeutic process.

The Cohesive Self

Sample activity	Description	
Life books	Suggested materials	Paper, construction paper (for covers), markers/crayons/writing and drawing materials, materials to decorate book, clips or ribbon to bind book, pictures of child and significant others (including pets), etc.
	Techniques	■ The goal of a life book is to help the child create and "own" a cohesive narrative of who she is, where he comes from, and significant life events. ■ Life books can be particularly useful for children who have been in multiple or disrupted placements, those who have not yet attained permanency in placement, and those who have been adopted or placed into a family that is not their family of origin. Life books are also often helpful for adolescents who are working to understand, make meaning of, and create a narrative about their life experiences and current identity. ■ For younger children, life books should ideally be done with the assistance of a primary caregiver and/or someone who has known the child over time (e.g., an ongoing social services caseworker, a school staff member). ■ There is no single best way to do a life book, and there are many existing models for their construction. In working with a child to construct a life book, consider the following: ■ *Timeline:* ◆ Begin with the basics: What happened, when, and who was involved? ◆ Help children create a timeline of significant life events. For example: Where were they born? How old were they when they started school? Who was their teacher then? What was their house like? ◆ For children who have experienced multiple placements, help them name the different homes in which they have lived and what they did and did not like about each of those homes. ◆ Is there a significant object (e.g., toy, blanket, piece of clothing) that a child has carried over time? If so, draw it or write about it. ◆ Fill in significant events that the child designates—for instance, the child's favorite memory, a birthday party, visits with caregivers or siblings, etc. ◆ Help the child fill in missing information. Elicit help from current caregivers, teachers (with consent), caseworkers, etc. ◆ Once significant life events are identified, place them in roughly chronological order. ■ *Thoughts and feelings:* ◆ Go back through the book with the child. Slowly (be aware of pacing) help the child add information about his or her thoughts and feelings in connection with specific events. Incorporate pictures, words, etc., into relevant places in the book. (*Note:* It is very important that children have ready access to basic affect regulation skills learned prior to beginning this task. These exercises may elicit strong feelings, and children must have a basic repertoire of coping skills.) ◆ For children who are able to do so, help them consider any changes in their feelings: Is how a child feels *now* about the event the same or different from how he or she felt *then*? Write or draw about both. ■ *Meaning and connections:* ◆ Primarily with older children and adolescents, a next step is to look at past events and experiences in connection with the present. Consider examining the following: ◆ How has each event impacted the present? Pay attention to both positive and negative impacts. ◆ How did the child or adolescent cope with or manage the events? What skills were used to survive or get through? How do these skills connect to skills the child or adolescent continues to use? How have these skills changed? ◆ Upon whom was the child or adolescent able to rely when those events happened? Are those people still in the child's life? If not, are there other people who fill similar roles? For people who are no longer present, are there ways for the child to concretely remember them or incorporate their qualities into present life? ◆ In what ways is the child or adolescent still similar to who they were when the events happened? In what ways has he or she changed?

Sample activity	Description	
Aspects of self	Suggested materials	Drawing supplies, paints, felt, popsicle sticks, magazines, masks, shoebox, posterboard, heavy cardboard, white T-shirts, papier-mâché materials, etc. (*Note:* Match materials to selected project.)
	Techniques	The goal of these techniques is to help the child concretely symbolize multiple aspects of self, and to create a single project that integrates the techniques. Note that many different projects could be used for this purpose; suggestions follow.

■ Each of these projects is generally nonverbal; however, it is important that the clinician provide some context for the selected activity. Consider the following teaching point to introduce the project: "We all have many different parts that make up who we are. In this project, we will explore some of those parts."

◆ *Personal crest:* Look up (in books, online, etc.) personal crests or shields so that children have a model. Help children create their own crest. (For younger children or those who have difficulty with unstructured tasks, it is often helpful to provide an outline of a crest as a starting point; see sample identity shields in Appendix D.) The crest should include several sections (this can be as simple as drawing a crosshatch to break the crest into four parts). Help children generate symbols that represent different aspects of self; incorporate these into each child's personal crest. Note that this activity can be as simple or complex as a child wishes.

◆ *Masks:* Create (or purchase) blank white masks and decorate according to selected goal. Many different variations on this task are possible, and clinician and child may choose to do more than one. For instance:
  ● How the child feels on the inside (inside of mask) versus what he or she shows on the outside (outside of mask)
  ● Different facets of the child on different sections of mask
  ● Different emotions: Where the child shows emotion; how often (or how much of) that emotion the child shows; how much of that emotion the child feels, etc.
  ● How different people see the child versus how the child sees him- or herself
  ● The child in different contexts

◆ *Ingredients of self:* Use a shoebox or other container to help the child symbolically represent the multiple aspects of self. Place in the shoebox pictures, objects, words, etc., that symbolize different qualities that the child selects to represent him- or herself. Child may choose to decorate the outside of the box or leave it blank.

◆ *Building blocks:* On thick posterboard trace a flattened three-dimensional block or have available ready-made foam blocks. Help the child decorate each block with symbols, pictures, or words that represent one facet of him- or herself. Put the blocks together.

◆ *Personal puzzles:* Prior to working with the child, cut a puzzle out from thick posterboard. Provide the child with individual puzzle pieces and ask him or her to decorate each piece with symbols, pictures, or words that represent one facet of him- or herself. Put the puzzle together and look at the different ways the parts intersect.

◆ *Parts of self—circles:* In talking about various aspects of the self, invite the child to depict them (e.g., as simple circles for each identified part or aspect of self) and apply simple labels or "names," using the client's labels—for instance, "mad," "caring," "protective," "vulnerable," or "superman," "hulk," "batman," etc.

◆ *The hand you deal—top five:* Invite children to write down different personal qualities on different index cards. For instance, a child might write "kind" on one card and "protective" on another. Encourage children to think of themselves in different contexts ("When you're upset," "When you're with your dad," "at school," etc.). Add to the deck over time. When talking about different experiences, invite children to re-sort the deck, pulling up their "top five." Notice which patterns of qualities tend to "cluster," and the ways in which other qualities or aspects of self may retreat in different situations.

◆ *Note:* This same activity can be used to explore relationships with others by picking an individual (e.g., "My dad") and listing different qualities that may emerge at different times. When used in this way, this activity may be very useful for helping youth explore fragmentation or different aspects of self displayed by key relationship partners (e.g., "Dad when he's drinking and Dad when he's sober").

Cohesive Self: Developing a Narrative around Traumatic Experiences

■ The processing or integration of specific memories and experiences into a broader narrative of self is often what is classically thought of as "trauma processing." This process involves careful exploration of aspects of memory and the intertwined/associated affect, physiological sensation, and cognition, both in the past and in the present. Through supporting the child in sitting with, tolerating, moving through, and observing his or her own experiences, the child is able (1) to integrate these experiences into a larger and more cohesive story of self; (2) to decrease the intensity and power of these experiences and therefore of their intrusive nature; and (3) to gain mastery over them.

■ In working with children who have experienced complex trauma, there are two types of more specific narratives related to creating a cohesive self that are likely to be relevant:

1. *Life narrative:* The development of a broader narrative that encompasses the many experiences of the child's life, across time and place, and includes traumatic exposures as well as more positive life experiences.
2. *Specific memories:* The processing and integration of specific memories, fragments of memory, or composite memories that are particularly distressing for the child and/or intrude into his or her life.

■ The development of a life narrative is clearly a process that takes place over time and includes, but is not specific to, trauma exposures. Work around the construction of life books or "All about Me" books, as described above, are an example of the process of constructing a cohesive life narrative.

■ Creating a narrative around specific memories is an important component of supporting children in developing a cohesive sense of self.

■ The following three factors—timing, what to target, and format—are among those to be considered when addressing specific memories with children.

Timing. When is it appropriate to target specific memories?

■ Historical experiences are incorporated into the language of skills development throughout this framework, and when treating a child who has experienced complex developmental trauma, these experiences are present in the room and named from early in the therapeutic process. This acknowledgment is often simple, such as, "When kids have really hard things happen, like what happened with your dad, it can be really tough to manage feelings."

■ This broader frame is distinct from the more detailed exploration encompassed in the processing of specific memories. The exploration of traumatic memory has the potential to elicit intense, potentially overwhelming affect, physiological sensation, and cognitive and behavioral dysregulation. It is crucial to consider the child's current functioning as well as current context when discerning whether to open, versus contain, traumatic memories. To safely explore memory, a child must have some capacity to modulate affect and physiology, must have developed some sense of safety in the therapeutic relationship, and must have a sufficiently stable context outside of the clinical space. In the absence of these factors, extensive exploration of the details of memory may lead to further harm and destabilization, rather than healing.

■ Having acknowledged the caution, the reality is that specific memories and experiences are likely to emerge in various ways and at many different times, regardless of whether we judge a child to be "stable" or not. Although some trauma processing work will be planned, a great deal will occur in the moment, in response to material the child presents. The professional's capacity to attune to the child and to be ready to respond to this material is crucial. The decision about whether to expand or contain material will depend on clinician judgment regarding the factors just delineated. Regardless of the decision, it is important to observe, acknowledge, and reflect the child's experience. Consider the following example.

> Delia is an 8-year-old girl who is in a short-term foster placement, having recently transitioned out of a longer placement that was disrupted. She has experienced a sharp increase in distressed functioning over the past several weeks, including statements about wanting to hurt herself. When meeting with her therapist, whom she has seen for several years, Delia positions two dolls in a sexual position and states, "That's how my dad liked to do it." The therapist responds, "It seems like you're thinking about your dad." Delia nods, then grabs the dolls and puts them in separate rooms in the dollhouse. The therapist states, "I know those can be scary thoughts when they come up. Have you been thinking about him a lot?" Delia shrugs and then nods. The therapist responds, "I'm sorry to hear that. It looks like you're feeling kind of sad and mad, just thinking about it now." Delia takes the male doll out of the dollhouse and throws it. "I don't like it!" The therapist validates Delia's current experience by stating, "Those are such big feelings you're having. What happened with your dad was really scary, and even though we've talked about the fact that you're never going to have to live with your dad again, I'm wondering if part of you might be scared about that." Delia shrugs but doesn't answer. The therapist says, "It seems like these are really important thoughts and feelings. Would you like to draw or write about some of the feelings and then find somewhere to put them so that you don't have to take them home with you?" Delia nods. The therapist works with Delia to do an energy and feelings self-check, and then to practice a modulation strategy, before drawing a picture of her feelings. When they have finished, the therapist lets Delia choose where to put the drawing; Delia selects a drawer in the therapist's desk she has used before for this purpose. The therapist and Delia then take several deep breaths, with the therapist guiding Delia in breathing in "calm" and breathing out any scary feelings or distress. The therapist makes sure there is sufficient time for less intense material (e.g., a game) before the session comes to a close.

In this example, the clinician is confronted with emerging intrusive material in a child who has experienced recent instability of living arrangements (placement disruption), along with destabilized presentation. Given these factors and the tenuous nature of the child's current relationship with her caregivers, the clinician chose not to explore in detail the child's intrusive memories; however, the clinician must still acknowledge and in some way explore the child's experience. By acknowledging the important nature of the memory, gently exploring the child's current experience, allowing the child to express a key component of the memory (i.e., the affect), and carefully containing the material, the clinician allows the child to achieve some mastery over her distress, without increasing the intensity of it beyond her capacity to manage. At another time, and in another context, the clinician might have further explored the details or nature of the child's memory or experiences.

What to Target. For children who have had many overwhelming experiences, it may be difficult to identify the focus of a trauma narrative. Consider the following.

■ *Specific emerging memories.* Some children will identify specific memories that are intruding into daily life. These memories, or memory fragments, are typically an important target for processing.

■ *Composite experiences.* When children have had multiple experiences of similar acts (e.g., repeated sexual or physical violence), memories may merge and overlay each other. In creating a narrative, it is likely that memory will encompass details of multiple experiences. It is possible to explore experiences in more thematic rather than specific ways. For instance, when working with a child who has a history of exposure to ongoing domestic violence, details explored may include memories of the father's voice, memories of noises, places in which the child hid, feelings in the child's body when hiding, or thoughts and fears while listening to parents fight. These details may encompass multiple experiences rather than a single one.

■ *High-impact experiences.* For many children who have experienced repeated and multiple early trauma exposures, the experiences that stand out may not be the ones we would anticipate. When asked about worst experiences, an adolescent may identify abruptly leaving a favorite foster mother and leaving a school without a chance to say goodbye to peers, as more distressing than early experiences of violence. Many of these experiences will emerge over the course of the therapy process, particularly in the context of constructing a larger life narrative (e.g., while identifying "significant events" or creating a timeline). These high-impact experiences are important to explore both in the details of the memory and in their influence on present systems of meaning.

Format. The mechanism for processing memories in childhood will vary depending on the child's age, developmental stage, and specific tolerance and preference. In the "Tools" section we discuss various techniques for exploring memory.

STEPS TOWARD PROCESSING SPECIFIC MEMORIES

In the following material we highlight five steps involved in the processing of specific memories. This work often proceeds over a period of time, with layers of detail and understanding added to narratives as the work progresses. Although each of these steps may happen in some way within a single session, it is likely that the creation and exploration of a narrative around an experience, and the integration of that experience into a larger narrative of self, will unfold over an extended time.

■ *Step 1:* **Support the child in self-assessment and modulation strategies.**

◆ To truly process and explore traumatic memory, a child must be able to sustain connection to the experience of exploring it. When entering into this work, invite the child to do a self-check regarding affect and physiological state (or reflect observed affect/ state). Number scales, such as those discussed in "Skill #1: Understanding Degrees of Feeling and Energy" (p. 207) in modulation (e.g., "How do you feel on a −1 to +10 scale?") are often helpful. Many therapies that focus on the processing of memory recommend the use of a "SUDS" (subjective units of distress) scale (e.g., 0–10 or 0–100) to assess a child's level of distress in relation to a memory, and to ensure that he or she is not shutting down or disconnecting. It is helpful to assess level of distress and arousal at the start of the work and in an ongoing way as the work progresses. Use modulation strategies to achieve a state that is tolerable for the child and effective for the work. Consider the range of coping skills developed with the child while building a "Feelings Toolbox" (see Chapter 11). Also consider specific strategies that may be useful in safely building a narrative, such as (1) helping the child achieve distance from the memory (e.g., "When you tell me this memory, tell me as if you are watching it from outside, like on a TV screen, instead of being in it"); (2) helping the child increase his or her sense of safety by introducing protective mechanisms (e.g., "While we talk about this, imagine that the little girl you're talking about has a safety bubble around her, so that no one can hurt her") or protective people/figures (e.g., "Imagine that your favorite superhero is standing right next to you"); and (3) increasing ties to the present (e.g., "While we're talking about this, I'm going to remind you every little bit to wiggle your toes against the floor, so you can remember that you're sitting here in the room with me, okay?").

- *Step 2:* **Guide the telling of the story in a careful, paced way.**

  - ◆ This step involves the telling of the story, whether through narrative, play, drawing, or other techniques. Support the child in the creation of a narrative: At what point does the child's memory start? What happened next? Work to create a narrative with a beginning, a middle, and an end. Move slowly in this work; allow the child choice in pacing and depth. Often, narratives are created over time. If returning to a previous narrative, review the work and add detail. In the "Tools" section of this chapter, we discuss examples of ways to facilitate the creation of narratives. Use SUDS or other concrete markers to explore the level of distress a memory evokes over time; an important goal of trauma processing is to diminish distress around specific memories as the child's exploration of them unfolds.

  - ◆ It is very important to be aware of indications that a child's processing or narrative is "stuck," or that the child is reexperiencing, rather than mastering, traumatic memory. In young children look for indicators of posttraumatic play, such as play with repetitive themes that may include literal or symbolic aspects of traumatic experience, and play that appears rigid and difficult to redirect, and in which the child's affect appears constricted or driven rather than enjoyable (Gil, 1991; Terr, 1990). With older children and adolescents be on the lookout for demonstrations of intense affect or sudden constriction, shifts in presentation (e.g., an adolescent who suddenly switches into a baby voice, or who speaks about him- or herself in the third person), and evidence that the child is reliving, rather than remembering, the experience (e.g., an adolescent who is shaking, crying, and pushing outward with his or her arms, as if to push someone away, and who appears unable to respond to clinician statements). If any of these occurs, the child is no longer "processing," and it will be important to focus on modulation, reestablishment of safety, and reengagement with the present.

- *Step 3:* **Facilitate self-appraisal and expand and explore the memory in context.**

  - ◆ Establishing the details of a memory is only the first step in creating a narrative. Over time, work with the child to go beyond the "facts" of the memory and facilitate the child's appraisal of his or her experience, including thoughts and beliefs, feelings, physiological sensations, and actions. Support the child in creating connections across elements—for example: "When they started to yell, I got really scared. My body just went all tense and my stomach got tight, like I was going to be sick. I wished I could stop them, but I was so scared I just couldn't move."

For very young children (or for children who are younger developmentally), this connection may occur through the reflected lens of the clinician or caregiver (with dollhouse play): "I can see that that little girl is hiding in the corner. So much scary stuff is happening, and she looks very scared. I wonder if her whole body is feeling scared, like her tummy hurting or her muscles feeling all tight." Over time, go beyond the specific memory and expand, at age-appropriate levels, on the larger context in which the experience took place. This may include incorporating (1) other experiences (e.g., was this experience representative of other times or distinct from them?); (2) nuances of relationship (e.g., acknowledging and exploring the range of feelings, including positive ones, a child may have about someone who hurt him or her; exploring the role of, and child's feelings about, other individuals who may or may not have been involved); and (3) other relevant and contributing factors (e.g., a parent's substance abuse or mental health issues).

- *Step 4:* **Engage in modulation to sustain connection to affect.**
    - ◆ As the work progresses, it is important to repeatedly revisit the child's level of arousal and affective state. Check in frequently and support the child in using modulation skills, as needed, to remain "present" and connected to the process.

- *Step 5:* **Explore and develop systems of meaning.**
    - ◆ In the final stage of processing, we work with the child to form a perspective on the past from the context of the present. This step involves observing past experience and its influence on the child's life, his or her sense of self, relationships with others, and systems of meaning. It is in this stage that we work with the child to explore not just past affect but also the thoughts and feelings that occur in the present moment when reflecting on that experience (e.g., "I just feel so mad at myself for not doing anything"). Psychoeducation and reality testing are often important components of this stage and may involve acknowledgment and exploration of the thought/feeling/wish in the moment (e.g., "It's my job to protect my mom"), as well as the building of more realistic appraisals from the present perspective (e.g., "Even though part of me still wishes I could have, he was just so much bigger than me, so there was no way I could have stopped him").

        Move beyond past and present to consider the future: In the past, for instance, no one may have helped; in the present and future, who might the child be able to trust? What skills, strengths, and resources does the child now have with which to protect him- or herself? In what ways has the child developed parts of self that go beyond this single (or multiple) experience(s)? Take note of ways to build cohesive links from past to present to future. Over time, we may link this memory to other behaviors and experiences and explore relevant ongoing patterns of response. Ultimately, an important goal is to *contextualize intense and fragmented memories into the larger narrative* of the child's life, so that various aspects of self and experience can be examined as part of a larger whole.

Target #4: Future Orientation

- **Overarching goal:** *Build children's ability to imagine self in the future and to build connections between current actions and future outcomes.*

- Keep in mind that "future" will be a different concept at different developmental stages; for young children, the future may be a week from now; for adolescents, the future may be 20 years from now.

- In addition to formal exercises, pay attention in the session to connecting current actions and experiences to future goals.

Future Orientation

Sample activity	Description	
Future self drawing	Suggested materials	Paper, drawing materials
	Techniques	■ The future self drawing is a concrete tool to help children begin to imagine themselves in the future. The technique can be more or less sophisticated, depending on each child's developmental stage. ■ Prompt children to imagine themselves in the future. Where will they be? What will they look like? Who else might be with them? What will they be doing? For children who have difficulty imagining a future self, prompts should be as concrete as possible (e.g., "What do you think you might want to be when you grow up?"). ■ Have children draw a picture of their imagined future self. ■ This technique is often helpful to repeat over the course of treatment. Note differences in children's ability to imagine a future self. ■ Older children may prefer to describe the future self in words rather than drawing a picture.
5 years, 10 years, 20 years in the future	Suggested materials	Paper, drawing materials
	Techniques	■ This technique is similar to the preceding future self drawing, but expands the concept to help children imagine the steps needed in reaching their future self. This technique is primarily geared toward older children and adolescents. ■ Separate a piece of paper into three sections (or use three sheets of paper). Sections represent increments of time (e.g., 5 years, 10 years, and 20 years in the future). ■ Prompt children to imagine future goals: Where would they like to be 20 years from now? Based on response, what goals would children want to accomplish in 5 and 10 years as steps toward achieving that goal. For instance: If a child states that he wants to be a professional baseball player in 20 years, what would help him get there in the immediate future? In 5 years? In 10 years? ■ Incorporate, to the degree possible, external sources of support. For instance, who in the child's life can help him reach his goal? What kind of person (or people) might the child want to have in his life in the future? ■ Draw (or write about) each of these stages. ■ Note that this task involves both anticipating and imagining the future, as well as goal-oriented planning and understanding the concept of goal-related steps.
Life book addendum	Suggested materials	Previously created life book, drawing and/or writing materials
	Techniques	■ This task is an addendum to the already created life book by adding "future" into previously examined "past" and "present." ■ Work with the child to imagine herself in the future (note that this can be done via the previous exercise). ■ Review the life book. What qualities has the child already developed that will help her reach the goal? What experiences has the child had that will prepare her for the future? What qualities or skills does child still want to build for the future?

🚶 Developmental Considerations

Developmental stage	Self-development and identity considerations
Early childhood	Early childhood understanding of the unique self is basic and often concrete. Help children build an understanding of individual qualities and unique attributes. Ask children's opinions: "What flavor do you like best?" "What color shirt would you like to wear today?" Work with caregivers to encourage children to have unique likes and dislikes and to express themselves (even if their clothing doesn't match).
	Children can start developing a sense of personal values from an early age. Work with children and caregivers to understand and build child and family values. Again, keep it simple. Work with caregivers to use age-appropriate language to explain personal choices (e.g., why the family goes to church), rationale for rules (e.g., why it is not okay to hit someone), etc.
	Help children begin to track changes in self over time. Concrete markers are useful. For instance, have a family designate a doorway on which to measure a child's growth at regular intervals, create a collage of school pictures from year to year, etc.
	Future orientation at this age is often fantasy- rather than reality-based. Encourage this; it is important for young children to have multiple possible futures and to engage their imaginations.
Middle childhood	Individuality becomes more nuanced as children become more independent. Work with caregivers to tolerate children's expression of independent preferences (e.g., decorating their bedrooms, hairstyle, clothing).
	Middle childhood is an age of vulnerability to peer influence. Help children identify unique qualities that make them stand out from other children, as well as ways in which they are similar to their peers.
	Understanding of values begins to be more sophisticated at this stage. Work with caregivers and children to identify personal values, familial values, and cultural values. Encourage children to act on their values. Work with caregivers to find forums in which children can concretely express personal and familial values (e.g., volunteer opportunities).
	Children in this stage are able to develop a basic understanding of short- and long-term goals and ways in which present choices impact the future. Work with children to identify goals and the steps with which to achieve them. Keep in mind that long-term goals often continue to be fantasy-oriented at this age (e.g., the child may still want to be a major league baseball player or a rock star), but short-term goals begin to be more grounded in day-to-day experience.
Adolescence	Identity is a primary task of adolescence. Keep in mind that adolescence is an age of extremes and exploration. Adolescents try on, experiment with, and discard various aspects of self. Help them do this in a meaningful way: What appeals to them about the people with whom they associate? The activities they are trying? What do these activities help them know about themselves? Continue to build cohesiveness in sense of self.
	Adolescents are often self-conscious; as they focus on exploration of their own identity, there is a belief that others are similarly focused on them. For teens who have experienced trauma, this self-consciousness can exacerbate feelings of damage, difference, and disconnection. This may be particularly true for teens who identify as being separate from the mainstream in some way (e.g., teens exploring sexual identity). Because of these additional challenges, it may be particularly important to work with adolescents to identify and celebrate aspects of the unique self.
	Adolescents with trauma histories often disconnect from their physical self, particularly as the developing body begins to change. It is particularly important at this stage to incorporate the physical self into identity development tasks. Help adolescents (re)connect to their bodies and tune in to their physical selves. Pay attention to self-care, physiological expression, and sexual identity. Psychoeducation and open discussion are essential.
	Adolescent values often grow beyond those of their family to encompass peer, iconic/cultural, and personal/independent values. Help adolescents explore and delineate values that are separate from those of their family.
	In normative development, adolescents are able to envision the future self in an abstract way while setting realistic goals. It is important to work with adolescent clients to build this ability as a primary developmental task.

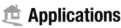 Applications

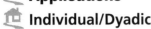 Individual/Dyadic

Self/identity activities are often integrated in different ways at different stages of therapy. Early in treatment, the self may be an area of focus as the therapist learns about the child. Particularly in trauma-focused treatment, it is essential that clinicians communicate an interest in the whole child, rather than in just the trauma experience. Over time, exploration of the self generally becomes deeper. Self and identity book activities, as described in this chapter, are good exercises to incorporate into routine check-ins (e.g., consider adding a weekly experience to the child's book). Self activities can be used to help the child build a cohesive narrative about the trauma experience as well as other life stories. Often, the focus on self and identity happens "in the moment": Listen for opportunities relevant to the targets of unique self, positive self, cohesive self, and future self, and build on these with conversation and activities. When possible and appropriate, integrate caregivers for a portion of this work. For instance, caregivers may be able to (1) provide additional information for a child's life story, (2) name and reinforce their child's strengths, and (3) help in building "action plans" for trying out new skills and interests.

Group

Group activities can easily be designed around and incorporate self and identity activities, particularly with adolescents. Activities can be both overt and subtle. For instance, consider incorporating questions relevant to identity into routine group "icebreakers" (e.g., all group members name their favorite car, the animal they would be). Icebreakers can be collected and may become part of individual "All about Me" books/projects and/or can be collected as part of a larger "All about Us" group book/project. Group identity activities should generally start by focusing on the external self and more concrete attributes before moving to the internal self, in order to allow group safety to build. Examples of group activities that incorporate identity concepts include paired interviews (e.g., children interview each other about individual attributes and report back to the group); creation of collages, masks, and identity shields; creation of physical value lines (e.g., group members identify a range of values; for each value, children physically place themselves between two points to indicate how important that value is to them); and creation of family sculptures (e.g., physical placement of group members in a frozen table to represent family dynamics). Examples of group activities relevant to this construct appear in Appendix C.

Milieu

A milieu system offers an excellent way to tap into and celebrate individual client identity as well as system identity. Consider incorporating visual displays that celebrate diversity, positive child accomplishments, and systemic philosophy and values. Build forums that tap into children's positive self, such as talent shows, as well as unique self, such as special holiday celebrations. Help clients concretely work toward their future selves by supporting goal setting and by teaching and supporting tasks relevant to success beyond the particular milieu program. Teach staff about the four facets of self and work with staff to recognize, explore, and reinforce key identity issues in day-to-day conversation.

⟳ Trauma Experience Integration: State-Based Skills Application

Distress Tolerance and Regulation

During early stages of treatment or when children/adolescents are experiencing more intense stress, it is important to anchor the work and foundational skills in positive and unique facets of self and identity. ARC intervention is grounded in our belief that individuals are resilient and that intervention should engage with the whole child rather than solely those aspects of the child connected with traumatic experiences. We set the stage for positive identity early on by normalizing experiences and adaptation to experiences and by supporting exploration of and reflection upon strengths. Identification of positive attributes often incorporates reframing identified "problem behaviors" as survival strengths. Attunement work with the caregiving system emphasizes the importance of understanding that child behaviors are functional strategies for meeting primary needs.

In addition, in this phase identity work provides opportunities for engagement. Exploration of unique characteristics and interests is often present during this phase. Techniques such as the "All about Me" activities provide a safe container for identity exploration as well as a template for relational connection over time (moving from interests and likes to more vulnerable content as the relationship progresses).

Curiosity and Reflection

As the child or adolescent is increasingly able to engage in reflection, and during more regulated states, self and identity work can focus on identification of more vulnerable self-states and the patterns of experience that are linked to those states. For instance, a child or adolescent may be able to identify a self-state that experiences and demonstrates anger and aggression. As the client develops greater coping resources and self-awareness, which allow sustained exploration over time, he or she may be able to begin to link that angry and aggressive state to a number of factors, including (1) specific triggers ("When my mom ignores me, I get so angry that I want to flip out—and sometimes I do"); (2) patterns of experience that emerge during that state ("Every time I feel ignored by my mom, I get so overwhelmed with anger that I can't think; I start yelling and screaming; I want to punch her; but I usually just throw things and call her names); and (3) awareness of the function of behaviors ("I think that when Mom ignores me, I am reminded of other times when she wasn't there for me, and I just want to push her away—literally").

In addition, children and adolescents who are able to reflect can begin to make some basic links between past (who I was), present (who I am), and future (who I want to be) within a familial and social context. Work can often focus on building a life narrative that includes those time periods and influential experiences that have occurred or may be imagined. A primary goal is increasing a child's or adolescent's understanding of and tolerance for a cohesive and integrated sense of self and personal identity.

Engaging Purposeful Action

Over time, as children and adolescents are increasingly able to tolerate connection to internal experience and have developed awareness of and language for internal self-states, they can begin to deepen their exploration of traumatic experience and to develop (with provider and/or relevant attachment figures) a trauma narrative within their broader story of self. Often a child's or adolescent's unique and positive sense of self contributes significantly to this process by informing the modality or technique that is used to construct the narrative. For instance, if art is a primary area of interest and competency, then the story may be told through art. An adolescent with whom we worked loves music used preferred song titles to construct her narrative. The family can also be encouraged to participate and to construct a family narrative that incorporates aspects of self-development (unique, positive, cohesive) as well as shared traumatic experiences.

Finally, during this phase, orientation to the future is supported and encouraged. This focus is often paired with executive function work where clear future goals are identified as steps toward goal attainment. When engaging purposeful action, clients are able to hold the idea that they are agentic, that the future holds possibility, and that they have the capacity to achieve desired goals and outcomes.

Real-World Therapy

Give it time. Many (if not all) of the children with whom we work have developed a strongly damaged sense of self. Tuning in to the positives is not only foreign but may be triggering, because the positive self is ego-dystonic. Be aware of pacing, and don't force something on children that they are not yet ready to accept. Be flexible; if a child cannot name any current positive qualities, for instance, can he or she imagine one he or she might someday have? Can you or the caregiver name one? Work *around* and *with* children's defenses.

Risks are scary. Much of the work described previously involves not just naming aspects of self but also exploring and trying them on. However . . . new exploration involves risks, and traumatized children have learned to minimize those. Go slowly and build internal and external resources that will help children manage the anxiety that comes with taking risks.

Whose business is it? Identity and self are, at core, often private domains. Sharing the self with another can create vulnerability. Be aware that clients may choose not to share aspects of self (particularly those they have learned to routinely hide from others) and/or may err on the side of sharing only "pleasing" aspects of self. It is important to validate the need for privacy and to acknowledge that we all have parts of self that we are more or less comfortable sharing. Look for ways to do this work that increase children's sense of safety. For instance, allow children to write or draw in a journal that only they see, create symbols without using words; allow children to choose which of the symbols or drawings they wish to share.

Part VII

Model Integration

15

Trauma Experience Integration Revisited

In Chapter 3 of this book, we define "trauma experience integration" as the sequential development of the capacity to first survive and tolerate moments of overwhelming distress and arousal brought on by both real and perceived experiences of danger in the world; to develop over time the ability to engage curiosity and reflect upon those states; and ultimately to be able to engage developmental capacities in service of purposeful action in the present moment. As described in Chapter 4 and throughout the book, we view the treatment process—and in fact, the human developmental process, regardless of traumatic exposure—as a fluid one that involves movement in and out of periods and moments of at times greater and at times lesser resourced functioning. As the child's (or adult's) developmental abilities grow and solidify, and as environmental safety increases and exposures to stress diminish, the individual is increasingly able to reliably harness developmental capacities in a purposeful and goal-oriented manner.

Throughout treatment, we invoke the foundational strategies of engagement, education, and routine to support the child, caregiver, and provider's ability to safely enter into, partner in, and feel empowered by the process of treatment or service provision, and to build an empathic understanding of those behaviors or experiences that have led the child or family to seek supports. We apply the eight core ARC targets in an integrated way, in support of system stability, caregiver and child safety, and increasing developmental capacities such as the abilities to tolerate experience, negotiate relationship, make active choices, and develop a healthy and cohesive understanding of self and other.

In Chapter 4, we first introduced Emma in the following brief vignette, as a means of illustrating the ways in which historical experiences emerge in and interfere with present functioning:

> Emma's aunt, who is her legal guardian, has picked her up from school and is driving her to an appointment. Emma, 13, begins to tell her aunt a story about something that happened at school that day. Her aunt is focused on the road, and midway through the story, fails to respond to a question Emma asked. Emma becomes enraged, yelling and calling her aunt an expletive. When the aunt begins to set a limit ("Calm down! I'm trying to drive") Emma shouts, "Stop yelling at me!" She then unlocks the car door and begins to open it, threatening to jump out even though the car is still in motion.

In this chapter, we return to Emma, describing through her history and treatment the fluid, synthesizing process of trauma experience integration.

Emma's Brief History

In the case vignette of Emma, we are given a glimpse of her in a moment in time. It is a moment in which her actions, behaviors, relational style, and emotional experience are partly about that moment, but are also very much about the combination of moments that came before. Throughout this book, we stress the importance of understanding the child, the caregiver, and the system in context, and of developing intervention approaches that are grounded in a formulation of the child and family system. An important part of that formulation is building an understanding—to the degree possible—of the child's story: the range of experiences that came before the present moment.

> Emma, a 13-year-old European American girl, is the only child of her father and mother, although she has learned from her aunt that she has three half-siblings on her father's side whom she has never met. Emma's father and mother both had significant mental health challenges and were active substance users, and during the 4 years that Emma lived with them, she was exposed to a chaotic and unpredictable living environment, frequent violence, and inconsistent caregiving. Emma's memories of her early childhood are hazy, but she has visceral memories of being hungry as well as a vivid memory of hiding in a closet in the dark while there were sounds of yelling and things breaking on the other side of the door.
>
> Emma was first removed from her parents when she was 4 years old, having been found walking alone on the street at night with no shoes. Over the course of the next 2 years, she moved through a series of foster homes interspersed with placement back with her mother; her father had since been incarcerated on charges of possession of opiates with intent to distribute. During her final removal from her mother, Emma was evaluated due to observed sexualized behaviors, and in that evaluation disclosed sexual abuse by her father and physical abuse by both parents. Emma's mother refused to engage with service plans set up by child welfare, and Emma's goal was changed at the age of 6 to adoption. Shortly after her goal was changed, Emma's maternal aunt, who had been estranged from her sister, Emma's mother, was identified as a placement resource, and Emma transitioned to her home. Emma was legally adopted by her aunt at age 9.

Emma's Early Treatment History

> Emma first entered into treatment when she was 7. She attended a short-term treatment group for sexually abused girls focused on body boundaries and safety, and participated in individual play therapy for 6 months. Her aunt was reluctant to engage in treatment and felt like she and Emma did "well enough." She pulled Emma from treatment when she was 8, although she agreed to let Emma see the school therapist as needed.
>
> When Emma entered seventh grade at age 12, her aunt's concerns escalated. Emma had always been a compliant, cooperative girl, albeit "needy"; however, with the transition into middle school she began to become moodier, defiant, and withdrawn. She spent time alone in her room, snuck out to see her friends, and could escalate quickly into arguing

with her aunt. Her aunt found cigarettes in a drawer and worried that Emma was using other substances. She also suspected that Emma was cutting herself, as Emma had recently begun wearing long sleeves even when it was warm out, and had reacted strongly, shouting and running out of the house, when her aunt asked where she had gotten what appeared to be a superficial cut on her arm. When she hadn't returned home an hour later, her aunt called the police. Emma was screened by an emergency team that night when she finally returned to her home at midnight, and had her first inpatient hospitalization at that time. Emma then spent 6 months moving through a series of hospitalizations and day treatment programs, before being referred for trauma treatment shortly after her 13th birthday.

The Course of Treatment: Trauma Experience Integration through Attachment, Regulation and Competency

Engagement and Relationship

As described in Chapter 5, engagement is a necessary foundation for any service provision process. In the absence of client "stake," even the best technique will fail. Engagement—the child, caregiver's, and/or provider system's belief that the process is meaningful, valid, and tolerable—is an ongoing process that begins when the child or family enters into relationship with the service provider, and it must continue to be cultivated by all players throughout.

> Emma's aunt was clear when she first called the outpatient therapist that she was leery about treatment. "We've been through pretty much everything," she reported, "And honestly, I don't know that it's done a bit of good."
>
> The therapist responded empathically, reflecting the aunt's experience. "I know that for so many families I've worked with, it can be really hard to find a treatment process that feels like a good match. I think this is especially true when your child or family has been through some really complicated experiences, like it sounds is the case for Emma. I can't promise that this treatment will feel perfect either, but when we all meet, we can talk through the ways that I usually work, see how good a match that is for you and Emma, and take it from there."

Treatment using ARC rests on a foundation of transparency, education, and empowerment of the client. Early meetings involve conversations about the ARC treatment approach and the role of all players (treatment system, child, caregiver); curiosity about child and family goals, and alignment of these with core ARC targets; education about and integration of the trauma lens, or the link between current behaviors and historical experiences; and enacting attunement processes by taking a curious, reflective stance about the child and family system.

> In early meetings with the therapist, Emma alternated between being quiet and withdrawn and actively challenging. In the second meeting, Emma confronted the therapist.
>
> EMMA: This is stupid. My aunt thinks she's going to fix me by sending me here. You don't know anything about me.
>
> THERAPIST: You're right, I don't know much. I do know that I wouldn't even begin to try to "fix you," because I don't think you're broken.

EMMA: Then you're just dumb.

THERAPIST: *(Laughs.)* I might be. But we've met a couple of times now, and I'm pretty impressed with you, to be honest.

EMMA: *(Quiet now, picking at her shirt sleeve.)* Then you're really stupid. Even my aunt thinks I'm a waste.

THERAPIST: *(Speaks quietly, mirroring Emma's body communication with her own energy and tone.)* I imagine it feels like that sometimes, though I don't really know for sure how you feel. It's really hard for anyone to feel like their feelings are all churned up, or like their body is out of control. I'll tell you this, though. I've known a lot of kids who have been through a lot of hard things in their lives, just like you have, and honestly, most of them are pretty remarkable. Even the things that make other people upset—like arguing, or running, or even hurting themselves—those are all things that kids do to try to help themselves, and I'm guessing that's true for you, too. I'm pretty sure that all the things you do make sense—even if they feel crazy sometimes, or they get in your way.

EMMA: I'm sick of talking. Can we just draw?

THERAPIST: Sure. *(Pulls out paper and markers.)* Can I just say one more thing, though, while we're drawing?

EMMA: I guess.

THERAPIST: I think you did something just now that's an example of how smart you are. You and I were talking about something kind of hard, and you had had enough, and you found a really good way to manage it by taking a break and asking to draw. I'm guessing you have all sorts of ways of managing the hard things.

EMMA: I guess.

THERAPIST: So a couple of things, okay? First, I'm really curious to learn more about the ways you've taken care of yourself, and figured out how to manage your world. And second, it's okay for you to say to me "I'm done" or "I don't want to talk about that stuff." Okay?

EMMA: Okay. I'm done, and I don't want to talk about that stuff.

THERAPIST: *(Laughs.)* See—I told you that you were smart!

In this example, the therapist brings in some important principles. First, the therapist enacts attunement strategies through the use of both verbal and nonverbal mirroring and reflection. She is actively curious about Emma, but explicitly respectful of Emma's observed boundaries and need for space. She accepts and validates Emma's feelings of damage, but also gently confronts them, bringing in education about trauma to reframe the behaviors as survival strengths. The therapist engages her own caregiver affect management, depersonalizing Emma's statements and managing her own reaction to the confrontation. Her early goal is to build relationship and reasonable therapeutic safety, and to bear witness to and begin to know the whole child while setting a preliminary frame for the work.

Developing Formulation: Provider Attunement

Our practice is guided by attunement and formulation: a belief that children and caregivers approach their lives in a manner that is reasonable and adapted to the world in which their development was shaped. By working to understand the range of influences (individual and collective history, cultural context, familial norms, child temperament, current stressors, etc.) and the link between these influences and ongoing behaviors, patterns of relationship, and patterns of arousal, we can try to understand the child's and/or caregiver's current needs and goals. In the absence of this attuned understanding, intervention efforts will be far less empathic and effective than they might otherwise be. It is no surprise that many children like Emma see themselves as "damaged" and broken: The communication from many systems is simply that their behavior is bad, wrong, and needs to change. Shifting that lens to one that incorporates an understanding of why the behavior makes sense, but may be getting in the child's way, is a far more empathic way to engage the child in the treatment process.

Through a review of records, conversations with Emma's aunt and previous treaters, and ongoing conversations with Emma, the therapist gradually pieced together the basics of Emma's early story of neglect, physical and sexual abuse, and multiple attachment losses and disruptions. The therapist knows that common triggers associated with these exposures include perceived rejection and deprivation, loss of control, boundary invasions, and perceived cues of physical danger. The therapist began to match up Emma's observed behavior patterns with likely triggers—for instance, shutting down and withdrawing when confronted, escalating to enraged when attention was withdrawn from her— and began to build them into an understanding of the functional nature of Emma's behaviors, her regulation patterns, and the ways that Emma has learned to protect herself and to get her needs met.

In working with children and adolescents who have experienced trauma, providers are simultaneously working with the embedded world in which the child lives; therefore, an attuned understanding of the caregiver or caregiving system is also critical to treatment success. Just as the clinician worked to learn more about Emma's story, she also expressed curiosity about the story of Emma's aunt, Kathryn. Although she is still hesitant to fully engage in the therapeutic process, Kathryn has shared a little bit about her family history. She has reported that she is the oldest of three children born to her mother and father, in what she describes as an Irish Catholic working-class family. When asked about her mother, Kathryn describes her as a quiet woman who tried really hard to "keep the peace." She indicated that she loved her mother and tried to help out with her younger siblings. She noted feeling protective of her younger siblings, particularly of Emma's mother, who she described as "always kind of the sensitive, moody one. She always seemed to take things harder and react more than the rest of us." Kathryn described her father as a hard worker who worked long hours and came home tired and in a bad mood, often yelling and screaming about "anything and everything." She did not report any history of violence or substance abuse in the home. Kathryn reported that her mother was diagnosed with cancer when she was 17 and that her youngest sibling, Emma's mother, was 12 and that things got "much harder" after that. She suspects that Emma's mom began using substances when their mother died 2 years later.

As the therapist learned more about Emma's aunt, she reflected on the ways Kathryn had learned to be a caregiver from her early experiences. The therapist expressed curiosity as to whether Kathryn saw herself as similar to her own mother in any ways, and Kathryn acknowledged that, much like her mother, she liked to "keep things peaceful," adding, "My sister [Emma's mother] was always such a wild child, and lately Emma just feels like that, too. I never liked all the yelling and screaming—I just want everything to be calm." Over time, the therapist observes the ways that Kathryn moves among nurturing, controlling, and disconnecting in response to triggers such as chaos and perceived loss.

‖‖ Developing Routines and Incorporating Predictable Structures

As described in Chapter 6, rhythm is a crucial foundation of both early and ongoing attention to safety and distress tolerance in trauma-informed treatment. As the basic rhythm of the service process is established—whether the rhythm of a treatment session, the predictable structure of a milieu program day, or the organizing elements of a classroom—specific structures can be integrated to support identified individual or programmatic goals.

Emma's therapist paid careful attention to building predictable rhythms in her work with Emma and her aunt. She made sure to reserve the same office each week in the clinic, and tried to have predictable materials available, tailoring these as she learned more about Emma's preferences (e.g., making sure to have drawing materials, specific sensory objects like clay, and small speakers that Emma could attach her phone to in order to play music while they met). She worked with Emma to transparently co-develop a routine, including checking in at the start of the meeting about Emma's week, her preferences ("Are you feeling in the mood to talk today or to do more drawing or something else?"), and establishing one goal for the meeting ("We've been experimenting with different ways to help your body feel settled and safe the last few weeks. Do you want to keep doing that today, or is there something else you'd like us to work on?")

As core treatment goals became clearer, the therapist began to integrate structures into the treatment to support those. Emma, her aunt, and the therapist identified three "big picture" goals for their work together: to help both Emma and her aunt develop some strategies for understanding and managing hard feelings (Caregiver Affect Management, Attunement, Identification, Modulation) ; to help Emma and her aunt build better communication with each other, especially when feeling stressed or upset (Attunement, Relational Connection); and to support Emma in getting to know herself, including understanding her family story (Self and Identity). The therapist and Emma gradually integrated ongoing structures into the work in support of these goals. For instance, self-reflective activities were used at the start of every meeting to support Emma in developing curiosity about and awareness of her internal experience (thoughts, feelings, energy state, body sensations). Experimentation with different modulation strategies (listening to music, doing yoga, engaging in deep breathing) was incorporated into some portion of every meeting, and reflection on shifts in energy states even during routine interactions became part of the "shared language" of Emma and the therapist. For instance, the therapist might name observed shifts in Emma's energy level when talking about hard topic areas and ask her to notice her internal experience; or might comment on her own internal state while reacting to their conversation. Emma's aunt was invited to join the closing portion of every other meeting. Early on, Emma, her aunt, and the therapist co-developed a meeting routine that emphasized a positive, strengths-based focus (e.g., talking about moments of pride or a positive accomplishment from the week) and, over time, incorporated more challenging topics such as processing difficult interactions and using these to troubleshoot future ones.

Foundational Work to Develop and Support Regulation Skills in Child and Caregiver

The ability to navigate daily experience in a purposeful manner in service of self-identified goals—our described ultimate goal of trauma experience integration—relies on the individual's capacity to actively regulate experience: physiology, emotions, actions, and relationships. For youth and adults impacted by chronic trauma, this capacity is strongly affected by repeated experiences of both real and perceived danger, which lead to frequent activation of the survival response, along with intense and often overwhelming experiences of affect and arousal. The capacity to understand, tolerate, and manage that arousal is a necessary foundation for present-oriented, healthy developmental functioning, and is often the early focal point of trauma-focused treatment.

Development of Regulation skills, described in depth in Chapters 10 and 11, requires both active experiential engagement in physiological strategies that shift and support effective and comfortable states of arousal (Modulation), as well as a development of reflective capacities that build awareness and capacity to identify states of both calm and of distress; awareness of internal state shifts; and gradually increasing understanding of states and the experiences that elicit them (Identification).

> Over time, Emma became comfortable experimenting with different strategies with her therapist. She particularly liked strategies she could control herself, like listening to music, drawing, or what she described as a "mental zone": "I sort of turn the volume down on everything and go inside, and if I stay focused on something, it's not like I really disappear like I used to. Like if I start dialing everything down, and I focus on my breathing, and then I start to count in my head, really slow. It helps me when I'm really jittery."

Much of this work happens initially in displacement: practicing and engaging in strategies outside of the distressed moment. However, there are numerous opportunities for engaging regulation strategies in the moments of crisis: the times when children and caregivers enter the treatment or service space actively experiencing overwhelmed arousal or distress. Crucial to this work is the role of attunement: witnessing, mirroring, and validating the youth's experience. Efforts to shift or reduce a child's arousal and affective state without first acknowledging, bearing witness, and recognizing the validity of it will often fail.

> The week after the incident in which Emma became enraged and then tried to jump out of a moving car when her aunt failed to respond to a question, Emma appeared shut down when she came into treatment. The aunt had already called the therapist to tell her about the incident, and the therapist acknowledged that she knew something had happened. Emma's face tightened, and she said angrily, "She always says we're supposed to listen to each other, and she can't even pay attention to what I'm saying!" The therapist acknowledged Emma's feelings, stating, "I can see how upset you still are. It's so hard to feel like we have something important to say, and someone isn't listening to us."

The work might continue with engaging modulation skills in the moment—for instance, experimenting with ways to manage observed or current distress/arousal or explore, over time, distress tolerance skills or external supports that might be accessed in similar distressed moments. However, when a child or caregiver presents in acute distress or expressing a strong emotional experience, the initial response should typically incorporate witnessing and mirroring that response and then affirming its validity.

A child is often only as regulated as his or her caregiving system, and so support for the caregiver's development of distress tolerance and regulation skills is also critical. As described in Chapter 7, the provider system works to support the caregiver's affect management through parallel attunement to and validation of the adult's affective response, support for development of internal resources and regulation strategies, and mobilization of external supports.

> Early in the engagement process, the importance of caregiver involvement in the treatment process was discussed with Kathryn. The therapist collaborated with her to determine where, when, and how she could participate as well as the frequency of contact with the therapist. For instance, would she be available by phone or for individual or joint sessions? The therapist normalized caregiver stress and described the opportunities for caregiver support within the context of ARC treatment, including individual meetings focused on her experience as a caregiver. Kathryn initially indicated that her work schedule made it very difficult to attend separate meetings with the clinician but agreed to weekly phone check-ins and participation in Emma's sessions as needed.
>
> However, 2 weeks after the car incident, the therapist received a call from Kathryn requesting a "private" meeting. Kathryn arrived for her meeting and was initially pleasant, thanking the clinician for taking the time. However, she quickly became distressed, expressing frustration and anger that Emma was still so challenging despite her work in treatment.
>
> "It's like we take two steps forward and then it all just blows up again. And over the stupidest things—it's like she needs me to be perfect or everything falls apart."
>
> The therapist acknowledged her frustration, saying, "I know how much most parents wish that things would just even out and stay that way. You've given Emma so much, and I imagine it must be so hard when it feels like it all falls apart, especially because I know how much you like things to be peaceful."
>
> Kathryn teared up, saying, "Everything just feels so stressful all of a sudden. I just don't understand why she seems to like the drama so much, and I don't know how to help her!"
>
> The therapist spoke quietly, leaning in toward Kathryn. "I can see you're feeling so frustrated and sad and kind of hopeless today, and I'm so glad you reached out. It's such a hard mix of feelings to hold all by yourself, though I know you're a strong woman and you've been doing it for a long time. I will say, though, that even though it feels like this is backward motion, it's not—you're not losing all the gains you've made. Even for kids who haven't been through everything Emma has, there are good days and hard days. You and I and Emma, too—we'll keep working on understanding and getting better at surviving the hard days, and trying to build more and more good ones."

In this interaction, as she does with Emma, the therapist bears witness to Kathryn's experience, mirroring, validating, and putting language to her affect. She acknowledges the feelings of hopelessness, while simultaneously normalizing them and beginning to provide education about the ebbs and flows of experience. She actively works to engage Kathryn in entering into a continued process of understanding and managing challenging experiences.

This empathic support for and acknowledgment of the caregiver's need for regulation—without working too quickly to engage the caregiver's reflective processes about the child—hinges on parallel attunement by the provider.

Cultivating Reflection by Child and Caregiver

In order to shift patterns of danger-based survival and need fulfillment, the child (or caregiver) must be able to harness effective regulatory strategies and other developmental capacities in the moment. In addition, the child (or caregiver) also must gradually build an understanding and attuned awareness of current adaptations and of his or her stake in and capacity to utilize alternative strategies. The ability to engage curiosity is built over time, during states of reasonable calm, through the cultivation of reflection on both self (Identification, Caregiver Affect Management) and other (Attunement). Early on, it is critical to pay attention to and understand current strategies used by the child or caregiver.

> Emma and her therapist began to keep track of the things Emma naturally did during the week when something felt hard—for instance, closing herself in her room when she was angry at her aunt. They started to try to identify what Emma might be needing in those moments (space? less stimulation? control?) and to match these to proactive strategies Emma could use. Whenever Emma was comfortable with it, they worked to share the information with her aunt so that she could support Emma's use of strategies—or at the least not interfere with them by, for instance, following Emma into her room when she needed space.

Reflection will often be held externally, by the provider, early in the work, or ideally (over time) by the primary caregiver. For instance, when working with a younger child, the primary observer may initially be the clinician: "I know there were lots of times when kids got yelled at in your house, and that it was kind of scary. It seems like when the teacher got mad, that felt kind of scary, too." If the child agrees, the clinician might observe, "It seems like something that feels pretty hard is people being mad."

Engaging curiosity and reflection can be done outside of the context of individual therapy as well. For example, after an adolescent reacts to a perceived space invasion in a residential program, the staff member might say, "I'm sorry, I think I just got in your space—one of the things I'm learning about you is that it makes you uncomfortable if people get too close." The more experience the caregiver (clinician or otherwise) has with the child, the easier it will be to jointly identify patterns. For example: "This kind of reminds me of the time you got upset when Gio sat right next to you on the bench in the break room without asking, and we were able to figure out that you felt like your space was really invaded. Does this feel similar to that?"

An important goal of reflection and curiosity is to build awareness not just of *current actions and adaptations*, but also an attuned understanding of the functions of behavior and regulatory needs in the context of historical experiences. This attuned understanding includes comprehension of triggers, patterns of adaptation (safety seeking and need fulfillment), and historical experiences and their influence on how current relationships and situations are viewed and evaluated. For an older child or a child with more experience in self-reflection, it is important to invite him or her to be the observer—for example: "From what you're describing, you started to feel this funny pit-of-your-stomach kind of feeling, and then got really down, really fast, and that it happened when your friend sent you that email. We've talked about different kinds of triggers, or things that push your buttons. I'm wondering if you think any of them were going on for you here."

> Emma and her therapist have been moving between activities focused on regulation, as described above, and building curiosity and reflection in moments that Emma shows she is able to tolerate it. The therapist has learned that Emma is often the best judge of this – if the therapist tries to engage too much curiosity when Emma is not ready, Emma will typically shut down or become angry. The therapist has learned to transparently acknowledge this as a "communication," naming the ways that Emma is now able to show—whether through behavior or words—that she needs time, space, or support to help her body feel comfortable.
>
> One week, Emma arrived for a meeting appearing shut down and reported having a "big blow-out" with her aunt that week. The therapist thanked her for sharing, and asked if she wanted to talk about it. Emma shook her head no. With Emma's permission, the therapist played some music that Emma had previously identified as helping her when she was feeling frustrated and upset. As they sat quietly together, listening to the music, Emma appeared to gradually relax, and eventually stated, "I'm feeling okay. We can talk about it if you really want to."

CLINICIAN: *(After eliciting Emma's description of the argument)* Okay, so let me just make sure I have this right. You were in a pretty good mood when you got home, because of the A– on your math test, and you knew your aunt had been waiting to hear about it. But then, when you went to tell her, she was kind of busy and wasn't really paying attention, and then it sounds like you started yelling at her. And then she started getting upset, and then you just felt angrier and more scared and like you had to get away, is that right?

EMMA: *(Nods her agreement.)* Yeah. It's like she wasn't even interested, even though she's been riding me about studying, and then she freaked out when I got mad. I just needed to take off, get some space.

CLINICIAN: Okay. So she got upset, and you got upset. But it was a pretty big upset—big enough that you ran out of the house and stayed out for over an hour. You weren't feeling upset when you got home, were you? *(Emma shakes her head no.)* Do you remember how we talked about the danger brain—how its job is to kick in really quickly whenever it thinks something is dangerous?

EMMA: Yeah, I actually thought that was kind of cool. Kind of like, "Super-brain." *(She sings.)*

CLINICIAN: *(Laughs.)* Yeah, well, I'm wondering if maybe your danger brain might have gone off, because you kind of went from 0 to 60 pretty quickly.

EMMA: *(Shrugs.)* Yeah, maybe, I guess.

CLINICIAN: I kind of think so too, from what you're describing. Maybe we can figure out what set it off.

EMMA: I know what set it off—my aunt was flipping out.

CLINICIAN: Yup, that was part of it, for sure—but you got pretty upset even before she started yelling. I know we've talked about a couple of things that get your danger brain going, because they're like the kinds of things that happened when you were little—like when things are chaotic, like people yelling or throwing things, or when you feel like people don't like you any more, or aren't paying attention to you. Do you think any of that could have been going on?

EMMA: I don't know. I guess maybe the not paying attention part, and then she got all angry. I just reacted really fast, you know? I just wanted to tell her about the test, and then everything just flipped out.

In this example, the clinician uses her attunement skills, in collaboration with Emma's own growing self-reflection skills, to monitor Emma's shifting need for *regulation and distress tolerance* and her increasing capacity to *engage curiosity and reflection*. As she makes use of in-the-moment coregulation support, and in the context of an increasingly safe therapeutic relationship, Emma is able to tolerate and build on an understanding of her own patterns, including acknowledgment of historical traumatic experiences and identification of triggers and danger responses.

Engaging the Caregiver's Reflective Awareness of Self and the Child

Because the caregiver's attuned understanding of the child is often a critical factor for supporting regulated action in the moment, treatment focuses on the development of the adult's understanding both of his or her own patterns of adaptation and of the child's.

Emma's Aunt Kathryn has begun to routinely connect with the therapist, typically by phone but occasionally in separate meetings. These individual meetings are in addition to the dyadic time that has been incorporated into the end of many of Emma's therapy sessions. Kathryn initially used the meetings "as a place to vent," as she described it, but as she begins to trust the therapist and to feel mirrored in her own feelings, she is increasingly able to accept the therapist's curiosity about Emma.

For instance, in one phone call Kathryn says, "I'm feeling kind of like a broken record, like all I do is call you and complain."

THERAPIST: *(Laughs.)* I bet I must sound like a broken record, too, with some of what I say back to you.

KATHRYN: I think I must need to hear it over and over again. I'm just feeling frustrated again this week. She took off, *again*, just ran out of the house even when I told her she'd be in big trouble if she did that again. It took everything I had not to flip out when she came home again 30 minutes later.

THERAPIST: So, I'm impressed here with two things. First, even though it's not great that she took off to begin with, it's fabulous that she came home just 30 minutes later. And second, how did you manage to keep from getting upset? I know it feels so scary to you when she leaves like that.

KATHRYN: Oh, I was upset. But I did some of what you and I talked about, like setting a timer so that I'd know when an hour was up so I could start making phone calls like we had talked about, and I kept reminding myself that she usually just goes to the park. And I made a cup of tea and made myself sit and drink it. If it had been much longer I would have gotten really upset, but just when I was working myself back up, she came home. And I didn't even yell, or scream—just told her I was upset that she had left and glad she had come home, and that I wanted us to talk to you about what had happened when we see you this week.

THERAPIST: Kathryn, you're amazing! I hope you felt proud of yourself. I know this is one of her behaviors that's just so hard for you.

KATHRYN: I just hate to think about something happening to her. I've lost too many people in my life already.

THERAPIST: I know you have, and I know you work so hard to keep her safe, and it's frightening when she puts herself in danger.

After talking for a few more minutes about Kathryn's feelings, her experiences of loss, and her fears, the therapist engages her curiosity about Emma.

THERAPIST: So we've been talking about how Emma sometimes gets so overwhelmed by even little feelings that she doesn't know what to do, and one of her instincts is to escape.

KATHRYN: I wish she wouldn't.

THERAPIST: I know you do, and when she's calm, Emma knows that too. But you know how we've talked about how even though Emma has been with you for a lot of years, she spent a long time not having anyone who could help her with her feelings, and sometimes her feelings still surge up and set off that old feeling of panic that we think she must have had when she was a little girl.

KATHRYN: *(quietly)* I get so angry at my sister when I think about that.

THERAPIST: I know. And I know we've talked a bit about some of the things we think Emma had to deal with and that get you so angry, and the ways she learned to manage those things, like hiding or doing everything other people wanted, and sometimes by taking off or escaping.

KATHRYN: Like yesterday.

THERAPIST: Exactly. And even though it's scary for you when she takes off, for Emma, it's a behavior that makes sense because it helps her calm down and feel safe again. What we need to keep working on is helping you and her to recognize those moments she's starting to feel that panic, so she can escape—if that's what she needs to do—but in a way that feels safer to everyone.

In this example, the therapist again moves fluidly between attunement, support for regulation, and curious reflection, building over time on the aunt's understanding of her own regulation responses and needs, her understanding of those responses, an increasing capacity to engage affect management skills in the moment, and a building empathic understanding of Emma's patterns of response.

The Dynamic Relationship between Reflection and Curiosity and Regulation and Distress Tolerance in Treatment

The treatment process is a fluid one, and capacity to engage in reflection will alternate routinely with the need for regulation and distress tolerance. Often, these states will bridge together. For instance, moments of dysregulation or distress in treatment provide an important opportunity to practice awareness of state shifts in the moment. As an example, as a child demonstrates a shift in states during a therapy session or other interaction, the provider might observe, "I'm noticing that as we're talking about this, your fists are clenching but your face is going kind of blank. What do you notice going on inside of you?"

The relationship may also bridge in the opposite direction. Because the process of engaging curiosity and reflection is itself often activating, the "work" of being curious may elicit the need for applied regulation. It is critical that clinicians and other providers explicitly set the stage for this regulation by supporting the child's or caregiver's awareness of his or her own clues of distress, and the ways these clues signal the need to pause and use established strategies for managing arousal. In the absence of this intervention, treatment runs the risk of inadvertently retraumatizing the child, requiring him or her to use older, danger-based strategies (e.g., compliance, aggression, escape) to manage clinical content. In contrast, with active application of self-awareness skills and regulation skills in the moment, and with the coregulatory support of the provider or other caregivers, the child or adult develops a visceral experience of mastery over managing and tolerating distress.

Emma's clinician checks in with her as they begin to talk about a hard interaction she had with a peer at school that week that escalated and led to Emma running out of the school midday and then cutting herself. "Emma, can you do a quick self-check and let me know where your energy is at right now?" Emma responds that she's feeling kind of spacy and that she's hovering in the "minuses" (on a –1 to +10 scale). The clinician states, "It makes sense to me that you might be feeling kind of shut down; it sounds like you had some really big feelings this week, and even talking about them may make your danger brain want to protect you."

She suggests that they take a few minutes before talking to use some of the strategies Emma has identified as helpful when she is feeling shut down. Emma agrees, and asks to use the modeling clay. The therapist and Emma sit quietly together, building a co-created clay structure. After a few minutes, Emma describes herself as feeling "mostly here now."

The therapist suggests that they continue to work on the clay together as they talk, to keep them grounded and connected. Once Emma agrees, the clinician states, "I think it's important that we talk about this, so we can figure out some of what happened. But you're in charge of how much we talk about it, and if your feelings start to get too big or too shut down, we can take a break or do something different to help get your energy back to a place that feels comfortable. We'll keep checking in as we go, okay?"

Building an Understanding of Patterns over Time

As the child and/or caregiver develop an increasing capacity to monitor internal experience and to engage or accept regulation support, opportunities to reinforce reflection and curiosity will increase. Ideally, over time this attuned understanding (of self, of other) will build into an awareness of patterns, as can be seen in the description of Kathryn's growing awareness over time of Emma's need to escape, and of her own activation when she is afraid of losing someone.

This empathic attunement incorporates an understanding not just of the "what," but also of the "why," through actively linking both traumatic experiences and other influential shapers of behavior with learned adaptations, needs, and developmental capacities. For instance, in speaking about Emma's experience with her aunt when she tried to tell her about the math test, Emma's clinician might state:

> "So when your aunt didn't listen, you got really upset, which makes sense to me, because I know we've talked about how, when you were a little girl, you felt all alone a lot of the time, like there was no one who would ever listen. With your mom, I think the only way you could get her attention was to get really big, and it seems like you tried to do that with your aunt. But then she got upset, and it hit your danger buttons even more, and your first instinct was to get out. And again, that makes total sense, because when your mom used to yell, things got really dangerous, really quickly. So even though we're trying to work on not just running out of the house, because something unsafe could happen, your brain really was doing its best to take care of you."

Supporting Developmental Capacities

Ultimately, the goal of our work with children and their caregiving systems is to support active engagement in present life: the ability to . . .

- Harness the range of developmental capacities that allow the child or caregiver to understand, manage, and cope with experience
- Understand needs and access resources
- Tolerate, build, and sustain healthy relational connections with others
- Develop an attuned and empathic self-concept, which includes a cohesive understanding of self over time
- Identify and work actively toward age-appropriate goals, either independently or with support
- Access and participate in moments of joy.

These developmental capacities are frequently derailed in trauma-impacted youth by the combination of what they are good at—highly sensitive danger-based patterns of response and adaptation (e.g., fighting, escaping, or finding ways to get needs met)—and of what has been negatively impacted by early and ongoing experiences of danger: those developmental capacities that require the luxury of safety (e.g., agency, cohesive sense of self, the ability to anticipate future possibilities).

Intervention will necessarily need to move over time between acknowledging, validating, and ultimately decreasing the frequency of and need for danger-based responses, and simultaneously supporting and engaging healthy developmental capacities.

From the start of treatment, the therapist integrated a focus on Emma's understanding of self and identity. This began with early acknowledgment of Emma as a "whole person" and exploration of the many facets of who she is: an adolescent who loved an eclectic mix of music, who disliked math but loved to express herself in words and images, who often reflected her mood with clothing and hairstyle. Emma's clinician encouraged Emma to capture her growing ability to claim self-attributes in a hardbound sketchbook she provided, and though additions to the book did not occur in every meeting, the book was regularly brought out as either the clinician or Emma identified a statement, experience, or behavior as reflective of Emma's values, goals, influences, and attributes.

As the relationship between Emma and her clinician strengthened and Emma was increasingly able to tolerate strong emotion, they began to talk about Emma's memories and her life story. Emma initially kept these stories separate from her "book of self," but eventually began to incorporate them in, saying, "It's kind of hard for the me-then and the me-now to be totally separate, you know? My mom and dad, they're a piece of who I am. I just don't want them to be all of it."

Exploration of those early relationships along with other influential relational experiences was a key part of supporting Emma's capacity to access resources and build relational connections. Although Emma clearly had the skill set to negotiate relationships, she was guarded and self-protective, and frequently saw others' intentions as hostile or judgmental. As a result, she reacted strongly or isolated herself. The clinician engaged her curiosity about the range of relational experiences she had had in her life, the "lessons" she took from those relationships, and ways those had influenced her current approach to connection. Gradually they began to concretely identify "possible connections" in Emma's life: peers she got along with at school and adults who she saw as "decent," and to consider the ways in which people might be supportive in meeting various needs. As Emma's regulatory capacity strengthened and she was more consistently able to identify and tolerate shifts in internal experience, she became increasingly able to access and enjoy moments of connection and interaction. In turn, these new connections allowed Emma and her clinician to integrate others as possible relational resources in Emma's "regulation plans."

The ability to engage relationship, to read and communicate effectively, and to tolerate missteps was addressed directly with Emma and her aunt. Clinical meetings frequently incorporated dyadic time at the start or end of session, and the clinician supported opportunities for attunement through a wide range of activities (guessing and sharing experience, identifying patterns of interaction, rhythmic games and shared experiences, and many others). Emma and Kathryn practiced communication around both positive and challenging experiences, and with support, actively identified and problem-solved challenges in their interactions. During times that Emma was actively focused on remembering and talking about her early life experiences, Kathryn often joined sessions and shared her own knowledge and memories of Emma's early life, and together they co-constructed a shared narrative about Emma's history.

Growing in-the-Moment Capacity to Act

The goal of our work with trauma-impacted youth is ultimately that of resilience: building each child's ability to act, at an age-appropriate level, in the present moment in service of self-identified goals. For children whose "moments" are frequently influenced and derailed by survival, the ability to access and utilize growing developmental capacities depends almost completely on the simultaneous ability to harness and "catch" the survival response as it occurs, so that they can purposely *act*, rather than simply *react*. The ability to do so is at the heart of children's ability to engage purposefully with their lives in the present context.

Building toward this stage involves many of the reflective strategies described previously, which can be utilized during times that the child is not overwhelmed by affect. Applying these skills in the moment will involve first helping the child notice and identify internal and/or external "clues" that previous experiences are driving a current response. These clues will be different for all children. For some, they may be sensory or physiological (e.g., "a funny feeling in my stomach"). For some, they may be cognitive (e.g., "I start thinking I'm really stupid"). Other children can identify specific emotions (e.g., "I just get really enraged, like as mad as I ever get") or lack of emotion (e.g., "I start feeling really shut down, like I can't feel anything at all"). Some children may be able to identify patterns of action or inaction (e.g., "I feel like I need to be moving, like I can't sit still and I have to get out," or "I kind of want to disappear, to not be seen or even exist"). Finally, some children may notice changes in how they interact (e.g., "Well, I usually really like being with my friends, but I suddenly start feeling like I hate them all, and like they don't really care about me anyway").

Over time, as you work with children to observe and reflect on their patterns of experience and response, try to help them identify the clues that signal that they have shifted from one self-state (e.g., calm and happy) to another (e.g., overwhelmed and shut down). Ideally, when possible and appropriate, caregivers can be important sources of support in this work as they are increasingly able to manage their own emotional responses and, as a result, observe and reflect the presence of these clues to their children.

As children and their caregivers develop increasing awareness and understanding of *distressed states* (triggers, needs, patterns of behavior) and of *state shifts* (signs that the child or caregiver is entering an overwhelmed state and losing access to developmental capacities), intervention can support the proactive pairing of specific modulation strategies with observations of clues of state shifts (i.e., patterns of response generated by previous experience), in the moment, so that the child is able to remain engaged in the present, rather than be driven by survival.

The ability to apply regulatory skills in the present moment increasingly *allows* the child to access developmental capacities such as relational skills and executive functions, and also *depends upon* the growing availability of these skills in anticipation of those moments. For instance, the child's ability to engage in this work may require *identification* skills to specify areas of distress (e.g., "What is it that's really bothering me?"), awareness of *self* and the values supporting the child in identifying his or her goals (e.g., "What is it that I really want?"), and *executive function* skills to support the child in identifying the range of possible solutions (e.g., "What is getting in the way of what I want? What is it that I can/want to do, and what will happen if I make choice A or choice B?").

The child may need to access *modulation* skills to explore, acknowledge, and process the range of feelings associated with moments of derailment, based on both past experiences (e.g., "I know that part of me is feeling really sad right now because I'm remembering sad things") and present ones (e.g., "Right now my feelings are just kind of hurt"). Embedded in this process is the development of a *narrative* around both discrete experiences of danger and more comprehensive life experiences. Children may need to identify areas of personal strength and *relational connection* resources they can harness to allow them to act in the present moment (e.g., "I don't like it when my friends are mean, but I know I still matter, and when I handle them without fighting and can speak to my grandma about it, I feel better"). Ultimately, our work is to support the child in applying solutions and observing and reinforcing the *act* of making active choices, rather than the outcomes. In other words, any instance in which the child makes an active choice, in the present moment, in the service of meeting a goal is a success—regardless of the outcome of the choice.

It is likely not necessary to state this, but actually harnessing developmental resources and engaging in action in the present moment are incredibly challenging; are derailed for all people during times of stress and distress; and for those children whose lives have been strongly impacted by trauma, generally occur only after a great deal of exploration, practice, and after-the-fact reflection. Successes may accrue slowly and will likely be reached in small, age-appropriate steps. It is important to recognize and acknowledge these successes as they occur, both with the child and with the child's caregivers

> The clinician works with Emma (1) to build her curiosity about her body's signals indicating that she needs something in the moment, and (2) to pay attention to the clues that her body gives her that she is shifting states, from feeling powerful and present to overwhelmed, angry, or afraid. In a careful, paced way they also spend a great deal of time exploring Emma's patterns of response and linking these to her early experiences and to her understanding of why various "danger signals" feel so hard for her. As part of this work, they gradually capture Emma's vague memories of her family of origin and her associated feelings about them through narrative, drawing, and expressive strategies like collage.
>
> Emma begins to express a desire "for things to be different—I don't want to be flipping out all the time, you know?" She names her goal of becoming a social worker one day, and says, "I can't be someone who helps people if I can't figure out how to get myself solid." The therapist and Emma's aunt are able to express to her both the acceptability of her harder responses and emotions, along with their faith in her ability to learn to shift these over time. With frequent reflection in the aftermath of difficult interpersonal experiences, particularly those leading to explosions or running off, Emma begins to identify "this ice-cold but kind of burning feeling—it's hard to describe—that shoots through me, like from the pit of my stomach straight up to my brain, when it feels like someone is ignoring me, especially Auntie K. When it happens, it feels like my energy just shoots up too, like crazy-quick."
>
> CLINICIAN: *(responding to Emma's self-identified clue)* So you get this "ice-cold but kind of burning feeling" that shoots through you, and it kicks up your energy really quickly. That's a tough one, because it sounds like your energy shifts so fast, it's hard to control. Do you think you notice that feeling when it happens?
>
> EMMA: I mean, yeah, I guess, but by the time I notice it, I'm like already pissed off and shouting.

CLINICIAN: Okay, so it's going to take a lot of practice, probably, for you to be able to catch it before it gets to that point—which makes sense because this is a new skill, and new things always take time to get good at.

EMMA: *(Nods.)*

CLINICIAN: So we've talked about some different things that bring your energy up and bring it down. It seems like we're looking for something to bring it down, is that right?

EMMA: Yeah, but it's got to be able to, like, bag the energy really quickly and then bring it down, because nothing's going to work that fast.

CLINICIAN: I'm not sure I know what you mean by "bag the energy."

EMMA: Like, if something was trying to run away from you, and you threw a bag over it to capture it, and it's still squirming inside, but you're keeping it from escaping, and then you can calm it down afterward.

CLINICIAN: Oh, okay—you mean like something to help you just get a hold of it first, without bringing it down, and then being able to take the time to bring it down?

EMMA: Yeah, exactly. It's almost like I just kind of have to take a breath and hold it, as soon as I feel that feeling in my stomach, and almost like—*(demonstrates throwing her arms around herself and holding herself tightly)*—like that, or something.

CLINICIAN: Do you think that would help you bag the energy, or grab hold of it, as a first step?

EMMA: Maybe.

CLINICIAN: It seems like when you do that, your aunt's going to need to know what's happening, so she doesn't say or do something to make it feel worse. Would it make sense for us to talk to her about this?

EMMA: Yeah, I guess so, otherwise she'll just think I'm nuts when I stop talking and start hugging myself.

CLINICIAN: Okay, so once you've stopped talking and start hugging yourself, what do you think you can do next to bring the energy down?

EMMA: I don't know. I liked that breathing thing we did, with that chant over and over, that kind of calmed me down. But if I do that, I'm really gonna have to tell Auntie K what I'm doing.

CLINICIAN: I think that'd be a good idea anyway. She might even know some clues that she sees from the outside when this kind of thing happens, and since it happens so fast, it might help to have an outside eye, also, so that she can help remind you to get your energy down.

Emma and her clinician continue to talk about and practice this strategy, and to engage Kathryn in understanding and supporting what Emma is trying to do. About 2 months after Emma first brings this idea up, and after several more escalations, outbursts, and explorations of these outbursts in therapy, she enters the therapy room, flops in the chair, and says, "So you'll never guess what I did." When the clinician asks what she did, Emma says, "I totally did the hold-my-breath-hug thing and didn't freak out!"

CLINICIAN: You mean, like you had that icy, burning feeling and you caught it?

EMMA: Yeah, I totally did.

CLINICIAN: So, what happened?

EMMA: I was with Leslie and Aisha—I told you about them, right? Anyhow, I was trying to talk, and they kept interrupting me and talking to each other, and then I said something, and Leslie did this thing with her hand, like, shut up, right? And I just got super-mad, really quickly—I could feel it just shooting through me. Normally I would have just exploded, which would have stunk, because Leslie and I just got back to being friends after we got mad last month. But then, before I said something, I just took a big breath and held it, and I didn't totally do the hug thing, but I like grabbed my shirt in my fists, and just kept thinking, "Bag it, bag it"—like the energy, you know? And I couldn't chant, because we were in the mall, but I did some deep breaths, and got my energy to go down, and then I was still irritated, but you know, not like crazy mad.

CLINICIAN: So then what happened?

EMMA: Not much of anything. It was fine, it really wasn't a big deal, you know? It just felt like it, for a minute. It was like that not-listening thing that we talked about—it just pushed my buttons.

CLINICIAN: I'm so, so impressed, I can't even tell you! I know you've been working on this, and it's really, really hard to catch it when it's happening. And not only did you catch it, but you did it all on your own, and without Leslie and Aisha even knowing what was happening. I'm so proud of you!

EMMA: Yeah, me too! Can we play on the computer today?

Transitioning and Anticipating the Future

Inevitably, our work with youth and families will come to an end, whether that ending is planned and anticipated or abrupt and unexpected. In most systems, a key part of our work in the now is anticipating and preparing for the time when we will no longer be a part of a child's or family's life. This is particularly true because the work that we do with any child or young person is generally only partly about supporting that child in the present; it is in equal if not greater part about the ways that the present will—we hope—facilitate an increasingly healthy and resourced future. This is true for the classroom teacher who builds skills and relationships that unfold into ever-more complicated mastery and confidence. It is true for the foster parent who provides the nurturing safety that allows the child respite from danger and a platform from which to enter a next relationship with greater internal resources. It is true for the juvenile justice program that acknowledges the factors and cumulative circumstances that led to an adolescent's current moment, and that holds and helps build a vision of future possibilities. And it is true for clinicians who bear witness to many past and present moments, while slowly collaborating in building the capacities that allow the child and caregiver to shape the future.

Emma and Kathryn continued to work with the clinician until Emma was 16. During those 3 years, both Emma and Kathryn had periods of confidence and periods of struggle. Emma continued to use strategies such as cutting and running away to manage her feelings until she was 14, but these gradually subsided as she felt safer in her body, had a wider range of strategies to draw on, and felt steadier in her relationship with Kathryn. She had one brief hospitalization during that time period, but none since turning 15.

The clinician worked with Emma and Kathryn to continue to identify their stake in making a positive life for themselves, their growing skills and capacities, a range of resources, and to simultaneously acknowledge their ongoing challenges. Each crisis moment was identified as a challenge to be addressed and learned from, rather than a setback, and with each successive experience of successfully navigating a "crisis moment," Emma and Kathryn grew in their confidence that they could continue to do so.

As Emma entered her junior year, she found her time increasingly taken by school, after-school activities, and peer relationships, and began to cancel and reschedule her meetings with her clinician. Following long experience of reading behaviors as communications, the clinician explored whether Emma might be ready to "take a break" from meeting with a therapist. Although Emma expressed sadness at not seeing her clinician, she acknowledged that she was feeling ready. The clinician, Emma, and Kathryn met and jointly set a timeframe to end treatment and a plan for termination. They used their final meetings to reflect back on their work together, and Emma organized and chose to take home a binder full of material; she asked the clinician to shred some of her earlier work, and to retain the remainder in her files. Emma and the clinician identified Emma's immediate and longer-term goals, and the ways in which she was already on the path to achieve them as well as potential roadblocks and pitfalls. They spoke candidly about clues that would tell Emma that she might need to seek support again, and the clinician normalized this as part of the journey.

In their final meeting, the clinician shared with Emma the ways that their work had influenced her, and the lessons she would take away from their time together. Emma brought the clinician a small anime character she had drawn and framed, saying, "I hope you'll keep this and think of me sometimes." The clinician assured her that she would not forget her, and gave Emma a new, blank hardbound sketchbook "for the self-story you're still creating."

Emma contacted her clinician via e-mail one last time, when she was 18, saying only, "I just thought you might want to know that I'm headed to college. Can you believe it?"

A Postscript

Over the years that we have been in clinical practice, we have had occasion to bear witness to the ultimate strength—as well as to the immense suffering—of children and families who must live with and negotiate layers of overwhelming stress.

During the year we worked on this book, within our own small clinical team we watched three families successfully negotiate the sometimes perilous route of "preadoption." Having held our collective breath the many times crises and stress threatened to lead to disruption, we have witnessed with great joy the growing confidence and attunement of the parents, the increasing comfort and competence of the children, and ultimately, were immensely moved as we celebrated the finalized adoptions of all six children.

We watched two other children languish in foster care, their futures and goals still bound in uncertainty, and while also advocating within the larger system for their needs, have worked to support our clinicians in the painful process of sitting with and providing protected space for children who remain in a state of constant crisis. For some children, we acknowledge that our successes come sometimes not in what we build and achieve in the present and for the future, but in what we are able to hold and protect during the time we are involved.

This year we have watched one young adult, whom we knew throughout her adolescence, transform her childhood and begin to build a new future, and we have watched another young adult struggle to transition from the known—as chaotic as it has been—into the confusing and somewhat frightening world of adulthood. We acknowledge the joy in watching seeds planted and watered begin to take hold and flower, and we acknowledge the awareness that this work often continues long past childhood, as the hurt children of yesterday negotiate new developmental stages, often without the protective resources of family and community.

Over the past year we have watched residential programs challenge themselves to build an understanding of trauma into their clinical and milieu teams, bring change to their systems in both small and large ways, and negotiate the very real-world constraints with which programs must struggle, while still trying to offer ethical, empathic, and comprehensive services. We have heard about the impact that a growing understanding of trauma has had on the attuned responses of foster parents, through programs that manage therapeutic foster homes, and we have seen the impact of this understanding in Head Start programs, preschools, and classroom settings.

We have learned at every step, and we continue to learn. We are struck, over and over, by the inventiveness and creativity, the positive intentions, and the impressive instincts of caregivers—both professional and familial—and the capacity of caregivers to thrive and to support the growth of children, once they are sufficiently supported themselves. We are struck, over and over, by the resilience of children, by their capacity to emerge from (and sometimes continue to negotiate) layers of stress, and still bring joy, curiosity, connection, and enthusiasm to their worlds, when given the foundation, resources, and permission to do so.

The successes we witness are sometimes small and sometimes large, and often come after long periods of plugging away, hanging in, and sitting with. Despite the setbacks, despite the crises and the pain, we leave this year with a great deal of hope. This is fitting, because in our own discussions of the ingredients of success, hope is among the strongest. Success is built on a faith in the potential of every child, every caregiver, and every system with which we work. It is built on an acknowledgment of the many strengths that already exist, on the belief that most people are doing their best with the resources that they have, and on the hope that our work will expand upon and foster new resources. Success is built on a foundation of support across levels: the child supported by the caregiver, the caregiver and child supported by the provider, the provider supported by a team. It is built on a respectful underpinning of partnership; an acknowledgment that empowerment lies in allowing the child, the caregiver, and/or the system to be the true agent of change; and an understanding that our role is as collaborator and team member, rather than sole orchestrator.

We are grateful for the opportunities we have had to enter into the lives of children and families, across settings and contexts, and we are immensely appreciative of the education we have received from the many clinicians, educators, program directors, milieu staff, nurses, child welfare workers, and foster/adoptive/biological parents who have shared their wisdom with us, and with the children whose lives they touch, as well as for the immense wisdom from the children themselves, who have been perhaps our most important teachers.

It is our hope that this book offers some small portion of that wisdom back, to support others in this journey. We look forward, with pleasure, to continuing our own.

APPENDIX A

Provider Materials

Session Fidelity Checklist/Tracking Tool

Client ID: _____   Therapist: _____

Date: _____/_____/_____   Session Number: _____

Modality (circle all that apply):   Individual   Caregiver   Dyad/Family

Session Component	X if Yes	Notes/Comments (optional)
FOUNDATIONAL STRATEGIES		
Routines and Rhythms		
Use of in-session routines		
Supporting familial routines		
Use of structure(s) to support identified goals		
Engagement		
Specific strategies to support child engagement in goal/treatment		
Specific strategies to support caregiver engagement in goal/treatment		
Psychoeducation		
Provide psychoeducation to caregiver(s)		
Provide psychoeducation to child(ren)		
ATTACHMENT DOMAIN		
Identify Caregiver(s):		
Caregiver Affect Management		
Psychoeducation, normalization, depersonalization		
Identify difficult situations		
Build self-monitoring skills		
Self-care/caregiver toolbox		
Identify support resources		

(continued)

From Margaret E. Blaustein and Kristine M. Kinniburgh (2019, The Guilford Press). Copyright © 2019 by the authors. Permission to photocopy this material is granted to purchasers of this book for personal use or use with clients (see copyright page for details). Purchasers can download additional copies of this material (see the box at the end of the table of contents).

Session Component	X if Yes	Notes/Comments (optional)
Attunement		
Parallel attunement/understanding caregiver perspective		
Engage caregiver active curiosity		
Observing/validating youth experience/mirroring skills		
Use of attunement to support youth regulation		
Positive dyadic engagement		
Effective Response		
Proactive identification of behaviors/active planning		
Use of attunement skills to understand behavior patterns and needs		
Use of regulation or addressing needs to prevent/reduce behaviors		
Support concrete skill building in behavior management strategies		
REGULATION DOMAIN		
Identification		
Language for emotions and energy/arousal		
Understanding trauma response/triggers/body's alarm system		
Connection (body/thought/behavior)		
Contextualization (Internal/external factors leading to emotions/energy)		
Modulation		
Understanding degrees of feeling and energy		
Understanding comfort zone/effective modulation		
Exploring/experimenting with regulation tools		

(continued)

Session Component	X if Yes	Notes/Comments (optional)
Identifying helpful strategies/building a toolbox		
Building external supports for modulation strategies		
COMPETENCY DOMAIN		
Relational Connection		
Explore goals of connection/relational history		
Identifying/establishing safe resources		
Create opportunities for connection and communication		
Build skills to support effective use of resources		
Teach appropriate physical/emotional boundaries		
Support effective verbal and nonverbal communication skills		
Executive Functions		
Support active recognition of choices/choice situations		
Support active evaluation of situations and goals		
Use of regulation skills to delay/inhibit responses		
Support in generating alternatives/identifying solutions		
Self-Development and Identity		
Help children identify personal attributes (Unique self)		
Build internal resources and identification of positive attributes (Positive self)		
Integrate self across states and time (past/present, multiple aspects of self (Cohesive self)		
Support capacity to imagine and work toward future goals/outcomes (Future self)		

(continued)

335

Session Component	X if Yes	Notes/Comments (optional)
TRAUMA EXPERIENCE INTEGRATION		
Identify client state(s) that guided intervention today		
Caregiver:		
Regulation and distress tolerance: Managing arousal		
Curiosity and reflection: Building attuned understanding of self/others		
Engaging present action: Supporting purposeful action		
Child:		
Regulation and distress tolerance: Managing arousal		
Curiosity and reflection: Building attuned understanding of self/others		
Engaging present action: Supporting purposeful action		

Goal Development Worksheet

Consider the core ARC treatment targets. Which feel most relevant to your client(s) currently? Which subskills might be the most important to work on? What might this work look like for the child/caregiver with whom you are working? Use this worksheet to link treatment targets to client-specific goals.

Core goal	Client-friendly language	Possible concrete goals	Examples of client-specific goal
Example: Caregiver Affect Management	Managing my feelings and actions	Recognize my push buttons Use an identified skill	Notice which of Johnny's behaviors make me the most frustrated. Count to 3 and tell myself "I can do this" before responding.
Example: Child Identification	Learning about my feelings and energy.	Recognize how much energy I have in my body.	Do a self-check with my therapist at the beginning and end of our meetings. Let my mom ask me where my energy is when I come home from school.

From Margaret E. Blaustein and Kristine M. Kinniburgh (2019, The Guilford Press). Copyright © 2019 by the authors. Permission to photocopy this material is granted to purchasers of this book for personal use or use with clients (see copyright page for details). Purchasers can download additional copies of this material (see the box at the end of the table of contents).

Concept-Driven Clinical Goal Development

My primary goals with the child are:

[ARC Concept]	by targeting	[Child-Specific Goal or Skill]	and by doing	[Child- or Family-Specific Strategy]
Examples				
1. Support **identification**	by targeting	a vocabulary for feelings and body states	and by doing	weekly check-ins
2. Build **caregiver affect management**	by targeting	awareness of push buttons	and by doing	review of hard and positive moments during the week.
3. Support **attunement**	by targeting	caregiver understanding of child	and by doing	dyadic meetings at start and end of session.

CURRENT GOALS

1. _____	by targeting	_____	and by doing	_____
2. _____	by targeting	_____	and by doing	_____
3. _____	by targeting	_____	and by doing	_____
4. _____	by targeting	_____	and by doing	_____
5. _____	by targeting	_____	and by doing	_____

From Margaret E. Blaustein and Kristine M. Kinniburgh (2019, The Guilford Press). Copyright © 2019 by the authors. Permission to photocopy this material is granted to purchasers of this book for personal use or use with clients (see copyright page for details). Purchasers can download additional copies of this material (see the box at the end of the table of contents).

Regulation Worksheet

OBSERVED PATTERNS

How would you describe your client's typical *energy level (constricted, highly aroused, fluctuating)?*

_____

_____

When does this client seem *most* regulated/organized?

_____

_____

When does this client seem *least* regulated? What types of situations seem to increase disorganization and/or distress?

_____

_____

What strategies is your client *already using* to support his/her/their regulation? Consider both "healthy" strategies as well as adaptive but potentially unhealthy strategies.

_____

_____

What might these strategies tell us about your client's energy state and regulation needs? For instance, is this person looking to bring down high arousal? To escape all feelings? To feel powerful? To express something to others? To feel present? Pick one or two examples and describe what the *need* might be.

_____

_____

Strategies

In what ways do **routines** seem supportive for this client? Are there other situations in which routines or predictability might be helpful?

_____

_____

What kinds of regulation strategies would seem helpful as **baseline/foundational** supports? (Consider gross motor, fine motor, sensory strategies, relational strategies, activities, etc.)

_____

_____

(continued)

From Margaret E. Blaustein and Kristine M. Kinniburgh (2019, The Guilford Press). Copyright © 2019 by the authors. Permission to photocopy this material is granted to purchasers of this book for personal use or use with clients (see copyright page for details). Purchasers can download additional copies of this material (see the box at the end of the table of contents).

Regulation Worksheet (page 2 of 2)

What are some regulation strategies that seem to help in **more challenging** moments? Try to define at least one challenging client state or behavior, and two or three useful and/or possibly useful tools.

_____

_____

What supports might be needed to help the client use these tools? Think about structures (e.g., regular check-ins, sensory toolkits, small "pocket tools") as well as relational supports and cuing.

_____

_____

APPENDIX B

Caregiver Educational Materials and Worksheets

Caregiver Educational Materials

Introduction: Children and Trauma

WHAT IS TRAUMA?

Many different things may be called "traumatic." *Trauma* refers to experiences that are overwhelming and may leave a person feeling helpless, vulnerable, or very frightened.

Trauma may include specific types of events, such as being in an accident or experiencing a natural disaster like a hurricane or an earthquake. Trauma may also include *ongoing stressors,* such as physical or sexual abuse.

For children, trauma is often about more than physical harm. For instance, separation from a caregiver, emotional neglect, and lack of a stable home (such as living in many different foster homes) are often very traumatic. Children may also be deeply affected by ongoing stressors such as poverty and racism, or repeated bullying/discrimination, particularly when related to characteristics of the child's social identity.

HOW DOES TRAUMA IMPACT CHILDREN?

Children who have experienced ongoing trauma may have many different reactions. Children may:

- Develop an expectation that bad things will happen to them.

  When children experience many bad things, they may come to expect them. They may overestimate times when they are in danger, or be fearful or withdrawn, even in situations that feel safe to other people.

- Have a hard time forming relationships with other people.

  Trauma often involves children getting hurt by others and/or not being protected by others. When early relationships are not consistently safe, children may develop a sense of mistrust in relationships.

- Have difficulty managing or regulating feelings and behavior.

  Because traumatic stress is overwhelming, children are flooded by strong emotions and high levels of arousal. Children may feel like they are unable to rely on others to help them with these feelings—for instance, they may believe that no one is safe, they may worry that other people will think they are bad, and so on.

  Without tools, children may try to overcontrol or shut down their emotional experience; to manage feelings and arousal through behaviors (such as being silly or getting in fights); or to rely on more dangerous, overt methods (such as substance abuse or self-injury).

- Have difficulty developing a positive sense of themselves.

  Children who experience trauma may feel damaged, powerless, ashamed, and/or unlovable. It is often easier for children to blame themselves for bad things happening, than to blame others. Over time, children may develop a belief that there is something wrong with them.

From Margaret E. Blaustein and Kristine M. Kinniburgh (2019). Copyright © 2019 The Guilford Press. Permission to photocopy this material is granted to purchasers of this book for personal use or use with clients (see copyright page for details). Purchasers can download additional copies of this material (see the box at the end of the table of contents).

Understanding Triggers

THE BODY'S ALARM SYSTEM

We all have a built-in alarm system that signals when we might be in danger. Evolution has helped human beings to survive by creating efficient systems in our brains that recognize danger signals and prepare us to respond. We become particularly efficient at recognizing signals that have been associated with past danger experiences. In the human brain, this system is known as the *limbic* system.

NORMATIVE DANGER RESPONSE

When the brain recognizes danger, it prepares the body to deal with it. There are four primary ways in which we can respond to something dangerous: We can FIGHT it, we can get away from it (FLIGHT), we can FREEZE, or we can SUBMIT/COMPLY.

What we choose to do often depends on the type of danger. So, for example:

- A large dog begins attacking your dog. You are bigger than the threat and motivated to help your dog. Response? FIGHT
- You are standing in the street and hear the squeal of brakes. You realize a car is speeding toward you. Response? FLIGHT
- You are a small child in a room where your parents are screaming and throwing things. You are not big enough to fight them, not fast enough to run away, and are trying not to be noticed. Response? FREEZE
- You are a young boy who has been threatened with harm if he does not engage in a sexual act with a teenager. Response? SUBMIT/COMPLY

Note: The "freeze" and "submit" responses are often the least understood and/or talked about, but may be the responses most accessible to young children. These are survival responses that are used when someone cannot fight the danger and cannot physically escape it (and, in fact, doing either one might increase the danger). The only options, then, are to become very still and try not to be seen or to yield to an aggressor and submit.

THE DANGER RESPONSE AND AROUSAL

When the brain labels something in the environment as dangerous, it must rapidly mobilize the body. The brain initiates the release of chemicals that provides our body with the energy needed to cope with danger (for example, to run from the car or to fight the attacking dog). The brain is remarkably efficient—within milliseconds of perceiving danger, the body's arousal level goes up, sensory perception shifts, and "nonessential functions" (such as digestion) shut down. Interestingly, higher cognitive processes—such as logic, planning, and impulse control—are considered *nonessential* in the face of danger. (Think about it—if a car is speeding toward you, do you want to be *thinking,* or do you want to be *running*?)

It is important to understand that this sequence will be initiated, whether the danger is *real* or simply *perceived.*

(continued)

From Margaret E. Blaustein and Kristine M. Kinniburgh (2019). Copyright © 2019 The Guilford Press. Permission to photocopy this material is granted to purchasers of this book for personal use or use with clients (see copyright page for details). Purchasers can download additional copies of this material (see the box at the end of the table of contents).

THE OVERACTIVE ALARM

Typically, when the danger signal first goes off, the "thinking" part of our brain evaluates the immediate environment. If there is no apparent danger (for example, it's a "false alarm"), the alarm system is shut off, and we continue with previous activities. For example: You are walking up a busy street and hear a car backfire. Within moments of your initial startle response, your brain will activate the sensory systems that scan your environment, assess the cause of the noise, and label it as nonthreatening. Almost immediately, you are able to continue on your way.

For some people, however, the brain's danger signal goes off too often. This generally occurs when there has been repeated danger in the past (remember, the more the brain engages in any activity, the more efficient it becomes at that particular activity). Children who have experienced repeated or chronic trauma often have *overactive alarms*—they may perceive danger more quickly than others and/or may label many nonthreatening things as potentially dangerous.

Consider again the example used above—you are walking down the street and a car backfires. Now imagine, however, that you have been in combat or have lived in an area that had frequent gunfire. As soon as the noise occurs, your body immediately prepares for danger. In this scenario, your "thinking brain" is less likely to get involved—or to take the time to assess whether the danger is real or not. This is because in the past, waiting would have put you at risk for being shot. In order to keep you safe, then, the "thinking brain" stays out of the way and lets the action brain take over. This overactive alarm is therefore adaptive: In times of actual danger, it kept you alive, but in the present, it may cause you to react too strongly to things that may really be safe.

WHAT TRIGGERS THE ALARM?

False alarms can happen when we hear, see, or feel something that reminds us of dangerous or frightening things that happened in the past, or even of dangerous things that are continuing to happen in our lives in other moments. Those alarm signals are called "triggers." Our brain has learned to recognize those signals because at other times when they happened, dangerous things also happened, and we had to respond quickly. A trigger acts as a signal to your brain that you might be in danger *right now,* and cues your brain to prepare for action.

Different children have different triggers, or alarm signals. For instance, for a child who has witnessed domestic violence, hearing people yell or watching adults argue might activate the alarm. For children who have not received enough attention, feeling alone or scared might turn on the alarm.

Often, these alarm signals, or triggers, are subtle. For example, trauma is often associated with unpredictability, chaos, or sudden change. As a result, even subtle changes in expected routine may activate a child's danger response.

Common triggers for children who have experienced trauma include:

- Unpredictability or sudden change
- Transition from one setting/activity to another
- Loss of control
- Feelings of vulnerability or rejection
- Confrontation, authority, or limit setting

(continued)

- Situations that are perceived as unfair, injustice
- Loneliness
- Sensory overload (too much stimulation from the environment)

Triggers may not always seem to make sense. For instance, some children may be triggered by positive experiences, such as praise, intimacy, or feelings of peace. There are many possible reasons for this. For example:

- A child who has experienced previous losses, rejection, or abandonment may be frightened or mistrustful of positive relationships.
- A child who has received praise or bribery while being sexually abused may fear ulterior motives.
- A child who has experienced consistent chaos may find calmness or routine unsettling.

It is important that children learn to tolerate these positive experiences, but it is also important for caregivers to be aware of the potential for distress.

HOW DO YOU KNOW YOUR CHILD HAS BEEN TRIGGERED?

The primary function of the triggered response is to help the child achieve safety in the face of perceived danger. Remember, there are four primary danger responses available to human beings:

FIGHT   FLIGHT   FREEZE   SUBMIT

What do these look like in children?

FIGHT may look like:

- Hyperactivity, verbal aggression, oppositional behavior, limit testing, physical aggression, "bouncing off the walls"

FLIGHT may look like:

- Withdrawal, escaping, running away, self-isolation, avoidance

FREEZE may look like:

- Stilling, watchfulness, looking dazed, daydreaming, forgetfulness, shutting down emotionally

SUBMIT may look like:

- Giving in too easily, denying the child's own needs like hunger or toileting, aligning with more powerful peers even when those peers are mean to the child

Emotionally, children may appear fearful, angry, or shut down. Their *bodies* may show evidence of increased arousal: trembling, shaking, or curling up.

Look for moments when the intensity of the child's response does not match the intensity of the stressor, or when a child's behaviors seem inexplicable or confusing. Consider: Might your child's alarm system have gone off?

Learning Your Child's Language

IT'S NOT WHAT I SAY . . .

Trauma can impact children's ability to understand, tolerate, and manage feelings. Even minor stressors can act as **triggers** that flood children with emotion. Often, children do not even know what it is that is upsetting them—only that there is a strong, bad feeling inside of them, and that *something* needs to happen to make it go away. In the face of these overwhelming feelings, and without strategies to cope with them, children will simply *react:* They work out the distress with their bodies and their actions.

Often, the only thing harder than dealing with feelings is talking to other people about them—especially for children who don't know themselves what they are feeling, or why they are feeling it. Furthermore, for children who have been hurt in the past by other people, or who did not have their needs met early in life, reaching out for help may feel dangerous or frightening.

WHAT I'M TRYING TO SAY IS . . .

Most children communicate through behavior to some degree; the ability to use words to share feelings and experiences grows naturally over the course of development, particularly as caregivers use their own words to reflect back experience. Consider these examples:

A 4-year-old returns home from preschool. She is quieter than usual, and when her mother asks if she wants to play, she shakes her head and curls up in a chair. Her mother sits next to her and says, "You're so quiet today. Do you feel sick?" The child shakes her head.

A 10-year-old comes home from school and slams the door. He throws his bag onto the kitchen table and says, "I'm never riding that stupid bus again!"

A 15-year-old has been nervous about her first date. She spends an hour in her room, trying on clothes, then finally comes downstairs, tearful. "Everything looks so stupid on me—I'm not going!"

Most caregivers are familiar with situations such as these, and—even if the precipitating event isn't yet known—will quickly recognize that feelings are driving these behaviors. Through their own words or actions, caregivers help children name and work through the emotion-inducing life events that they experience day to day.

The experiences driving trauma-impacted children's behaviors may be less obvious, and the feelings may be bigger, stronger, or more sudden, but at core, the emotions are the same: fear, sadness, anger, anxiety, and even joy.

(continued)

From Margaret E. Blaustein and Kristine M. Kinniburgh (2019, The Guilford Press). Copyright © 2019 by the authors. Permission to photocopy this material is granted to purchasers of this book for personal use or use with clients (see copyright page for details). Purchasers can download additional copies of this material (see the box at the end of the table of contents).

TUNING IN

Attunement is the ability to "read" (understand) your children's cues and respond in a way that helps them manage their emotions, cope with distressing situations, and/or make good choices. When a caregiver is attuned, he or she can respond to the emotion underlying a child's actions, rather than simply reacting to the most distressing behavior.

Consider two different scenarios for one of the above examples:

> *A 10-year-old comes home from school and slams the door. He throws his bag onto the kitchen table and says, "I'm never riding that stupid bus again!"*
>
> *Scenario 1: His mother is going through mail in the kitchen and looks up as he enters the house.*
> MOTHER: How many times have I told you not to slam that door!?
> CHILD: (*Kicks his bag.*) What's the big deal—it's just a stupid door!
> MOTHER: That's it—if you can't be polite, you can just go to your room!
>
> *Scenario 2: His mother is going through mail in the kitchen and looks up as he enters the house.*
> MOTHER: Whoa—you seem pretty mad. Did something happen on the bus?
> CHILD: (*Looks down, kicking his bag gently.*) Stupid bus driver hates me—he won't let me sit with my friends. I'm not riding it anymore!
> MOTHER: (*Pulls out a chair.*) C'mere. Why don't you tell me what happened, and we'll see if we can figure it out?

In the first scenario the child's mother responds to the behavior—slamming the door—and the emotion escalates, leaving both mother and child frustrated. In the second example the mother responds to the emotion—anger? frustration?—and provides the child with support, calming the situation.

Most situations aren't quite this straightforward, and no caregiver can be attuned at all times. The goal is not to be the "perfect parent," but to try—more times than not—to understand the feelings driving children's behavior.

PUTTING ON YOUR DETECTIVE HAT

Attunement requires caregivers to be "feelings detectives." Every child gives cues that help signal what might be going on.

Learn your child's individual communication strategies. Pay attention to the following areas and consider: How does your child look when he/she is angry? Sad? Excited? Worried? For each of these emotions, ask yourself the following questions:

(continued)

Facial expression	What does your child show on his face? Does his expression change? This may include being very expressive or appearing shut down.
Tone of voice	Does your child's voice become louder? Softer? Higher-pitched?
Extent of speech	Does your child suddenly have more to say than usual? Does she become quiet? Do her words seem like they come out in a rush, or sound more hesitant?
Quality of speech	Do your child's words become disorganized? Is he rambling or having a hard time getting words out? Do his words seem more babyish or regressed than usual?
Posturing/muscular expression	What does your child's body look like? Is she curled up? Are her fists clenched? Are her muscles tense or loose? Is her posture closed or open?
Approach versus avoidance	Does your child become withdrawn and retreat? Does he become overly clingy? Does he seem to want to do both at the same time?
Affect modulation capacity	Does your child seem to have a harder time than usual being soothed, and/or self-soothing? Does she start to need more comforting from you or someone else? How receptive is she to comfort—does this change in the face of stress?
Mood	Does your child's mood overtly change? For instance, is he normally even-tempered, but becomes more reactive in the face of intense emotion? If so, pay attention to signs of moodiness—it can serve as a warning sign that something is going on.

(continued)

NOW WHAT?

When your detective skills tell you that something is going on with your child, it's time for action. But what kind of action? Often, we rush to solve children's problems for them or try to help them "solve" things themselves. Sometimes, though, the most important action is simply to be there, to provide support, and to help children name, understand, and regulate their feelings. Only after doing that can children move toward solving problems.

Consider a possible example from your own life: You've had a hard day, your boss is irritating you, people are making demands, and you come home ready for a little sympathy. Your spouse notices that you are upset and asks what is going on. You begin to unload: "My boss is so unreasonable! Can you believe he asked me to . . . ?" Your spouse listens to your story, then shrugs, and says, "Well, you could have . . ." (or "Why don't you just . . . ?").
Do you feel more frustrated, or less?

Most of us want people to *listen to* us before they solve our problems or tell us what we could have, should have, or what they would have done. When people listen to us, understand us, and give us empathy, it validates our experience, shares the burden, and often helps us begin to feel better.

Mirroring

Validate: To demonstrate or support the truth or value of

Reflect: To bear witness

SEARCH FOR WHAT'S UNDERNEATH THE BEHAVIOR

Kids primarily communicate their emotions in nonverbal ways such as through behavior. Often adults get caught in the trap of addressing the surface behavior before considering what is underneath the behavior or what is driving the behavior, so to speak. The "driver" is commonly the emotional experience.

PROVIDING LABELS

Many young children do not have words for their emotional experience. It is adults who provide young children with the words/labels for their experience. We do this through **Reflection** and **Validation.**

"IT SEEMS LIKE . . ." WORDING

It can be helpful to begin validating statements with the phrase "It seems like . . . ," which allows the child to correct us if we are wrong.

"IT MAKES SENSE THAT . . ." WORDING

Sometimes it can be very normalizing to use this beginning phrasing when we are aware of the precipitant to the problem, like a change in schedule, a disappointment, tough day, etc. This type of phrasing affirms that the child's reactions are valid and reasonable.

OTHER EXAMPLES OF MIRRORING STATEMENTS

Reminder: Link labels with cues.

- "That kind of thing can make kids feel really bad."
- "It looks like you are feeling really happy and proud!"
- "Your energy looks very high and uncomfortable."
- "Wow, how hard that must be."
- "That stinks!"
- "Boy, you just got really quiet all of a sudden. I'm guessing I hurt your feelings."
- "It makes sense that that might make you feel really sad."
- "You look so excited right now!"
- "I bet you feel disappointed."
- "I'm sorry. I know how much that meant to you."
- "Tell me more." (Shows interest.)

From Margaret E. Blaustein and Kristine M. Kinniburgh (2019, The Guilford Press). Copyright © 2019 by the authors. Permission to photocopy this material is granted to purchasers of this book for personal use or use with clients (see copyright page for details). Purchasers can download additional copies of this material (see the box at the end of the table of contents).

Understanding the Trauma Cycle

	Youth	Parent/Caregiver
Cognitions	"I'm bad, unlovable, damaged." "I can't trust anyone."	"I'm ineffective." "My child is rejecting me."
Emotions	Shame, anger, fear, hopelessness	Frustration, shame, anger, fear, worry, sadness, hopelessness/ helplessness
Behavior/ Coping Strategies	Avoidance, aggression, preemptive rejection	Overreacting, controlling, shutting down, being overly permissive
The Cycle	"I'm being controlled; I have to fight harder."	"He keeps fighting me; I better dig in my heels."

From Margaret E. Blaustein and Kristine M. Kinniburgh (2019). Copyright © 2019 The Guilford Press. Permission to photocopy this material is granted to purchasers of this book for personal use or use with clients (see copyright page for details). Purchasers can download additional copies of this material (see the box at the end of the table of contents).

Behavior Strategies: What Are Your Tools?

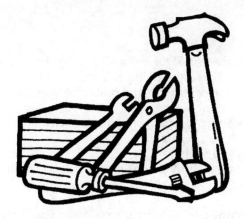

PRAISE AND REINFORCEMENT

- **Why?**
  - ♦ To build children's awareness of their successes and positive capacities
  - ♦ To shift the adult frame from negative ("bad behavior" focused) to positive ("strength and success" focused)
- **When?**
  - ♦ Any time a child is engaging in a behavior you want to increase (including ending a negative behavior)
- **How?**
  - ♦ Verbally (with words), nonverbally (showing pride and appreciation), and/or concretely (reinforcement charts or tangible rewards)
  - ♦ Be specific; label the behavior. For example:
    - • "I'm so proud of you for trying to use your tools and calm down."
    - • "You just did such a good job listening when I asked you to clean up."

PRAISE AND REINFORCEMENT: TRAUMA CONSIDERATIONS

- Be aware that praise can be triggering for trauma-impacted children.
- If kids reject or ignore your praise, try not to take it personally, and don't engage in a power struggle. It's okay for the child to disagree with, or not respond to, your statements.
- With children who seem triggered by praise, it may be helpful to focus on the *positive behavior,* rather than on the *whole child,* and to be selective (don't praise everything!).
  - ♦ *"You worked so hard on that drawing" versus "What a good artist you are!"*
- Keep noticing the positive things. Even for a child who seems distressed or unresponsive, over time the positives will matter.

(continued)

From Margaret E. Blaustein and Kristine M. Kinniburgh (2019, The Guilford Press). Copyright © 2019 by the authors. Permission to photocopy this material is granted to purchasers of this book for personal use or use with clients (see copyright page for details). Purchasers can download additional copies of this material (see the box at the end of the table of contents).

PROBLEM SOLVING

- **Why?**
  - ◆ To help children build awareness of having and making choices, and the ability to get in front of challenges, instead of just reacting to them
  - ◆ To help children feel more in control of, and powerful over, their lives
- **When?**
  - ◆ In calm states, in anticipation of or following distress, challenges or other "problem" situations
  - ◆ When the child is asking you for help
  - ◆ Regularly, through building skills by practicing and addressing the many small challenges that arise day-to-day
- **How?**
  - ◆ Communicate your willingness to support the child and your belief in a solution ("Let's figure this out").
  - ◆ Help the child identify what the problem is ("What is it that you're trying to solve?").
  - ◆ Identify goals or outcomes ("What do we want to have happen?").
  - ◆ Identify choices ("What kinds of things might we be able to do?").
  - ◆ Identify consequences ("What might happen if we do that?").
  - ◆ Make a plan and troubleshoot it. Be sure to pay attention to the adult support role.

PROBLEM SOLVING: TRAUMA CONSIDERATIONS

- Ability to engage in this process will depend upon:
  - ◆ *Agency:* the child's belief in his or her ability to make choices and be successful
  - ◆ *State:* which part of the brain is online
  - ◆ *Stage:* developmental capacity; problem-solving ability increases over time
- The adult's calm approach, appropriate timing, and ongoing support are crucial; very few children can do this on their own.

LIMIT SETTING

- **Why?**
  - ◆ To establish an understanding of boundaries, expectations, and a safe world
  - ◆ To help children contain and shift negative behaviors and identify positive alternatives
  - ◆ To help children learn where the "lines" are drawn regarding inappropriate behaviors
- **When?**
  - ◆ When behaviors cross established boundaries: threat to safety, harm to others, harm to self
  - ◆ Thoughtfully, and not for every behavior

(continued)

- **How?**
  - ◆ In a calm adult state, whenever possible
  - ◆ Thoughtfully: Work to identify appropriate limits in advance of behaviors occurring.
  - ◆ Provide age-appropriate responses.
  - ◆ If naming consequences, do so when child is reasonably calm, after regulation tools have been used.
  - ◆ Less is more: Be concise and clear in naming consequences, and link them to the behavior (not to the child).
  - ◆ Move on: Allow space for the child's distressed affect (it's okay for a child to be angry about a consequence), but also create space for repair. Try to let go of your own anger, and use your tools.

LIMIT SETTING: TRAUMA CONSIDERATIONS

- Any limit can be a potential trigger for a trauma-impacted child.
- Be thoughtful about history when choosing and naming consequences (time-out may escalate distress for a child with a neglect history; yelling is likely to trigger a child who has experienced violence).
- Bring in attunement: Validate and name child affect, even when you have identified a consequence for the behavior ("I understand how angry you were, but we use our words, not our hands, when we are mad").
- Separate the behavior from the child.

Building Daily Routines

Morning	The morning transition is often difficult for everyone, but particularly when families are coping with stress. Think about whether you and your family have a consistent morning routine. If not, are there ways to make the morning process more consistent?
Mealtimes	Meals are often a great opportunity for communication and a place for family together time. For children (and their caregivers) family meals can build social skills, turn taking, manners, and interest in each other's activities. Consider building family meals into your daily routine, as often as possible. *Note:* Food choice is a common place for children to exert their need for control. Try to avoid power struggles. Find a middle ground between too much flexibility and too much control. For instance, provide a predictable alternative (for example, child can eat family meal or eat a peanut butter and jelly sandwich).
Play	Play is a child's natural means of expression. Try to find time to play with your children. Consider building time into the week for "family play" as well as solitary and peer-to-peer play. *Although often mistakenly considered less important than chores, homework, etc., play is a crucial part of healthy development.* In addition, play also provides a forum for socialization and skill building. ■ Together time should *not* be tied to rewards or consequences (for example, "If you don't clean your room, you don't get to spend time with Mom"). For children with histories of neglect and abandonment, in particular, this can be triggering. ■ Try to build one-on-one time with each child in the family, as well as full family time.
Chores	Chores help to build a sense of responsibility and self-efficacy. Of course, chores should be age-appropriate, but it is okay for even very young children to expect to be responsible for certain (however small) chores. This distribution of chores builds in the idea that all family members are integral to the successful functioning of the family, and that the child makes an important contribution. Try to develop child-appropriate and realistic daily expectations.
Homework	School achievement and success are important areas of competency building for children. Caregivers can contribute here by emphasizing the importance of homework, providing an appropriate environment to support homework completion, being available to offer help and encouragement, and emphasizing effort over success.
Family Together Time	It is important to build into family daily routines a formal or informal time for caregivers and children to come together to share experience. For instance, some families may consider holding a weekly "family meeting" in which to share significant events, or together time could be incorporated into mealtime, bedtime, etc. Regardless of the forum, it is important that family members have opportunities to share experience on a routine basis.

(continued)

From Margaret E. Blaustein and Kristine M. Kinniburgh (2019). Copyright © 2019 The Guilford Press. Permission to photocopy this material is granted to purchasers of this book for personal use or use with clients (see copyright page for details). Purchasers can download additional copies of this material (see the box at the end of the table of contents).

EXPANDED EXAMPLE: BEDTIME ROUTINES

Teaching Points	Bedtime is often a difficult time for children and adolescents who have experienced trauma, particularly those whose abuse occurred at a similar time in the day/night or in the place where they are now expected to sleep.	
	For children whose arousal is high during the day, it may be hard for them to calm their bodies in preparation for sleep.	
	Bedtime routines help children decrease their arousal and learn to transition into sleep.	
Things to Consider	■ *Develop a consistent bedtime routine.* Have your child put on pajamas, brush teeth, have quiet time, etc. Pay attention to the location where your child is sleeping; try to help your child sleep in the same place each night. ■ *Troubleshoot.* How can you keep bedtimes and their routines as consistent as possible? What might (or sometimes does) interfere with a regular routine? Think about how you will handle any such interference. ■ *Identify nighttime boundaries and ways to cope with nighttime fears.* For example, what will you do if your child awakens during the night? Try to be consistent in follow-through. ■ *Minimize your child's engagement in highly arousing activities near bedtime.* Decrease your child's involvement in activities such as video games, overstimulating television shows, loud music, active play, etc.	
General Activities	Nurturing	Read a story, cuddle, or listen to soft music together.
	Bathing	Have your child take a bath or shower about an hour before bed; this may help bring down arousal. Pay attention to issues of privacy, boundaries, and the possibility of this area being a trigger.
	Safety check	Help children feel safe. Leave on a nightlight, hang a dream catcher, check under beds or in closets, reassure children of your own location, etc.
	Relaxation/ quiet time	Allow child to read, listen to quiet music, etc.
Bedtime Routines: Developmental Considerations	**Early Childhood**	Routines at this age should include caregivers. Nurturing activities (for example, reading a bedtime story) are a good way to build attunement and relax the child.
		Night is a time when generalized fears often emerge. Predictable nighttime routines are particularly important during this developmental stage.

(continued)

	Middle Childhood	Although children at this age will desire greater independence, bedtime is a natural place for nurturance, and children who have experienced trauma may show some developmental regression around bedtime.
		Developmental changes may shift the mechanics of bedtime: For example, caregivers may now read *with* their children instead of *to* them; may include independent activities (child brushes teeth, showers, gets into pajamas) as well as together time (caregiver enters room to say "good night").
	Adolescence	Balance is very important at this developmental stage. The important areas to balance include: ■ *Independence versus nurturance:* Adolescents need privacy. However, like younger children, they may also experience developmental regression around bedtime. Check in with your teen before bed—does he or she want a hug good night? Etc. ■ *Flexibility versus limits:* Although adolescents are independent, don't lose sight of the need for limits. Maintain expectations around bedtime (for example, must be in room by 10:00 P.M.), but allow flexibility (for example, can have quiet time—read, listen to music—and turn off lights when ready).

What Are Your Self-Care Tools?

First set of tools: Prepare yourself. Before going into a stressful situation:

- Use self-talk.
- Have a plan.
- Bring a support person.
- Get a good night's sleep and make sure you're not hungry.

Second set of tools: Have tools "in your pocket," such as:

- Deep breathing
- Relaxing your muscles
- Counting to 10
- Walking away for a moment
- Thinking of self-affirmation statements

Third set of tools: Have recovery tools, such as:

- Calling a friend
- Making a cup of tea or coffee
- Exercising
- Doing something you enjoy
- Trying to remember one good thing that happened today

Fourth set of tools: Ongoing self-care strategies, such as:

- Having and using a team
- Making time for yourself
- Finding something that is about you, and not about you as a parent
- Ensuring your basic self-care needs, such as sleep, food, and health

From Margaret E. Blaustein and Kristine M. Kinniburgh (2019, The Guilford Press). Copyright © 2019 by the authors. Permission to photocopy this material is granted to purchasers of this book for personal use or use with clients (see copyright page for details). Purchasers can download additional copies of this material (see the box at the end of the table of contents).

Five-Minute Connection Activities

The following table provides examples of ways to build connection that can be easily built into daily routine.

Five-Minute Connection Activity Examples					
Physical activities	Games	Creative/music	Self-care	Chores	"Talk" games/ activities
Balance feather Basketball Dance off Dancing to a song Going outside (walk, bike ride, throw a ball) Jump in puddles with rain boots Jump rope Pillow fight Play with balloon Playing with pets Push ups/ jumping jacks Red light/green light Skipping Swinging Take the dog out Throw Frisbee back and forth Workout video Yoga	20 questions Alphabet game Bubbles Card games Come up with a special handshake Feelings charades "Guess what's different" Hand-clapping game Hide and seek Hot and cold game I spy Interactive game on phone Legos Lincoln logs Make up a game Mirror game Playdough Screaming contest Shapes of clouds Silly Simon Says Staring contest (who laughs first) Thumb war Tic-tac-toe	Co-create a story (take turns saying a word/sentence) Coloring Coloring a mandala Do a puzzle Finger painting Gong/singing drum Listening to a song Make a collage Make a stress ball Name that tune Origami Paper airplanes Read comics Read short book Rhythm band Take selfies	Bake Bath time Brushing hair Braiding hair Cook Cuddle Apply lotion Make a smoothie Make an after-school snack Make lunch Get a massage Paint nails Pick fruit Have tea, coffee, hot cocoa	Clean an area Do a piece of homework together Do chores in a playful way Gardening Get the mail together Getting-ready race Job application/ visit a college website Laundry folding train Prayer/ devotions Set the table together Take care of a pet together Unload dishwasher in a funny way	"Book of questions " Cat videos Current events discussion Highs/lows Make a list of favorite things (movies, animals, etc.) Name three good things about your day Plan birthday Share a positive affirmation Rose/thorn or sun/cloud Sign language Switch roles Talk about something you look forward to Talk about upcoming holiday Tell jokes Time to vent Watch a YouTube video together

From Margaret E. Blaustein and Kristine M. Kinniburgh (2019, The Guilford Press). Copyright © 2019 by the authors. Permission to photocopy this material is granted to purchasers of this book for personal use or use with clients (see copyright page for details). Purchasers can download additional copies of this material (see the box at the end of the table of contents).

Make a Regulation Toolbox

Build regular tools into your child's life to support baseline regulation.

Provide ongoing activities, such as:

- Playtime (alone or together)
- Sports
- Expressive arts/dance/theatre
- Yoga
- Reading
- Listening to music

Find ways to soothe by providing:

- Sensory activities
- Gross motor activities
- A dedicated, calming space
- Opportunities for engagement and connection

Develop creative daily routines and rhythms.

- Routines are the rhythms, structures, and predictable moments that build safety, skill, and support.
- Routines are not about rigidity—they are about creating a rhythm
- Routines should decrease rather than increase distress. If your routine is making things harder, change it.

Use routines to:

- Target challenge points, such as transitions, hygiene, expectations (homework, chores)
- Provide natural soothing opportunities at bedtime, playtime, bath time, etc.
- Provide engagement and connection points, such as check-ins, asking about the day, solving problems together.

Be a detective—read your child or teen's patterns.

- What sorts of activities or experiences lead to feelings or energy that seem more or less organized or in control?
- How do you know your child or teen is comfortable or uncomfortable in his or her body and with his or her feelings? What are the clues?
- What patterns of strength and challenge does your child or teen show? When does your child or teen do best—and worst? Target soothing routines for the challenging times.
- Actively track clues each time your child or teen has a hard time. These clues will come in handy next time.

From Margaret E. Blaustein and Kristine M. Kinniburgh (2019, The Guilford Press). Copyright © 2019 by the authors. Permission to photocopy this material is granted to purchasers of this book for personal use or use with clients (see copyright page for details). Purchasers can download additional copies of this material (see the box at the end of the table of contents).

Modulation Activities

There are many ways to support your child or teen with *regulation,* or bringing energy and feelings to a comfortable and effective level. Some activities can be used in moments of distress, but many may be useful to build into daily routines. Support your child in experimenting—every child is different!

Choose activities that are naturally modulating, such as:

- Play (alone or together)
- Sports
- Expressive arts, dance or theater
- Yoga
- Reading
- Listening to music
- Crafts

Use sensory strategies, such as:

- **Sound:** Listen to music, use headphones or noise machines to drown out noise.
- **Touch:** Provide hugs, weighted blankets, soft pillows, stuffed animals, cool stones, things to fiddle with, chewable jewelry.
- **Smell:** Provide lotions, use air fresheners, fill the air with the scent of cooking.
- **Taste:** Share a favorite food.
- **Sight:** Provide pictures of safe people and favorite places. Minimize visual stimulation.

Provide gross motor opportunities, such as:

- Small trampolines
- Opportunities to run, jump, and play
- Exercise balls or yoga balls
- Balance beams
- After-school dance parties

Create a dedicated comfort zone:

- Make it in a safe place, preferably just for the child or teen.
- Fill it with materials that are safe, comforting, and sensory.
- Have the child or teen practice using it when he or she is calm.

(continued)

From Margaret E. Blaustein and Kristine M. Kinniburgh (2019, The Guilford Press). Copyright © 2019 by the authors. Permission to photocopy this material is granted to purchasers of this book for personal use or use with clients (see copyright page for details). Purchasers can download additional copies of this material (see the box at the end of the table of contents).

Additional activities to support modulation include:

Breathing activities, such as:

- *Deep breathing with movement and sounds.* You be the model. Say: "We are going to practice deep breathing with movement and sounds. When I raise my arms up [*demonstrate*], I am going to take a deep breath in. When I bring my arms down, I am going to exhale, making a sound, like this: oooooooooooooooooh. You can make any sound that you wish to make. Okay, on the count of 3, let's practice together. . . ."
- *Bubble breathing:* You be the model. Use a jar of bubble mixture and a wand. Breathe slowly into the wand, emphasizing breathing slowly to make a large bubble.
- *Deep breathing with a straw.* Remind your child or teen that deep breathing is the fastest way to send a message to the brain that everything is okay. Give him or her a straw and a small piece of paper. On the count of 3, ask the child or teen to take a deep breath in (expanding the belly out so that it looks and feels like it is filling with air). The goal is to hold the small paper on the end of the straw. After a count to 4, prompt the child or teen to exhale, allowing the paper to fall to the floor.
- *Pillow breathing.* Have child or teen lie on floor with pillow or stuffed animal on stomach. Teach him or her to breathe so that pillow or animal rises and falls with each breath.
- *London Bridge breathing.* Have children or teens raise their arms (like in game London Bridge). Breathe in as arms go up; breathe out as arms come down. See how slowly they can move their arms up and down.
- *Breathing with imagery.* Have children or teens imagine taking a deep breath and blowing out birthday candles. Or have them try to paint the opposite wall with their breath, or smell flowers, then blow a dandelion puff.

Focus activities, such as:

- *Focus bell.* Explain that you will be ringing a bell. Ask the children or teens to focus on the sensory experience of sound and encourage them to practice their deep breathing while listening. Notice the change in sound as time passes. Say, "Raise your hand when you no longer hear the sound."
- *Memory game.* Ask the child or teen to be mindful of his or her environment and study all the things in the room. Then ask, "Please close your eyes. Now recall an item in the room that is white." You can modify this by selecting a few items (toys, pens, objects, etc.) and placing them in the middle of the table. Have the child or teen focus on the items for 1 minute. Then say, "Close your eyes," while you remove one item. The final step is to give the child or teen an opportunity to guess the missing item.
- *Grounding.* Have children tune in to their senses, using concrete, easy-to-hold stimuli, such as:
  - ◆ Magic wands
  - ◆ Magic rocks
  - ◆ Worry stones
  - ◆ Piece of velvet cloth
  - ◆ Small stuffed animal
  - ◆ Glitter cream
  - ◆ Pleasurable smell
  - ◆ Stress balls

(continued)

Movement activities or games, such as:

- *Dice game.* The goal is to practice breathing or light movement. You roll the dice, then choose a movement for you and the child or teen to sustain to the count indicated on the die. For example, roll your shoulders to the count of 10, or wiggle your nose to the count of 7.
- *Stretching.* Lead the child or teen in gentle movement and stretches.
- *Simon says.* Review the rules to Simon Says. Remember that in this game, there is a leader (Simon) and followers. The follower is to follow the leader's actions—but only when the leader says "Simon says. . . ."
- *Head, shoulders, knees, and toes.* Play this game with younger children to expose them to music and movement at the same time.

Music activities, such as:

- *Relaxation with music.* Play some relaxing music and have the children or teens listen to it mindfully and remind them to breathe while listening.
- *You've got the beat.* "We are going to create music together today. Each of us is going to have a turn creating a beat using our hands and body. We will take turns being the leader or creator of the beat. The rest of us will follow the leader." You can do this exercise with movement, too.
- *Musical instruments.* Gather several types of musical instruments and demonstrate the sound of each. Say, "Close your eyes or turn your back (if comfortable)." Ask the child or teen to identify the sound and link it to a specific instrument.

Supporting Modulation

Consider a scenario in which your child's emotion escalates.

Steps toward supporting modulation:

1. **Be attuned:** Notice the feeling (tune into the energy).
2. **Keep yourself centered**: Check in with yourself.
3. **Ask yourself:** Where is your child's energy? Where does it need to go (up or down)?
4. **Reflect (simply) what you're seeing** (e.g., "I can see you just got really mad. Let's see if we can calm it down a bit so we can talk").
5. **Cue child in use of skills** (e.g., breathing, sitting quietly, calming down space, stress ball).
6. **Reinforce use of modulation skills** (e.g., "I'm really proud of you for trying to calm down your energy").
7. **Invite expression**/communication when child is calm.

From Margaret E. Blaustein and Kristine M. Kinniburgh (2019). Copyright © 2019 The Guilford Press. Permission to photocopy this material is granted to purchasers of this book for personal use or use with clients (see copyright page for details). Purchasers can download additional copies of this material (see the box at the end of the table of contents).

Tuning In to Yourself

Situation: _____

Using the following questions as a guide, write down observations about yourself during difficult interactions or situations. Fill in any additional observations at bottom.

Domain	Prompt Questions	Caregiver Observations
Body	What are you experiencing in your *body*? Pay attention to cues such as heart rate, breathing, muscle tension, temperature, and feelings of numbness or disconnection.	
	What warning signs does your body provide of "losing control" or hitting a danger point?	
Thoughts	What do you *think* in this situation? Consider both thoughts about yourself (for example, "I can't handle this" or "I should have _____") and thoughts about your child (for example, "He's doing this on purpose" or "She'll always be this way").	Thoughts about self:
		Thoughts about child/adolescent:
Emotions	What do you *feel* in this situation? Consider anger, guilt, shame, sadness, and-helplessness.	
Behavior	What do you *do* in this situation? Do you freeze? Withdraw? Dig in your heels? Scream?	
Other	What else do you notice about yourself? Consider your ability to cope with emotion, ability to use supports, unhealthy (or healthy) coping responses, etc.	

From Margaret E. Blaustein and Kristine M. Kinniburgh (2019). Copyright © 2019 The Guilford Press. Permission to photocopy this material is granted to purchasers of this book for personal use or use with clients (see copyright page for details). Purchasers can download additional copies of this material (see the box at the end of the table of contents).

What Makes a Hard Day?

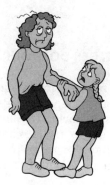

What pushes your buttons or leads to big feelings in you?

_____

_____

_____

_____

This week, try to notice if any of these things happen and how they affect your mood or responses. Ask yourself:

What is my body telling me?

_____

_____

_____

_____

What am I feeling?

_____

_____

_____

_____

What am I thinking?

_____

_____

_____

_____

What do I want to do?

_____

_____

_____

_____

From Margaret E. Blaustein and Kristine M. Kinniburgh (2019, The Guilford Press). Copyright © 2019 by the authors. Permission to photocopy this material is granted to purchasers of this book for personal use or use with clients (see copyright page for details). Purchasers can download additional copies of this material (see the box at the end of the table of contents).

Body Map for Caregivers

WHAT CLUES DOES OUR BODY GIVE US ABOUT OUR ENERGY?

All of us have energy in our bodies. Energy can tell us something about how we are feeling. Sometimes our energy feels comfortable, sometimes uncomfortable and it can show up in our thoughts, behaviors, feelings, and in the ways that we interact with our children.

Our bodies give us clues about the level of energy that we are having. For example, if we pay attention to the pace of our breathing, the rate of our heartbeat, the temperature of our bodies, the amount of tension in our muscles, we can gather a lot of information about our energy.

Breathing:

☐ Fast   ☐ Medium   ☐ Slow

Heartbeat:

☐ Fast   ☐ Medium   ☐ Slow

Muscles:

☐ Tense like uncooked spaghetti

☐ Relaxed like cooked spaghetti

Body Temperature:

☐ Hot   ☐ Warm   ☐ Cold

Other Body Cues: _____

_____

_____

_____

_____

_____

_____

_____

From Margaret E. Blaustein and Kristine M. Kinniburgh (2019, The Guilford Press). Copyright © 2019 by the authors. Permission to photocopy this material is granted to purchasers of this book for personal use or use with clients (see copyright page for details). Purchasers can download additional copies of this material (see the box at the end of the table of contents).

Self-Care Worksheet

Consider a challenging interaction or experience you have had in the past few weeks with your child or in another relationship.

Briefly describe the situation: _____

_____

_____

_____

_____

_____

What do you remember *feeling*? _____

What do you remember *thinking*? _____

What do you remember *doing*? _____

What happened in your *body*? _____

When you think about that situation now, what comes up for you (thoughts, feelings, body sensations, action urges)?

_____

_____

_____

Is there something about this situation that's particularly hard for you, and that might come up at other times? If so, what is it? (Consider specific behaviors, your own state–for example, feeling tired, reminders of previous experiences.) _____

_____

Are any of your reactions ones that are "typical" when you are feeling stressed or upset? Which ones? _____

_____

Look at the previous two questions and circle anything that might be a "clue" for you in future situations. These elements (whether in situations or in your own reactions) are the cues that you might need to do something to take care of yourself.

Now . . . think about this type of situation. What is/are your *immediate* goal/s? (Consider . . . to keep calm, to stay present, to be able to express yourself, to get through until the situation is over, etc.) _____

_____

_____

_____

(continued)

From Margaret E. Blaustein and Kristine M. Kinniburgh (2019, The Guilford Press). Copyright © 2019 by the authors. Permission to photocopy this material is granted to purchasers of this book for personal use or use with clients (see copyright page for details). Purchasers can download additional copies of this material (see the box at the end of the table of contents).

Given those goals and the realities of the situation, brainstorm a few possible coping strategies. These may be:

- *Advance preparation,* or something you do before entering the situation (for example, mental rehearsal, relaxation strategies, seeking support)
- *"In-the-pocket" strategies,* or something you do *in* the situation (for example, deep breathing, muscle relaxation, self-mantra)
- *"Recovery" strategies,* or something you do *after* the situation (for example, reaching out to friends, enjoyable activities, taking down time)
- *Ongoing self-care*

Write at least two or three possibilities down: _____

_____

_____

_____

_____

_____

Taking Care of Yourself

Situation: _____

Use the following techniques for ideas and consider possible self-care strategies you might apply in difficult or challenging situations. Fill in any additional ideas at bottom.

Self-Care Strategies		
Technique	**Tips**	**Might this technique work in this situation? Describe when and how you might use this:**
Deep Breathing	**When?** ■ Well, hopefully always! ■ Particularly when faced with surging or intense emotions **How?** ■ In through the nose, out through the mouth ■ Through the diaphragm, not your chest or shoulders ■ Pair with a calming visual image, verbal mantra, or saying	
Muscle Relaxation	**When?** ■ When the tension is building up . . . ■ As an alternative focus for energy (instead of exploding) **How?** ■ As big or small as you want it to be ■ Under-the-table methods (tense and release) ■ Progressive muscle relaxation	
Distraction	**When?** ■ Dealing with a problem you can't solve immediately. ■ Caught in a negative mental thought cycle. **How?** ■ *Self-soothe*: Consider your five senses. ■ *Find alternatives*: Switch activities.	

(continued)

From Margaret E. Blaustein and Kristine M. Kinniburgh (2019). Copyright © 2019 The Guilford Press. Permission to photocopy this material is granted to purchasers of this book for personal use or use with clients (see copyright page for details). Purchasers can download additional copies of this material (see the box at the end of the table of contents).

Technique	Tips	Might this technique work in this situation? Describe when and how you might use this:
Self-Soothing	**When?** ■ As an ongoing tool, to prevent stress build-up ■ When you want to pamper or reward yourself ■ When you are upset or stressed and need to calm down ■ When you are feeling disconnected and need to reconnect **How?** ■ *In-the-pocket techniques*: Carry small objects that feel soothing or pleasurable; consider all five senses (for example, a pleasant lotion, a small stone or piece of velvet, a picture of a favorite place). ■ Identify and incorporate pleasurable activities into daily routine (for example, a long, hot bath; going for a walk; listening to music).	
Time-Outs	**When?** ■ In the moment, to delay a negative response ■ Preventive, as an ongoing measure to "charge the batteries" **How?** ■ In the moment: For example, go for a walk, go to your room, go to the bathroom. ■ Preventive: Build in self-care time daily/ weekly/monthly.	
	Ask yourself: Is this a safe situation in which to take a time-out?	
Other Techniques?	What other techniques can you think of? Describe **when** and **how** you might use these techniques:	

Learning Your Child's Emotional Language

Emotion: _____

Using the following questions as a guide, write down "clues" that tell you that your child is experiencing the selected emotion. Fill in any additional clues at bottom.

Domain	Prompt Questions	Caregiver Observations
Facial expression	What does your child show on his/her/their face?	
Tone of voice	Does your child's voice become louder? Softer? Higher-pitched?	
Extent of speech	Does your child suddenly have more to say than usual? Does your child become quiet? How pressured (in a rush) is your child's speech?	
Quality of speech	Do your child's words become disorganized? Rambling? Stilted? Regressed?	
Posturing/ muscular expression	What does your child's body look like?	
Approach versus avoidance	Does your child become withdrawn? Clingy? Both?	
Affect modulation capacity	Does your child seem to have a harder time than usual being soothed, and/or self-soothing?	
Mood	Does your child's mood overtly change?	
Other?	What other clues are there that your child is experiencing a given emotion?	

From Margaret E. Blaustein and Kristine M. Kinniburgh (2019). Copyright © 2019 The Guilford Press. Permission to photocopy this material is granted to purchasers of this book for personal use or use with clients (see copyright page for details). Purchasers can download additional copies of this material (see the box at the end of the table of contents).

What Does Your Child Look Like When Triggered?

It may be hard to identify a specific trigger, but you can learn to read signs that your child is showing the danger response

Fight Response:

Description: Signs of high arousal levels, which often appear sudden: for example, irritability, swearing, sudden anger, hyperactivity

Your child's behaviors that may indicate "fight":

_____

_____

_____

_____

_____

Flight Response:

Description: Physical withdrawal or escape: for example, avoiding contact with others, isolating self from friends or family, refusal to do homework

Your child's behaviors that may indicate "flight":

_____

_____

_____

_____

_____

Freeze Response:

Description: Shutting down or disconnecting from experience: for example, child looks numb; blank stare; child appears dazed

Your child's behaviors that may indicate "freeze":

_____

_____

_____

_____

_____

(continued)

From Margaret E. Blaustein and Kristine M. Kinniburgh (2019). Copyright © 2019 The Guilford Press. Permission to photocopy this material is granted to purchasers of this book for personal use or use with clients (see copyright page for details). Purchasers can download additional copies of this material (see the box at the end of the table of contents).

Submit/Comply Response:

Description: Overly compliant behavior, giving in too easily, denying needs like hunger or thirst, false reassurance (for instance, saying "I'm fine" when it is clear that the child isn't)

Your child's behaviors that may indicate "submit/comply":

_____

_____

_____

_____

_____

Identifying Your Child's Triggers

Name: _____ Date: _____

Example of Trigger	May Remind Child of . . .
1. Hearing people yell in loud tone of voice	Times when child was yelled at a lot
2. Feeling alone or being ignored	Times when child did not get enough attention when he or she was little
3. Smell of smoke	A bad fire
4. _____ _____ _____ _____	_____ _____ _____ _____
5. _____ _____ _____ _____	_____ _____ _____ _____
6. _____ _____ _____ _____	_____ _____ _____ _____
7. _____ _____ _____ _____	_____ _____ _____ _____
8. _____ _____ _____ _____	_____ _____ _____ _____

From Margaret E. Blaustein and Kristine M. Kinniburgh (2019). Copyright © 2019 The Guilford Press. Permission to photocopy this material is granted to purchasers of this book for personal use or use with clients (see copyright page for details). Purchasers can download additional copies of this material (see the box at the end of the table of contents).

Being a Detective: Understanding a Child's Patterns

Emotional reaction/body state/problem behavior: Identify/describe a concerning behavior, emotional response, or physical state observed in the child or teen _____

In-the-moment clues: What does the child or teen look like *in that moment/in that state* (feeling expression, behavior, response to relationship, etc.): _____

_____

_____

_____

_____

The buildup: What does the child or teen look like *before* that moment? What clues do I have that the child or teen might be headed into a hard time? _____

_____

_____

_____

_____

Triggers/situation: What sorts of situations/experiences are most likely to lead to that behavior/ body state/reaction? Think of both environmental stressors (things that happen around and to the child or teen) as well as inside experiences (like being hungry, tired, or upset about something else):

_____

_____

_____

_____

Needs: What do the behaviors suggest the child or teen might need in those moments? For instance, yelling and screaming might be *attention seeking behavior,* or might signal a *need for space*. What kinds of reactions do the child or teen's behaviors tend to elicit, and what might those behaviors mean in terms of the underlying need? _____

_____

_____

_____

_____

(continued)

From Margaret E. Blaustein and Kristine M. Kinniburgh (2019, The Guilford Press). Copyright © 2019 by the authors. Permission to photocopy this material is granted to purchasers of this book for personal use or use with clients (see copyright page for details). Purchasers can download additional copies of this material (see the box at the end of the table of contents).

Effective responses: What helps in those moments? Think of what the child or teen does or responds to, what adults are able to do, and the immediate environmental structures (like routines or available tools). What have you found helpful? Does that give you any other information about the child or teen's needs? _____

_____

_____

_____

_____

_____

_____

Adult reactions: When this behavior happens, what does it do to *you?* How does it affect you or other adults/caregivers? (It's important to pay attention to this, because our own experience is both a clue about the child or teen's experience, as well as a factor in how well we're able to respond). _____

_____

_____

_____

_____

_____

_____

Adult needs: Are there any tools or strategies for managing or addressing your own reactions, which *you* (or other caregivers) might need to pay attention to, in order to be effective in responding to your/this child or teen? What type of tools or strategies might you need? Be sure you're thinking realistically, given the typical situation in which the child or teen's behavior occurs. _____

_____

_____

_____

_____

_____

_____

Approaches to Behavior Worksheet

Pick one behavior a child or teen in your home is displaying that you find challenging or that you want to increase. Use this worksheet to try to identify patterns and needs and to develop a plan.

1. What behavior do you want to address?

   Behavior: _____

   Do you want this behavior to . . .   Increase   Decrease

2. Identify patterns: What do you think *leads* to this behavior? What are some of the triggers (situational, environmental, internal)?:

   _____

   _____

   _____

   _____

   _____

   What do you think the child is trying to do? What is the *function* or *need* that the behavior is addressing?

   _____

   _____

   _____

   _____

   _____

3. "Go-to" strategies to address this behavior:

   a. How else might you be able to meet the needs identified in question 2? Be specific: when, how, who?

   _____

   _____

   _____

   _____

   b. What regulation, deescalation, or crisis management strategies can you support in the moment if the child is dysregulated?

   _____

   _____

   _____

   _____

(continued)

From Margaret E. Blaustein and Kristine M. Kinniburgh (2019, The Guilford Press). Copyright © 2019 by the authors. Permission to photocopy this material is granted to purchasers of this book for personal use or use with clients (see copyright page for details). Purchasers can download additional copies of this material (see the box at the end of the table of contents).

4. Which of these additional behavior response strategies do you think might work? Remember: Each of these might be used for the same behavior in different moments.

   Praise and reinforcement (use to increase a behavior or a desired alternative behavior).

   Problem solving (use when child is in regulated state to support control/choice and identify alternatives).

   Appropriate limits (use to contain and address negative or dangerous behaviors).

   _____

   _____

   _____

   _____

   _____

5. *After* the behavior occurs, how might you and the child continue to learn from it? Consider timing, method, and approach to revisiting behaviors, with a goal of shifting the behavior the next time. What can you plan to do? Be specific:

   With my child, I can (When? How?):

   _____

   _____

   _____

   _____

   By myself or with my caregiving partner, I can (When? How?):

   _____

   _____

   _____

   _____

   _____

My Child Makes Me Smile When . . .

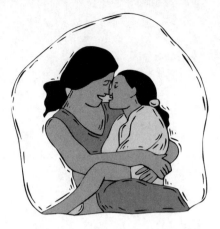

Please write down three things that your child does that puts a smile on your face.

1. _____
   _____
   _____
   _____

2. _____
   _____
   _____
   _____

3. _____
   _____
   _____
   _____

As you think about those three things, what kinds of feelings are you experiencing?

_____
_____
_____
_____
_____
_____
_____
_____

From Margaret E. Blaustein and Kristine M. Kinniburgh (2019, The Guilford Press). Copyright © 2019 by the authors. Permission to photocopy this material is granted to purchasers of this book for personal use or use with clients (see copyright page for details). Purchasers can download additional copies of this material (see the box at the end of the table of contents).

APPENDIX C

Group Activities

Sample Group Activities

ACTIVITY: GUESS WHO?

- **ARC Target(s): Relational Connection, Identity; Icebreaker activity**
- **Purpose:** Increase group members' awareness of/attunement to other members and awareness of ways in which they already know each other. Have fun.
- **Materials:** Preprinted slips of paper with questions (see examples).
- **Directions:** Each group member receives five slips with prompts on them (e.g., "What is your favorite movie?"; "What is your favorite song?"). Each member writes answers to each prompt and puts the folded slips in a hat. Members take turns picking a slip out of the hat and guessing whose answer it is. If they guess right, they get a point. If short on time, you can leave slips out of hat after all guesses, right and wrong, so the hat goes around five times, and then those that were guessed wrong can be claimed by those who wrote them. If you have more time, you can put wrong guesses back in hat and keep going around until all have been guessed.
- **Sample Prompt Topics:** favorite type of pet, favorite food, favorite movie, favorite song, favorite actor or actress, favorite TV show, favorite color, favorite band or musical artist, place you'd most like to travel to, favorite book.

ACTIVITY: BODY DRAWING

- **ARC Target(s): Identification**
- **Purpose:** To increase participant ability to tune in to ways that feelings are expressed in the body.
- **Materials:** Silhouette drawing of body (e.g., *"Where Do I Feel . . . "* in Appendix D), crayons or colored pencils (preferable to markers).
- **Directions:**
- Provide participants with body drawings and six colored pencils or crayons each.
  - ◆ Ask participants to create a key, selecting colors to represent the following feelings: happy, angry, sad, scared, excited, worried.
  - ◆ For each identified feeling, participants should use crayons/pencils to color . . . *where in their body they feel.*
  - ◆ **Discussion:** Following completion of this activity, discuss with participants:
    - "How easy/hard was this to do?"
    - "Were some feelings easier than others to locate in your body? Which feelings were the easiest? Which were the hardest?"
    - "Did any feelings overlap in location? Which ones?"
    - "Which feeling was the most distinct—that is, the only one held in a particular part of your body?"

DISCUSSION: THE FUNCTION OF FEELINGS AND "MASKING" FEELINGS

- **ARC Target(s): Identification, Modulation, and/or Relational Connection**
- *Ask:* "What function do feelings serve?" Elicit ideas from the group.
  - ◆ If group members are not able to think of reasons, provide examples: "Fear may tell us we need to run, and it helps us survive; anger may help us feel powerful in a difficult situation"; and so on.
  - ◆ *General idea:* Feelings provide us with information about the external world and our internal experience) and pull us toward specific actions or responses.

(continued)

From Margaret E. Blaustein and Kristine M. Kinniburgh (2019). Copyright © 2019 The Guilford Press. Permission to photocopy this material is granted to purchasers of this book for personal use or use with clients (see copyright page for details). Purchasers can download additional copies of this material (see the box at the end of the table of contents).

- *Ask:* "Are feelings always accurate? In other words, is what we're *AWARE* of feeling always the true feeling we are having?"

Teaching points:
  - One feeling sometimes acts as a "mask" for another. This can happen for many reasons:
    - To decrease feelings of vulnerability (e.g., anger substituting for sadness or fear).
    - Because past experience made it dangerous to exhibit or acknowledge a particular emotion (e.g., showing fear might increase vulnerability, *or* showing anger might increase abuse).
    - Cultural or family norms: How acceptable it is to show particular feelings, as well as different ways feelings are expressed.
- *Ask:* "Are there feelings that you don't like to show? Do you know why?"
- *Ask:* "How do you know when feelings are 'true feelings' versus 'mask feelings'?"
- *Ask:* "Is there any risk that comes with consistently masking your feelings?"
  - ◆ *Teaching point:* Feelings that don't come out in one way will often come out in other ways (e.g., held in the body, interfering with sleep or eating, irritability)
- *Ask:* "Why might you want to shift your feelings?"
  - ◆ *Teaching point:* Feelings may be too intense, interfere with current activities, be inappropriate to the situation, lead to impulsive behavior, etc.
- *Ask:* "How do you shift to a different feeling?"
  - ◆ Review or discuss skills associated with managing feelings (e.g., relaxation, breathing, music).
- *Ask:* "What skills do you use?"

ACTIVITY: FIGHT, FLIGHT, FREEZE, SUBMIT GAME, PART 1
Identification of Danger Response

- **ARC Target(s): Identification (Advanced)**
- **Purpose:** To facilitate application of the learned concept of the body's alarm system and the human danger response.
- **Materials:** Scenarios listed on the next page, or similar.
- **Directions:**
- The group facilitator reviews the body's alarm system and the trauma response. See the teaching points that follow:
  - **The Body's Alarm System:** *"We all have a built-in alarm system that signals when we might be in danger. One reason why human beings have been able to survive over time is because our brains recognize signals around us that tell us that danger might be coming. This helps our bodies prepare to deal with danger when it comes."*
  - **The Human Danger Response:** *"When our brains recognize danger, they prepare our bodies to deal with it. We can deal with something dangerous in four major ways: We can fight it, we can get away from it (flight), we can freeze, or we can give in to someone more powerful than us (submit or comply)."*
  - **Our Responses May Be Different in Different Situations:** *"What we pick to do sometimes depends on the kind of danger. So, for example, if a really small squirrel is attacking you, you might fight it, because you're bigger and stronger than it is. If a car comes speeding at you, and you're standing in the street, you'd probably run, because you can't really fight it, and if you stand still, you'll get hit. If you saw a big bear or some other animal nearby, you might freeze, because you can't really fight it, and you're probably not fast enough to run away. If someone really powerful is forcing you to do something, you might submit or comply – even if you don't want to – so that you can get through the situation without getting hurt"*

(continued)

- **Our Bodies Give Us the Fuel/Energy That We Need to Survive:** *"When it's time for our bodies to fight, or run, or freeze, we need a lot of energy to do those things. So, once the brain recognizes danger, the "action" or "doing" part of our brains sends a signal to our bodies to release a bunch of chemicals, like fuel for a car. That gives us the energy we need to cope with the danger."*
- ◆ Following review of the concepts, the group leader facilitates the "Fight, Flight, Freeze, Submit Game." Each member takes a turn listening to one of the scenarios below. The task is to identify whether the person in the scenario is actively engaged in the *fight*, *flight*, *freeze* or *submit* response. Group members can earn points for guessing the correct response (the goal should be cooperative, rather than competitive).

FIGHT, FLIGHT, FREEZE, SUBMIT GAME, PART 1—SAMPLE SCENARIOS

1. Joey is crossing the street and all of a sudden a car comes racing toward him. Without thinking, he runs to the other side of the road as fast as he can. *(flight)*
2. Bobby is taking a nature walk and all of a sudden he sees a bear standing 10 feet away looking at him. He has learned that bears react to sudden movement and noise. He stays as still as he possibly can until the bear finally moves away. *(freeze)*
3. Jennifer is in school and one of her peers calls her a name and starts to threaten her. She starts screaming and yelling as loud as she can "NO, NO, NO . . . you don't threaten me." *(fight)*
4. Holly just started a new program. One of her roommates is having a difficult time and starts slamming things around the room. Holly bolts out of her room and out of the front door of the building. *(flight)*
5. Liza's classmate tells her that if she wants to be friends, she has to let him cheat off of her test. She feels really uncomfortable with the idea, but agrees anyway. *(submit)*
6. Gage is at the hospital waiting for news about a family member who is in surgery. He sees the doctor walking toward him and then everything feels as if it were in slow motion: He can't move, he can't talk, and time stands still. *(freeze)*
7. Nate is walking down the street and a small dog begins to attack his leg. Nate starts screaming at the dog and kicks his leg back and forth, over and over again, until the dog finally lets go of him. *(fight)*
8. Betty is walking down the street and a large, large dog starts to walk toward her. Without thinking, she starts running toward the nearest building and is able to narrowly escape the dog. *(flight)*
9. Bobby just left the movie theater after watching a scary movie. Walking down a dark road, he hears a weird noise nearby. His heart starts beating, his body feels jumpy, his arms go up, and his fists are ready to strike. *(fight)*
10. A deer is crossing the road and a car starts coming toward it. The deer just stands there—"a deer caught in the headlights." *(freeze)*
11. Marie is really hungry, but in her last home she wasn't allowed to eat between meals. When her foster mother asks if she wants a snack, she says, "No, I don't get hungry a lot." *(submit)*
12. Joey's dad comes home in a really angry mood and starts calling for him. Joey runs into his room and hides under the bed. *(flight)*
13. Lilly is sitting in class and one of her classmates starts to throw things at the teacher. Lilly gets up from her desk, grabs her classmate's arm to stop her, and puts a book in front of the object that is being thrown. *(fight)*
14. Johnny is tiptoeing out of his room, trying to sneak down the hallway to get some water, even though he does not have permission. All of a sudden he hears a staff member calling his name. Johnny tries to stay as still and as quiet as possible because he is very scared of getting in trouble. *(freeze)*

(continued)

ACTIVITY: FIGHT, FLIGHT, FREEZE, SUBMIT GAME, PART 2: RECOGNIZING TRIGGERS

- ■ **ARC Target(s): Identification (Advanced)**
- ■ **Purpose:** To facilitate application of the learned concept of triggers, or "false alarms."
- ■ **Materials:** Scenarios
- ■ **Directions:**
- ■ The group facilitator reviews the concept of triggers, or "false alarms," using the teaching points outlined in the following:
  - ◆ **False Alarms:** *"False alarms can happen when we hear or see or feel something that reminds us of bad things that have happened to us, either in the past or in other situations. Those reminders are called* triggers. *Our brains have learned to recognize those reminders, because at other times when they were around, dangerous things happened, and we had to react pretty quickly. Different people have different reminders. So, if someone got yelled at a lot, hearing people yell might activate the alarm and make the 'doing' part of the brain turn on. If someone didn't get enough attention paid to him or her when little, feeling all alone or scared might turn on the alarm."*
  - ◆ **What Happens When the Alarm Goes Off?:** *"Once our alarm turns on, our brains prep our bodies for action. When that happens, our body fills with 'fuel' to prepare us for dealing with danger. This is really important if it's real danger (like a bear, or a speeding car, or a really mean squirrel), but not so helpful if it's a false alarm, and there isn't really any danger around. Imagine if you were in math class, and something felt dangerous—suddenly, your body is filled with fuel."*
  - ◆ **How Our "Danger Energy" Affects Us:** *"Remember that the fuel gives us the energy to fight, or get away, or freeze. Even when we submit or comply, our bodies are full of energy. When our bodies have all that energy, we have to do something. So, some kids suddenly feel really angry, or want to argue or fight with someone. Other kids just feel antsy or jumpy. Some kids want to hide in a corner or get as far away as they can—and sometimes they don't even know why. Still other kids suddenly feel really shut down, like someone flipped a switch and turned them off. All of these are ways that the body tries to deal with something it thinks is dangerous."*
  - ◆ **The Problem with the False Alarm:** *Sometimes, though, what sets off the alarm isn't really dangerous—it's just something that feels bad or reminds us of something bad that happened or still happens. When kids have a false alarm like that, it can be hard for other people to understand what just happened, and to help. Sometimes, kids even get into trouble."*
  - ◆ **Recognizing Triggers:** *"It's important to learn about what kinds of reminders might feel dangerous to you, and how your body reacts when those reminders are around. Everyone has different triggers and different ways to respond when the alarm goes off. If we know what sets off your alarm, and how you respond, we can get your thinking brain on board to help figure out when the sense of danger is coming from something that is real in the moment, and when it's a false alarm.* **Triggers can be people, places, sounds, smells, touch, change, etc."**
  - ◆ Following review of these concepts, the group leader facilitates the "Recognizing Triggers Game." Each member takes a turn listening to one of the scenarios provided in the following material. The task is to identify the current trigger that reminds the person in the scenario of past experiences. Group members can earn points for figure out the correct response (goal should be cooperative, rather than competitive).

(continued)

RECOGNIZING TRIGGERS GAME—SAMPLE SCENARIOS

1. Lavert grew up in a neighborhood where there was a lot of violence. He often heard scary sounds outside of his window at night, including the sound of gunshots. One day Lavert was in school and someone dropped a book on the floor. He reacted quickly by yelling and then crying. *(sound of book dropping)*

2. Francisco's dad was really strict and often became very, very angry at home when Francisco broke a rule or made a mistake. Francisco learned to be very good at following rules, and he worked very, very hard to *never* make mistakes. He couldn't even have fun because he always had to think and plan to make everything in his life perfect. He would not do things that felt good if they broke one of his rules. *(mistakes)*

3. Tammy's mother used to hit her a lot when Tammy lived with her. Her mother's perfume smelled like oranges. At snack time Tammy started to peel an orange. All of a sudden she appeared frozen. She didn't say or do anything and couldn't answer staff's questions about whether or not she was okay. *(orange scent)*

4. When Debbie did something wrong at home, like break the rules or fail to do her chores, she would get into trouble and her dad would hit her. One day at her school Debbie was told that she was in trouble for breaking a rule and was going to earn a consequence. Debbie stopped talking, did not move, and appeared frozen. *(being in trouble)*

5. When Jimmy was a little boy, his mother always promised to do something special with him on Saturday afternoons. But, every Saturday afternoon Jimmy's mother would drink too much and break her promise. Jimmy would feel so disappointed and scared when his mom would drink. Yesterday, Jimmy's mom cancelled a visit. Jimmy started yelling at a female staff person, saying, "You are the worst staff person! You don't want me to see my mother! It's all your fault!" *(being let down/canceled visit)*

6. Vivian had three younger sisters in her home growing up. Her mom wasn't around to take care of the younger kids, and they often took Vivian's things without asking. When Vivian complained, her mom always took her sisters' side. One day at the program, Vivian's roommate picked up one of Vivian's CDs and put it in the radio to play. Vivian ran over to her and punched her as hard as she could, screaming, "That's not yours!!!!!!!!!!" *(taking CD)*

7. When Evan was 8 years old, he was taken suddenly from his parents' home by DCF because his home was not a safe place for him. He didn't get any warning and was so, so scared, not knowing what was going to happen next. One day at the program he was living in, Evan learned that one of his favorite staff members had to leave the job suddenly for personal reasons. Evan found this out and went immediately to his room. He crawled under his bed and refused to come out. *(sudden departure/change)*

8. Gerald's dad used to hit him in the head with an open hand all the time. Gerald can't really remember why this happened—just that it did. One day one of his friends came walking up to him and started to move his arm and hand to give Gerald a side hug. Seeing the hand moving toward him, Gerald flinched and ducked his head. *(raised hand)*

9. Briana loved making things for her grandmother, with whom she lived as a little girl. She would spend all day working on cards, drawings, and other nice things to give to her grandmother when she returned home from work. Most of the time her grandmother, returning from work, would glance at the artwork that Briana gave her and say "What's this? I can't even tell what it is. Do you call this a drawing?" She would often throw it away. Briana usually won't even try to make things now that she is living with a foster family, but

(continued)

one day she did participate in an art project at school. She handed it to her foster mom when she got home, who started to ask a question about it. As soon as Briana heard the word *what,* she grabbed the paper back, ripped it up, and said, "I suck at doing art." (*the word* what)

10. Benjamin's mother had a boyfriend who often hit his mother when angry. Benjamin was scared and angry watching his mother get hurt by someone so much bigger and stronger than she, and he would often try to help her/protect her. Now, in his program, Benjamin always makes sure that he pays attention to helping smaller animals or kids when they need it. Like at home, Benjamin feels that his job is to be the protector. One day one of the other kids was having a hard time and started threatening to hurt the program dog. Benjamin, without thinking, jumped in between the dog and the other student and started fighting back. *(threatened dog)*

ACTIVITY: TUNING IN TO YOUR BODY/CHANGES IN PHYSIOLOGICAL AROUSAL

- **ARC Target(s): Modulation**
- **Purpose:** To increase participants' awareness of their own level of physiological arousal, and the ways in which various activities might increase or decrease arousal level.
- **Materials:** Worksheet for measuring pulse rate. *(See worksheet, "Checking My Pulse," Appendix D.)*
- **Teaching Points:**
  - ◆ "In order to regulate your body, you need to be able to tune in and know where you're at."
  - ◆ "Although your body responds automatically to different cues in the environment, and to internal and external experiences, there are things you can do to change your own arousal level."
  - ◆ "What kind of cues does your body give that you're in a comfortable or uncomfortable state of arousal?"
- **Measure Your Heartbeat:**
  - ◆ **Baseline pulse:** Teach participants how to take their own pulse by placing their index and middle fingers on the wrist or neck; be sure participants are not using their thumbs. Have each participant measure his or her pulse for 20 seconds and multiply by 3 to get the baseline pulse rate. Write down the baseline pulse on the worksheet.
  - ◆ **Exercise pulse:** Have participants do 10–15 jumping jacks (and/or other brief strenuous activity—e.g., jogging in place for at least 20–30 seconds). Immediately after stopping, have participants remeasure their pulse and write down the results on the worksheet.
  - ◆ **Resting pulse:** Have participants take five deep breaths while seated. Show participants how to breathe slowly in through the nose and out through the mouth. Immediately after completing the deep breaths, have participants remeasure their pulse and write down the result on their worksheets.
- **Discussion:** Ask participants: "How did your heart rate change across the three measurements? What other changes did you notice in your body? How effective was deep breathing in slowing down your heart rate? If not, why do you think this is? When else do you notice that your heart rate speeds up? Slows down?"
- **Note:** Other activities or exercises can be substituted or added at the discretion of the group leader; it is helpful to teach multiple exercises for each component (up-regulation, down-regulation).

(continued)

ACTIVITY: BALL TOSS/GROUP JUGGLE

- **ARC Target(s): Relational Connection, Attunement**
- **Purpose:** To build awareness of key skills involved in effective communication.
- **Materials:** For every six participants, four to six small balls (ideally, round Nerf balls, beanbag balls, or similar)
- **Directions:**
  - ◆ Participants should stand in a circle. The group leader explains: "We are going to make a pattern using this ball. I will throw to someone, saying his or her name first. That person should then throw the ball to someone else. Make sure that you throw the ball to someone who has not yet received it. The rules are simple: We are going to make a pattern with our throws. Everyone should get the ball once, and no one should get it more than once. The last person to get the ball should throw it back to me, completing the pattern. Every time you throw the ball, say the name of the person you are throwing it to first. There are no winners or losers in this game. If you drop the ball, just pick it up and keep going."
  - ◆ The group leader should then start the pattern, making sure that all participants receive the ball once. When the group leader receives the ball back, practice the pattern several times to make sure all participants remember from whom they receive the ball and to whom they throw the ball.
  - ◆ Once the group has become comfortable with the pattern, the group leader explains: "We are going to introduce more balls into our pattern, one by one. Our goal is to see how many balls we can throw at the same time, and keep the pattern going."
  - ◆ Make sure the group is comfortable with adding more balls, and then slowly add additional balls into the pattern. The group should be comfortable with two balls before a third is added, with three before a fourth is added, and so on.
- **Postactivity Discussion:** Start with open-ended questions: Ask group members what they noticed about the activity, whether they liked it or not, etc.
  - ◆ Specific questions:
    - "What did you notice about what made it easier or harder to be effective in this game? What helped keep the pattern moving smoothly?"
    - If not mentioned, tune in to the following ideas:
      - ○ Making eye contact with the person who is throwing to you, and with the one who is receiving from you.
      - ○ Saying the person's name (that is, offering a cue that you are about to throw the ball).
      - ○ Not throwing too hard or too softly.
      - ○ Indicating with body language, eye contact, etc., that you are ready to throw/receive.
      - ○ Tuning out distractions, concentrating only on the person who is throwing to you, and the person to whom you throw.
      - ○ Lack of pressure: If you drop the ball, you can pick it up and continue the pattern.
    - Discuss with the group: "All of these skills were important in being successful at this activity. These skills are also all important in communicating effectively." Ask, "How does each of these skills play into good communication?"

(continued)

ACTIVITY: CIRCLES

- **ARC Target(s): Relational Connection, Identity**
- **Purpose:** To build awareness of relationship resources; to build awareness of variations in intimacy across relationships.
- **Materials:** "Circles of Trust" worksheet (see Appendix D); pencils/pens
- **Directions:** Participants are given worksheets (concentric circles) and asked to consider the various relationships in their lives. The center circle represents them; each participant is then asked to place names/initials of significant people in their lives in the remaining circles, with distance from the center circle indicating strength/closeness of the relationship.
- **Postactivity Discussion:** Questions/discussion points may include: "Notice how many/few people are in your circles, and notice where people tend to cluster. What does this tell you about your pattern of relationships? Do you tend to keep many people close? Most people at arm's length? Are you comfortable with the number of people in your life? Are there resources that you forgot about?"

- **Examine Specific Relationship Types:**

- Have participants circle or mark in different colors, who in their circles are . . .
    - People with whom they have fun?
    - People to whom they speak about important decisions?
    - People to whom they turn for emotional support?
    - People whom they consider family?
    - People who really know them?

- **Using arrows, have participants indicate people to whom they would want to be closer, or from whom they would want more distance.**
    - ◆ **Discuss:** "Notice who in your life fills which functions. Are there any functions that are missing?"

DISCUSSION: "I STATEMENTS"

- **ARC Target(s): Relational Connection**
- **Purpose:** To teach participants about "I statements" and how these are linked to effective communication.
- **Materials:** None

- **Directions:**
    - ◆ Provide participants with an example of two statements, such as:
        - "I can't believe you did that! You're such a jerk!"
        versus
        - "I'm really angry about what you did. I need some space from you right now."
    - ◆ **Ask:** "What is different about these two statements? What kind of reaction might there be to the first one? To the second one?"
    - ◆ **Teach:** "I statements" are an effective way to communicate:
        - Rather than blaming, insulting, being aggressive, or putting someone on the defense, "I statements" focus on our own feelings and reactions.
        - Someone can challenge a "you statement" (the obvious answer to "You're such a jerk" is "No, I'm not, you are!"), but it's harder for someone to challenge an "I statement" (if I say I'm angry, it's hard for you to tell me I'm not!).
        - "I statements" express how we feel and why we feel that way. They allow us to work on solutions and resolve conflicts. "You statements," in contrast, often increase conflicts or negative situations.

(continued)

394

ACTIVITY: CRAZY "I STATEMENT" TRANSLATION

- **ARC Target(s): Relational Connection**
- **Purpose:** To provide practice in using "I statements" rather than "you statements."
- **Materials:** Prompts for "I-statement" translation; large Post-its (or any brand of sticky notes) and markers for Part 2, application/discussion.

- **Directions:**
    - ◆ *Part 1:* Demonstration: Crazy "I Statements"
    - ◆ Ask participants if they have ever seen movies in which words are translated from one language to another. Tell them: "In this activity you will act as the translators for people speaking in the foreign 'You language'; your job is to translate each statement from *you* into *I*."
    - ◆ Group leaders demonstrate:
        - • One leader reads a crazy "you statement." For example: "You yellow-bellied, no-good rotten horse's pimple! You're a sniveling good-for-nothing who couldn't get something right if your life depended on it!"
        - • The second leader offers a translation: "I'm very frustrated with how you did that." *Note: Leaders should play up the humor/contrast between the two statements.*
    - ◆ Participants are then asked to translate further statements. This activity may consist of dialogue between the two group leaders or individual statements by the two, with translations offered by two participants. **(See below for sample statements.)**
    - ◆ *Part 2:* Application: "You" versus "I Statements"
    - ◆ Ask participants to generate a list of "you statements." These can be statements they've heard or ones they find themselves making. If participants have difficulty, offer examples (e.g., "You're such a jerk," "You make me so mad," "You ruin everything"). The goal is to generate a list of *realistic* "you statements" that are commonly experienced.
    - ◆ For each "you statement" generated, ask the group to offer translations: "What kind of 'I statements' might go with these? Write these next to the 'you statements.'"
- **Postactivity Discussion:** Ask: "How did the statements change when they were *you* versus *I*? Which statements seemed more respectful? Which ones were likely to make the situation worse versus lead to solution? How would you rather be talked to?"

"I STATEMENTS" TRANSLATION GAME—SAMPLE PROMPTS

"You statement":
"You yellow-bellied, no-good, rotten horse's pimple! You're a sniveling good-for-nothing who couldn't get something right if your life depended on it!"
   Sample "I statement":
   "I'm very frustrated with how you did that."
"You statement":
"This school assignment is lame! It's only for stupid pea-brain donkeys! Your directions stink! And I already did this last year!"
Sample "I statement":
   "I don't know how to do this assignment."/"I don't like doing this type of work."

(continued)

"You statement":
"You must be a complete and utter moron, if you think I am so stupid/insensitive/dumb/worthless/inconsiderate/hopeless that I wouldn't know already that I shouldn't have done that!"

> *Sample "I statement":*
> "I already feel really bad about what happened."/"I'm sorry."

"You statement":
"You're getting on my last, worn-out, overstretched nerve! You annoying, pestering, aggravating, irritating, bothersome turnip head! Cut it out!!!"

> *Sample "I statement":*
> "I want you to stop that."

"You statement":
"You brainless, dim-witted, moronic nincompoop! You make me absolutely, certifiably, completely insane! You big baboon! How does someone get to your age without a brain!?"

> *Sample "I statement":*
> "I'm really angry with you."/"I'm feeling frustrated."

"You statement":
"You're so pushy and annoying. Why are you always shoving into my business? You don't know what you're doing. You can't help me. You're always getting involved in stuff you don't know anything about."

> *Sample "I statements":*
> "I need some time alone."/"I'd like some space."/"I don't want to talk about that."

"You statement":
"Like your life is so big and important—you're just sooooo busy, and then you don't want to do anything, and here I am just twiddling my thumbs having nothing to do because you're just a stupid jerk!"

> *Sample "I statement":*
> "I want you to spend more time with me."

ACTIVITY: OWN YOUR ZONE

- **ARC Target(s): Relational Connection**
- **Purpose:** To recognize personal "comfort zones" with physical boundaries and to practice asserting personal preferences around boundaries.
- **Materials:** Strips of paper or masking tape, marker
- **Directions:** Participants can either be paired with each other or paired with a group leader one at a time.
  - ◆ Participants should face their partner at a 10-foot difference (distance should be great enough that it is larger than most individuals' spatial needs).
  - ◆ One partner should begin to walk slowly toward the other. The person who is not moving should say "Stop" when the partner reaches a distance that feels comfortable.

(continued)

♦ Once stopped, the partner should be directed to "check in" with the other person, asking whether the distance is comfortable or whether he or she should move in/out. Once a comfortable distance is reached, the group leader should measure the distance with a strip of paper or piece of tape, and mark it with the participant's name. This is his or her "physical comfort zone."

♦ For each participant, introduce at least one novel variable (e.g., "Pretend that your partner is your best friend" [mother, therapist, school principal, kid you hate, etc.] *or* "You are in a . . . great mood" [terrible mood, feeling sick, feeling jumpy, etc.]. Redo the distance and ask: "How do these different variables change your comfort zones?"

♦ Each participant's comfort zones (primary plus added variables) should be hung on the wall.

■ **Postactivity Discussion:**
  ♦ "What are *physical spatial needs*? How do you understand these needs?"
  ♦ "What kinds of factors influence our spatial needs?" (If not done previously, introduce concepts such as relationship to other person, current mood state, family norms about space, cultural norms about space, current situation, etc.?)
  ♦ "How do you know if your spatial need is different from other people's?" Group leaders can demonstrate physical cues: "What does it look like if you step into someone's personal space? Pay attention to cues such as the other person stepping or leaning back, avoiding eye contact with you, looking pained, and so on."
  ♦ "How do you or *should* you handle people's different spatial needs?" *Teaching point:* In interpersonal interactions, boundaries are generally determined by the person with the furthest/greatest boundary need.
  ♦ "Are you ever in situations where people inadvertently violate your boundaries—for example, in a crowded train? How do you deal with this?"

ACTIVITY: EMOTIONAL BOUNDARIES

■ **ARC Target(s): Relational Connection**
■ **Purpose:** To explore personal "comfort zone" with emotional boundaries, and to illustrate differing boundary needs across interaction partners.
■ **Materials:** List of interview questions (see sample questions, below) with increasingly intimate questions
■ **Directions:** Participants are paired up and given the following instructions:
  ♦ "Each of you is being given a list of interview questions to ask your partner. The questions start out broad but become increasingly personal. Each of you gets to choose which of these questions you answer. The person being interviewed may answer whichever questions he or she is comfortable with; once you reach a question you do not feel comfortable answering, let your partner know you are ready to stop."
  ♦ Once the first partner has had an opportunity to act as interviewer, the roles should switch, and the second person should be interviewed.

■ **Postactivity Discussion:**
  ♦ How many questions were you willing to answer?"
  ♦ "Were your boundaries the same as your partner's, or different—that is, did you stop on the same question?"
    • *Teaching Point:* Often, we reciprocate social intimacy needs—we go only as near or far as our social partner.

(continued)

◆ "What factors influenced how many questions you were willing to answer? Consider who your partner was, the setting, the mood you were in, etc. Is there anyone you can think of for whom you would have answered all of the questions? Any situations where you might answer none?"

◆ General boundary discussion point: "How do you know when something has intruded upon your boundaries? What internal cues do you have that your boundaries are being pushed?"

SET YOUR BOUNDARIES: SAMPLE INTERVIEW QUESTIONS

1. What is your favorite color?
2. Who is your favorite musical artist?
3. How many people are in your immediate family, or what you consider immediate family?
4. What book or books have influenced you?
5. Who is the person that you admire the most?
6. Who is the person that you feel closest to in your family?
7. What is the best experience you ever had in school?
8. What is a dream you have for your future?
9. If you could have three wishes, what would they be?
10. What is one of your earliest memories?
11. What is the worst experience you ever had in school?
12. What is something you don't like people to know about you?
13. Who is the person in your family you feel most disappointed by?
14. What is the scariest thing that ever happened to you?
15. What is something that you're ashamed of?

DISCUSSION: HEALTHY RELATIONSHIPS

- **ARC Target(s): Self andIdentity, Relational Connection**
- **Purpose:** To distinguish healthy from unhealthy relationships.
- **Materials:** Large Post-its (or any brand of sticky notes), markers

- **Discussion Points:**
  ◆ "What does it mean to have a 'healthy' relationship? What qualities do you think are seen in healthy relationships? Write your responses on Post-it notes.
    • If not listed, include qualities such as *respect, not exploitive, appropriate to role.*
  ◆ "How do you know you are safe in a relationship? What does it mean to be 'safe' in a relationship?

ACTIVITY: RELATIONSHIP CONTINUUM

- **ARC Target(s): Identity, Relational Connection**
- **Purpose:** To distinguish healthy from unhealthy relationships
- **Materials:** Sheets of paper or preprinted handouts with horizontal lines forming a continuum, anchored at each end by the labels *Healthy/Unhealthy*; relationship description prompts (see below); pencils; large Post-its with continuum lines; marker

(continued)

398

■ **Directions:** Read participants the "Relationship Description Sample Prompts," one at a time, in the next box (select four to six, depending on the group, or generate appropriate scenarios based on group composition). After reading each one, have participants mark whether they think the relationship is healthy or unhealthy by placing a vertical line on the continuum and marking it with a rating number—for example, from 1 to 5, where 1 is the healthiest and 5 is the unhealthiest.

■ **Postactivity Discussion:** After all prompts have been read, go back to each description and survey the group. Mark on a large sheet of paper how the group rated each scenario. Note differences in group ratings, and elicit why group members made the ratings they did.

■ **Possible follow-up questions:**
  - "How can you tell if a relationship is healthy or unhealthy? What struck you about these descriptions?"
  - "What do you think influences your perception of whether a relationship is healthy?" (Help participants to consider family norms, cultural norms, past experience in relationships, etc.)
  - "How can you make a relationship healthier? Do you always have control over this?"
  - "Is there ever a reason to stay in an unhealthy relationship? If yes, why? Are there things you can do to protect yourself in less healthy relationships?"

RELATIONSHIP DESCRIPTION SAMPLE PROMPTS FOR RELATIONSHIP CONTINUUM

1. Joshua and Tanya have been going out for 6 months; they are both 16. They started spending all their free time together right away. Josh gets really jealous if Tanya spends time away from him, whether with her girlfriends or even with her family. He wants her to prove that she loves him, and he suspects that she is cheating on him. Sometimes he accuses her of cheating and calls her names. Recently, he got so angry that he pushed her into the wall. Later, he apologized and said that he really loved her and didn't want to hurt her.

2. Kenny has always looked up to his father. His dad spends time with him and has taught him how to do many things, like drive a car (when he was 13 years old) and fix things around the house. A lot of times, Kenny's dad is funny and fun to be around. However, at other times, Kenny's dad will get angry with him for little things. When Kenny doesn't understand how to do things right away, his father calls him "stupid" and an "idiot." Kenny tries really hard to do things the right way so that he will stay on his father's good side.

3. Jamie and Maria have been friends since they were small; they grew up next door to each other. They like to do things together, such as go to the mall or just hang out. Sometimes they argue and get angry with each other, but usually they work it out pretty quickly. When Jamie is upset about things at home, she sometimes talks to Maria about it. Maria doesn't say much, but she knows Jamie very well, so she understands.

4. Larry is 15 and lives with his mother and younger sister, Amelia, who is 13. He works after school until 10 o'clock every night at the supermarket, bagging groceries. Half of his paycheck goes to his mother to help pay the rent, and he brings food home every night when he gets off work. Amelia has been getting into trouble at school and was suspended today for getting into a fight with another girl. When Larry came home and found out about Amelia's suspension, he became upset and began to yell at her and took away her cell phone as punishment.

(continued)

5. Joe and Mark have been friends forever. They both graduated high school and Mark went off to college 100 miles away. Joe works a steady job, owns a car, and lives at home with his mother and father. Every weekend, Joe drives over to Mark's school and hangs out with Mark and his friends, often staying over in Mark's dorm on Saturday nights. Sometimes Mark has schoolwork to do but is unable to get it done because Joe wants to hang out and party.

6. Jennifer and Tommy have been going out for a few months. Jennifer is 17 and graduating this year. Tommy is 18 and going to GED classes along with working. Jennifer loves sports and has joined a team each season and spends all her extra time studying or seeing Tommy. Tommy expects her to be home in the evenings when he calls to talk. Jennifer has had the opportunity to go out with the girls on her team after practice but doesn't do this because she doesn't want to miss Tommy's calls.

7. Johnny and Lindsey have been dating for about a month. It is the first time that Lindsey has had a boyfriend. She is excited that Johnny calls her a dozen times a day, both at home and at her after-school job. He says that he really loves her and is concerned about her, so he just wants to check to make sure she's okay. Recently he has wanted to spend a lot of time with her and asks her to cancel any plans that she has made with her friends. Lindsey's parents are concerned because she doesn't help out with her younger sister anymore.

8. Ryan lives with his mother, stepfather, and younger brother Joey. Ryan gets along with his family okay, but would rather spend time with his friends. He usually does the chores he is supposed to do at home. He has a curfew of 11 on weekdays and 12 on weekends, and he usually follows it, but sometimes he doesn't. When he comes home late, his mother and stepfather are angry and they ground him or take away his electronics or something else that he likes to do. He thinks he should have more freedom, since he is 16, so sometimes he gets angry at his parents, especially his stepfather, who, after all, isn't his "real" father. But he also knows that his parents are usually there for him when he needs them, and last year when he got in trouble in school for something he really didn't do, they went to bat for him.

9. Jordan is 13 years old; his next-door neighbor, Ray, is 17. Jordan has always looked up to Ray, but Ray has barely paid any attention to him. Lately, Ray has allowed Jordan to hang out with him and his friends, as long as Jordan does them favors, like go and get them cigarettes or beer out of Jordan's house when his parents aren't looking. Sometimes Ray pushes Jordan around and laughs with his friends about it, but Jordan knows it is all in fun. Recently, Ray suggested that Jordan might help him and his friends out with some other things; for example, Ray and his friends are planning to break in to a house where they know there is a lot of money, and Ray says Jordan might be able to help.

10. José and Marie have been hanging out together for about 9 months. José is 18 and Marie is 17. They spend a lot of time together, but also have other friends, too, so sometimes they might go several days or even a week without seeing each other. They each get along with each other's families as well, which is nice. They are having sex together but do use condoms, even though they trust each other, because they don't want Marie to get pregnant.

11. Jim is having trouble understanding his math homework. He has sat in the study hall for almost an hour without getting more than two problems done. Other people can see him getting more upset over not knowing how to do the math. Finally, Armand walks in and notices what is happening. Armand walks over to find out how Jim is doing. After seeing what Jim is working on, Armand shows Jim how to come up with the answer to the next problem, and later, Jim gives Armand a good idea for a story he has to write for English class.

(continued)

12. Rihanna practiced for many months to get ready for volleyball tryouts. When the tryouts were over, she found out that she did not make the freshman team. Rihanna went home feeling very angry with the coaches and was disappointed in herself. When she walked in the house, her older sister Juleesa asked Rihanna if she made the team. When Rihanna said no, Juleesa laughed at her and said, "What can you expect from a klutz?"

ACTIVITY: GIVING COMPLIMENTS TO OTHERS

- **ARC Target(s): Relational Connection, Self and Identity**
- *Note:* See worksheet, "Giving Others Compliments," in Appendix D.
- **Purpose:** To build group members' ability to tune in to and name positive qualities in others; to build understanding of how other people see them.
- **Materials:** "Giving Others Compliments" worksheet, crayons or markers
- **Directions:** *(Group leader says:)* "Most of us like the feeling that we get when people say nice things to us or recognize what we do. Today we are really going to practice giving compliments to each other in order to celebrate things about each one of us that we really like or see as positive." Group participants should be invited to list one positive quality about each group member on their worksheet. Participants then share these compliments with other members. *Note:* Participants may need to have adults write their answers or may choose to verbalize answers without writing.

ACTIVITY: ALTERNATE VERSION—GIVING COMPLIMENTS TO OTHERS

- **ARC Target(s): Relational Connection, Self and Identity**
- **Purpose:** To highlight competencies and positive aspects of self; to build group members' ability to tune in to and name positive qualities in others; to build understanding of how other people see them.
- **Materials:** Giant Post-it notes (one per group member, with member's name written on top); smaller Post-its on which members write comments; pens/markers
- **Directions:**
  - ◆ Group members are handed a stack of smaller Post-its and a pen/marker.
  - ◆ Members are asked to write at least one positive comment about each member of the group. Comments *must* illustrate something positive about the other person. Comments can be anonymous, or group members may sign their names to the Post-it.
  - ◆ When all group members have written their comments, they should attach their Post-its to the giant Post-it sheets; all comments should be attached. Group leaders should ensure that all comments are appropriate/positive.
  - ◆ Group leaders then read aloud each member's list.

(Alternative directions: Group members may write directly on other members' giant Post-its, with a rule that no two comments should be the same.)

- **Postactivity Discussion:** Possible questions include: "Did anything surprise you in what other people wrote about you? What is it like to hear all of these positive things about yourself?"

(continued)

ACTIVITY: POSITIVE SELF-RECOGNITION

- **ARC Target(s): Self and Identity (Positive Self), Relational Connection**
- ***Note:*** Complete this activity in association with the worksheet, "Giving Myself Compliments", in Appendix D.
- **Purpose:** To highlight competencies/positive aspects of self
- **Materials:** "Giving Myself Compliments" worksheet, crayons or markers

- **Directions:** *(Group leader says:)* "Sometimes it's hard to focus on what we like about ourselves, or what we're proud of. Today we want to practice giving ourselves compliments. This is important to do because it helps us to feel good about ourselves. We are going to hand out a worksheet for you to complete. The worksheet focuses on things that you think you do well in different areas of your life, such as school, activities, relationships, the residence [or other group venue], etc. After you complete the worksheet, you can choose whether or not to share your self-compliments with the group."
  - ◆ Distribute worksheets and writing materials to all group members. When all participants have completed their worksheets, invite members to share.
  - ◆ *Note:* Participants may need to have adults write their answers, or they may choose to verbalize answers without writing.
- **Postactivity Discussion:** Possible questions include: "What was it like to give yourself compliments? Were there some areas where it was easier to compliment yourself than others? Were there areas where it was harder? Is it comfortable to compliment yourself? Why, or why not?"

ACTIVITY: DESERT ISLAND

- **ARC Target(s): Executive Functions, Relational Connection**
- **Purpose:** To apply skills, including problem solving, negotiation, "I statements," conflict resolution, etc., to a group problem-solving task.
- **Materials:** Forty index cards listing an array of objects, including essentials (e.g., food, matches, bedding), personal items (e.g., shampoo, toothpaste), and "luxury" items (i.e., iPhone, tablet, radio, deck of cards)

- **Directions:**
  - ◆ Participants are told that they are members of a group that has been stranded on a desert island. As a group, they are able to select 10 objects out of those listed on the provided index cards; these will be the objects that have also been stranded with them. The group must negotiate which 10 objects to select, and figure out and agree upon a process for making the selection.
  - ◆ After the initial selection, group leaders should generate a "challenge" scenario. For example: A big storm is coming that will last two days (meaning, participants can't leave shelter to gather food), and the temperature will drop (meaning, participants need to find a way to stay warm). Ask: "Based on the objects you have selected, how will you survive?" The group is given a 5-minute period to consider their items, to renegotiate selected objects, and to exchange them for other items in the stack.
  - ◆ At the discretion of the group leaders, further challenge scenarios may be provided. After the first selection, group members are no longer allowed to exchange cards and must use problem-solving skills to describe how they will address the challenge using only the selected items.

(continued)

- Sample challenge scenarios:
    - "You are being attacked by a group of people from another island."
    - "Wild monkeys steal all the food you have gathered."
    - "Half of your group develops a nonfatal but uncomfortable illness, like serious poison ivy."
- **Postactivity Discussion:** "How was the negotiation process? Did everyone feel able to express their opinions? Did it feel like someone 'won' and someone 'lost'? How well do you think, as a group, you did with selecting objects? What factors did you consider? Do you think you considered different alternatives, or did you impulsively select certain objects? Which of the skills we have learned in the group do you think you applied to this challenge?" (Group leaders should note any skills not mentioned by the group.)
- **Sample Items for Desert Island Game:** iPhone, flashlight, tablet, or other electronics, batteries that are halfway rundown, six-pack of bottled water, sunflower seeds, vegetable seeds, 20 yards of rope, Swiss army knife, tarp, toothpaste, bar of chocolate, toilet paper, matches, bubble gum, balloon, machete, duct tape, potatoes, camera, five large pizzas, big bag of assorted Chinese food, dictionary, encyclopedia, compass, popular book series, Boy Scout manual, binoculars, hammer and nails, magnifying glass, sunscreen, one set of extra clothes per person, deck of cards, waterproof blanket, one pillow, metal bucket, soap

ACTIVITY: INFLUENCES ON SELF

- **ARC Target(s):Self and Identity**
- **Note:** Complete this activity in association with the worksheet "What Has Influenced My Identity?" in Appendix D.
- **Purpose:** To individually examine the relative importance of influences on identity, and to concretely represent those influences.
- **Materials:** Small plastic bottles with cork stoppers, sand in different colors (at least six colors), small funnels, measuring cups/spoons in various sizes, paper and pencil
- **Alternative Version:** Modeling clay can be used instead of sand. In this case, color of clay and relative amount will correspond to values. The prompt may instruct participants to make a specific item (e.g., an "identity stone") or leaders may choose to leave the sculpture choice open-ended.
- **Directions:** Group members are asked to select up to six key factors that have influenced them; group leaders should give examples (e.g., family, religion, neighborhood, life experiences). Members should pick a color of sand to represent each of these values or beliefs. Using the measuring spoons, members should select amounts of sand to represent how strong/important these values are to them (e.g., the most important belief or value would correspond to the largest measuring cup). Members then use the funnels to fill their bottles with the different-colored sand.
- **Postactivity Discussion:** "How well do these influences represent you? What's missing? Was it hard to select what to include? Do you see any commonalities across group members? Any differences?"

ACTIVITY: IDENTITY SHIELD

- **ARC Target(s): Self and Identity**
- **Note:** Complete this activity in association with the worksheet "Identity Shields" in Appendix D.
- **Purpose:** To examine multiple aspects of self; to acknowledge that all people have facets of identity that change in different contexts.

(continued)

- **Materials:** Paper, colored pencils/markers/crayons
- **Directions:** Group members are provided with an outline drawing of a shield divided into four sections. Instruction is to complete sections of the shield using prompts such as the following (select four):
  - ◆ "Something that symbolizes you as you are with your friends"
  - ◆ "Something that symbolizes you as you are with kids you don't know"
  - ◆ "Something that symbolizes you as you are with your family"
  - ◆ "Something that symbolizes you as you are when you are alone"
  - ◆ "Something that symbolizes you as you are in school"
  - ◆ "Something that symbolizes you as you are in this program"
  - ◆ "Something that symbolizes your hopes for yourself"
  - ◆ "Something that symbolizes an important part of you"
  - ◆ "Something that symbolizes your culture"
- **Postactivity Discussion:** Possible questions include: "What reactions do you have to this activity? Were there sections of the shield that were easier to complete? Sections that were harder? What similarities and what differences were there across shield sections? How do each of these sections capture different aspects of your identities? Do any sections feel 'truer' than others?"

ACTIVITY: VALUE LINE (PHYSICAL)

- **ARC Target(s): Self and Identity**
- **Purpose:** To examine one aspect of self that may differ across group members: that is, personal values.
- **Materials:** None
- **Directions:** Group leaders stand in opposite corners. One group leader represents "very important"; the second group leader represents "not at all important." Group leaders provide different prompt values (e.g., importance of education, importance of family, working hard, fairness, being tough, being strong, having friends). Group members are asked to place themselves on the invisible "line" between group leaders to represent how important that value is to them.
- **Postactivity Discussion:** Possible questions include: "Were you surprised by what you discovered about your vales or those of others? Did you find yourself closer to or farther from other group members than you expected? Was it hard/easy to rank your values? Were some easier than others? Which ones? What kinds of things might affect how you rank your values?"

ACTIVITY: VALUE LINE (DRAWN)

- **ARC Target(s): Self and Identity**
- **Purpose:** To individually examine relative importance of personal values
- **Materials:** Paper, pen or pencil
- **Directions:** Students are asked to draw a line down the middle of a piece of paper. Group leaders provide a list of values (e.g., importance of education, importance of family, working hard, fairness, being tough, being strong, having friends). Members are asked to place the words on the line in order of relative importance.

(continued)

- **Postactivity Discussion:** Possible questions include: "Were any of these hard to rank? Do any feel like they're equally important? Do any feel completely unimportant? Completely important? Where do you think these values came from? What kinds of things affect your values?"

ACTIVITY: QUALITY OF INFLUENCE

Note: This activity is based on a technique taught by Janina Fisher, PhD.

- **ARC Target(s): Self and Identity**
- **Purpose:** To explore past influential relationships and to build awareness of important qualities for future relationships.
- **Materials:** "Quality of Influence Pyramid" worksheet (see Appendix D); pens or pencils
- **Directions:** Participants use the worksheets to identify past influential relationships and the qualities they want to develop or avoid in future relationships:
  - ◆ "Using the worksheets, identify five people who have most influenced you in your life, either in a positive or a negative way." *Note:* If participants do not want to write actual names, they can use initials or some other "code" to identify the person.
  - ◆ In the space next to that person's box, write one quality that was important within that relationship, either as something you would want to experience in future relationships, or as something you would want to avoid.
- **Postactivity Discussion:** "How hard or easy was it to identify the people who have most influenced you? Did you find yourself purposely leaving out some people who were probably influential? How easy/hard was it to identify the key qualities? How many relationships do you have in your life right now that capture these qualities? What kind of relationships do you think you might want/need to build in the future?"

Feelings Toolkit Creation

ACTIVITY: FEELINGS TOOLKIT—INTRODUCTION

- **ARC Target(s): Modulation**
- **Purpose:** Ongoing project; goal is for each participant to build a "toolkit" for use in managing feelings and emotional experience over time.
- **Materials:** Cardboard boxes, markers/paint, other decorative materials
- **Directions:** Ongoing project is introduced. Participants are each given a cardboard box, which they can decorate in any way they like. One thing will be added to the toolkit at each subsequent session.

ONGOING INSTRUCTIONS

- **Materials:** Toolkit objects
- **Directions:** At end of group sessions, provide a variety of materials within each category (e.g., several scents of lotion, several types of stress balls, several picture postcards). Each participant may choose one object for his or her toolkit.

FEELINGS TOOLKIT: SAMPLE ITEMS

- Biofeedback dots
- Cedar squares/balls
- ChapStick tube (flavored)
- Cloth swatches (fabric, felt, velvet, etc.)
- Feathers
- Hard candy
- Index cards (participants to write positive self-statements on cards)
- Mini bottles of lotion
- Mini bottles of bubbles
- Mini glitter wands
- Mini thought-for-the-day book
- Mini stuffed animals
- Picture postcards
- Plug-in lights (nightlights)
- River stones (or other small polished stones)
- Plastic Slinkys
- Scented sachets
- Stress balls/other textured balls (e.g., Koosh balls, stretch balls)
- Water snakes
- Wikki stix

From Margaret E. Blaustein and Kristine M. Kinniburgh (2019). Copyright © 2019 The Guilford Press. Permission to photocopy this material is granted to purchasers of this book for personal use or use with clients (see copyright page for details). Purchasers can download additional copies of this material (see the box at the end of the table of contents).

Progressive Muscle Relaxation Technique

Note: Wording as follows is directed toward participants who are lying on their backs. For participants who are seated, modify language accordingly.

"Get into a comfortable position and relax. Now begin by clenching your right fist, tighter and tighter, studying the tension as you do so. Keep it clenched and notice the tension in your fist, hand, and forearm. Now relax. Feel the looseness in your right hand and notice the contrast with the tension. Repeat this with your right fist again, always noticing, as you relax, that this is the opposite of tension—relax and feel the difference. Repeat this entire procedure with your left fist and then with both fists.

"Now bend your elbows and tense your biceps. Tense them as hard as you can and observe the feeling of tightness. Relax, straighten out your arms. Let the relaxation develop and feel that difference.

"Turning your attention to your head, wrinkle your forehead as tight as you can. Now relax and smooth it out. Let yourself imagine your entire forehead and scalp becoming smooth and at rest. Now frown and notice the strain spreading throughout your forehead. Let go. Allow your brow to become smooth again.

"Close your eyes now, squint them tighter. Look for the tension. Relax your eyes. Let them remain closed gently and comfortably.

"Now clench your jaw, bite hard, notice the tension throughout your jaw. When your jaw is relaxed, your lips will be slightly parted. Let yourself really appreciate the contrast between tension and relaxation.

"Now press your tongue against the roof of your mouth. Feel the ache in the back of your mouth. Relax. Press your lips now, purse them into an *o*. Relax your lips. Notice that your forehead, scalp, eyes, jaw, tongue and lips are all relaxed.

"Press your head back as far as it can comfortably go and observe the tension in your neck. Roll it to the right and feel the stress; roll it to the left. Straighten your head and bring it forward, pressing your chin against your chest. Feel the tension in your throat and the back of your neck. Relax, allowing your head to return to a comfortable position. Let the relaxation deepen.

"Now shrug your shoulders. Hold the tension as you hunch your head down between your shoulders. Relax your shoulders. Drop them back and feel the relaxation spreading through your neck, throat, and shoulders—pure relaxation, deeper and deeper.

"Give your entire body a chance to relax. Feel the comfort and the heaviness. Now breathe in and fill your lungs completely. Hold your breath. Notice the tension. Now exhale, letting your chest become loose, letting the air hiss out. Continue relaxing, letting your breath come freely and gently. Repeat this breathing pattern several times, noticing the tension draining from your body as you exhale. Next, tighten your stomach and hold. Note the tension, then relax. Now place your hand on your stomach. Breathe deeply into your stomach, and notice how your stomach pushes your hand up. Hold—then relax. Feel the contrast of relaxation as the air rushes

(continued)

From Margaret E. Blaustein and Kristine M. Kinniburgh (2019). Copyright © 2019 The Guilford Press. Permission to photocopy this material is granted to purchasers of this book for personal use or use with clients (see copyright page for details). Purchasers can download additional copies of this material (see the box at the end of the table of contents).

out. Now arch your back, without straining. Keep the rest of your body as relaxed as possible. Focus on the tension in your lower back. Now relax, deeper and deeper.

"Tighten your buttocks and thighs. Press down on your heels as hard as you can. Relax and feel the difference. Now curl your toes downward, making your calves tense. Study the tension. Relax. Now bend (flex) your toes toward your knees, creating tension in your shins. Relax again.

"Feel the heaviness throughout your lower body as the relaxation deepens. Relax your feet, ankles, calves, shins, knees, thighs, and buttocks. Now let the relaxation spread to your stomach, lower back, and chest. Let go more and more. Experience the relaxation deepening in your shoulders, arms, and hands. Deeper and deeper. Notice the feeling of looseness and relaxation in your jaw and all of your facial muscles.

"Let the tension dissolve away. . . . "

Icebreaker Prompts
Group Opening Activity

OPENING CIRCLE

- *Purpose:* Build group cohesion and attunement; share information; create a consistent routine/ritual
- Ask each group member to respond to the icebreaker question of the day (e.g., "If you were any car, what kind would you be?")

CLOSING CIRCLE

- *Purpose:* Build group cohesion and attunement; create a consistent routine/ritual
- Go around the circle and ask "Who can remember from the check-in what car _____ would be?" for each member
- Ask: "What is one thing you learned about this person today in group?"

IDENTITY-FOCUSED ICEBREAKER SAMPLE PROMPTS

- "If you were any musical instrument, what kind would you be?"
- "If you were any form of weather, what kind would you be?"
- "If you were any magazine/book title, what would you be?"
- "If you were any animal, what would you be?"
- "If you were any celebrity, who would you be?"
- "If you had any type of magical power, what kind would it be and why?"
- "If there was one activity you had to do every day, what would you want it to be?"
- "If you could be any age, what would you be?"
- "If you were guaranteed success at any job in the world, what would you do?"
- "If people could use only one word to describe you, what would you want that word to be?"

RELATIONAL-FOCUSED ICEBREAKER SAMPLE PROMPTS

Name . . .

- "One quality you are proud of that you bring to your friendships"
- "One quality that you would want in a friend"
- "One quality you have improved in yourself that is important to relationships"
- "One quality that you appreciate in authority figures"
- "Something that you like to do for fun with friends"
- "One quality you are proud of that you bring as a son/daughter [or in other family relationships]"
- "One quality that you would want to have as a father/mother"
- "One quality that you would look for in a spouse or intimate partner"
- "One quality that you want to work on in yourself that affects relationships"

(continued)

From Margaret E. Blaustein and Kristine M. Kinniburgh (2019). Copyright © 2019 The Guilford Press. Permission to photocopy this material is granted to purchasers of this book for personal use or use with clients (see copyright page for details). Purchasers can download additional copies of this material (see the box at the end of the table of contents).

- "One quality that you would *not* want to have as a father/mother"
- "The number of friends you feel you need in your life"
- "Something you like to do with your family"
- "Something you would rather *not* do with your family"
- "One quality important to you in your parents/program staff/teachers/therapists/adults"

AFFECT-FOCUSED ICEBREAKER SAMPLE PROMPTS

Name

- "Something that you really love to do"
- "Something that relaxes you"
- "Something that you like to do when you're mellow"
- "Something that you like to do when you're really excited"
- "Someone you like to talk to when you're annoyed"
- "Something that makes you really frustrated"
- "Something that you're proud of"
- "Something that you think is scary"
- "Something that puts you in a good mood"
- "Something that puts you in a bad mood"
- "Something that you like to do when you want to think"
- "Something that you like to do when you don't want to think"
- "Something that brings your energy down"
- "Something that brings your energy up"
- "A way that other people could tell if you were really happy"
- "A way that other people could tell if you were really angry or upset"
- "A way that other people might know you wanted to be left alone"
- "A way that other people might know you wanted company"

Sample Group Session
Learning about the Connection between Behavior, Feelings, and Energy

GOALS

1. To practice advanced identification skills: connecting behavior to affect and energy states
2. To continue practicing self-appraisal and modulation
3. To continue to work on self-development skills

MATERIALS

Paper "leaves"

Markers

Lunch bags

Different objects/materials for guessing game (one for each group member)

"Going on a Vacation" script

OVERVIEW

1. Review program rules and group expectations.
2. Opening modulation activity: "Guess what's in the bag using your sense of touch."
3. Process the opening check-in; invite each member to share his or her experience (energy check-in).
4. Group members fill out their identity leaf.
5. The group facilitators lead discussion and worksheet activity that focuses on the connections between affect, behavior, and energy, building on previous group activities.
6. Closing mindfulness activity: Conduct relaxation exercise using imagery ("Going on a Vacation" script).
7. Process the closing check-in; invite each member to share his or her experience (energy check-in).

GROUP ACTIVITIES

Opening Circle: The facilitator leads the opening energy check-in by asking each group member to identify the level of arousal that he or she is currently experiencing: *high*, *medium*, or *low*. Group members are also asked to determine whether their energy is *comfortable* or *uncomfortable*.

Opening Modulation Activity: Following the initial energy check-in, the facilitator leads the opening modulation activity, "Guess what's in the bag":

> "We are going to practice using our sense of touch today to figure out what the item is that's in each of these bags. You are each going to have your own bag. Reach into the bag, without looking in it, and try to figure out what the object is that is in your bag. When you feel like you have figured it out, give the bag back to [facilitator]. There is going to be a

(continued)

From Margaret E. Blaustein and Kristine M. Kinniburgh (2019). Copyright © 2019 The Guilford Press. Permission to photocopy this material is granted to purchasers of this book for personal use or use with clients (see copyright page for details). Purchasers can download additional copies of this material (see the box at the end of the table of contents).

time limit of 2 minutes. When finished, each of you is going to have a chance to share your guess with the group. The goal is to focus on the shape, texture, and weight of the object to determine what it is. Good luck." The group facilitator repeats the opening energy check-in and observes and discusses any notable changes in energy following the modulation activity.

Competency Activity: The group facilitator leads this identity activity, Personal Leaves. (Leaves should hang on the "All about Me Tree" in the group room.) The question for today's group is "Tell us about something that you are good at in school."

Self-Regulation Activity: The group facilitator leads a discussion about the connection between affect, energy, and behavior:

> "Last week we talked about how feelings are very important because they help us learn many things about ourselves. We played a game to learn about how feelings are connected to the different kinds of behaviors that we all have. Today we are going to take it one step further. We have been teaching you about your energy since the very beginning of this group. The reason that we have been doing that is because your energy is connected to everything that you think or don't think about, say, feel, and do. Today we are going to go back to the behaviors that we talked about last week and we are going to connect those behaviors not only to feelings but also to the energy that we feel in our bodies."

Each group member is given a worksheet "Connections: Learning about Our Energy, Feelings, and Behavior." *See the worksheet below.*

Closing Circle: The group facilitator leads the closing mindfulness activity: relaxation using imagery (see "Going on a Vacation" script below), ending with a final energy check-in. Group facilitator observes and discusses any notable changes in energy.

The facilitator praises the members for their participation in the group and hands out the practice worksheet for homework.

(continued)

Connections: Learning about Our Energy, Feelings, and Behavior

1. **Behavior:** Staying alone in my room

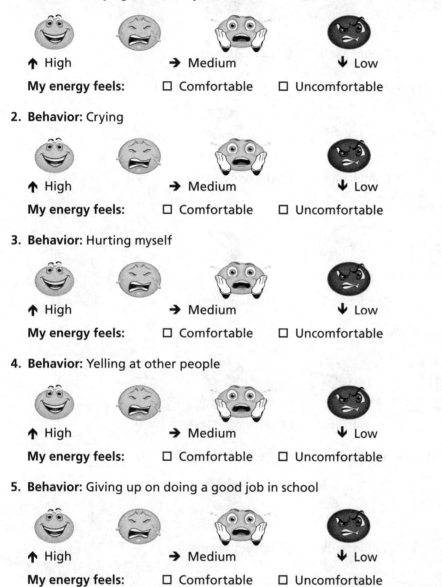

↑ High   → Medium   ↓ Low

My energy feels: ☐ Comfortable   ☐ Uncomfortable

2. **Behavior:** Crying

↑ High   → Medium   ↓ Low

My energy feels: ☐ Comfortable   ☐ Uncomfortable

3. **Behavior:** Hurting myself

↑ High   → Medium   ↓ Low

My energy feels: ☐ Comfortable   ☐ Uncomfortable

4. **Behavior:** Yelling at other people

↑ High   → Medium   ↓ Low

My energy feels: ☐ Comfortable   ☐ Uncomfortable

5. **Behavior:** Giving up on doing a good job in school

↑ High   → Medium   ↓ Low

My energy feels: ☐ Comfortable   ☐ Uncomfortable

(continued)

6. **Behavior:** Hitting or throwing things

↑ High   → Medium   ↓ Low

My energy feels: ☐ Comfortable   ☐ Uncomfortable

7. **Behavior:** Not wanting to go to bed because I think something bad might happen

↑ High   → Medium   ↓ Low

My energy feels: ☐ Comfortable   ☐ Uncomfortable

8. **Behavior:** Sharing with a peer

↑ High   → Medium   ↓ Low

My energy feels: ☐ Comfortable   ☐ Uncomfortable

9. **Behavior:** Trying to run away

↑ High   → Medium   ↓ Low

My energy feels: ☐ Comfortable   ☐ Uncomfortable

10. **Behavior:** Provoking other people so they get mad

↑ High   → Medium   ↓ Low

My energy feels: ☐ Comfortable   ☐ Uncomfortable

(continued)

"Going on a Vacation" Script

Close your eyes and make yourself comfortable. We are going on a vacation, and this will require you to use your imagination and your senses to try and experience the trip.

Imagine yourself at the beach. You are barefoot walking on the sand. Notice the feeling of the soft, hot sand on your feet. Are your soles sensitive? Does the sand tickle? Can you feel the sand between your toes?

Look around to find a perfect spot on which to lay your towel. You spread out your towel and notice the color of the stripes— red, blue, green, and black. Look out at the ocean. Can you see the horizon? What color is the water? Is the surf calm or choppy? Notice the ocean breeze on your skin and the smell of the tide? Do you taste the ocean air?

Take out your sunscreen and begin to rub it on your skin. How does it feel? How does it smell? Does the fragrance remind you of anything?

Lie down and get your body comfortable in the sand. How does the sand feel under your back? Notice your body relaxing. How does the sun feel beating on your skin?

Listen to the surf hitting the shore and the sounds of nature around you.

Enjoy the peacefulness and quiet for a few minutes . . .

(continued)

ARC Practice Sheet: Tracking Positive Behaviors and Energy

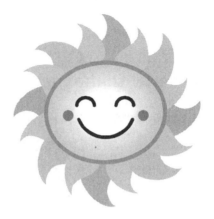

Name: _____   Date: _____

1. I participated in a group activity.   _____
                                              (Staff check-off and initial)

2. I gave someone a compliment.   _____
                                              (Staff check-off and initial)

3. I gave myself a compliment.   _____
                                              (Staff check-off and initial)

4. I encouraged someone to do well.   _____
                                              (Staff check-off and initial)

5. I helped someone out with   _____
   chores or something else.   (Staff check-off and initial)

APPENDIX D

Youth Educational Handouts and Worksheets

Tracking My Energy

- This worksheet supports Modulation by providing a tracking mechanism of a child's arousal response and comfort level before and after engaging in various activities.

Making My Energy Comfortable

- This worksheet supports a child in practicing a "feelings toolbox" (Modulation) skill for making energy comfortable.

Circles

- This worksheet helps a child to identify interpersonal resources (Relational Connection) through use of the "Circles" exercise.

Starting a Conversation

- This worksheet helps a child anticipate and evaluate the process of initiating communication (Relational Connection) with an identified other.

Giving Others Compliments

- This worksheet supports positive interactions with others (Relational Connection) by helping a child identify/describe positive attributes of others. This worksheet may be particularly useful in a group context.

Giving Myself Compliments

- This worksheet supports positive esteem/efficacy (Self and Identity) by helping a child identify positive self-attributes.

What Has Influenced My Identity?

- This worksheet should be used in conjunction with the "Influences on Self" group or individual activity described in Appendix C. This worksheet and associated activity support a child in exploring influences on identity (Self and Identity—Unique Self).

Quality of Influence Pyramid

- This worksheet helps the child identify specific people who have had an influence on the child, whether positive or negative, and the qualities of those individuals which have been most influential. This worksheet may be used in conjunction with the "Quality of Influence" group or individual activity described in Appendix C.

Identity Shields

- This worksheet provides templates for completion of identity shields (Self and Identity—Cohesive Self).

About My Feelings

Name: _____ Date: _____

Please come up with examples of times when you have felt the following emotions during the week and why. Notice what was happening in your body and what was going on around you.

This week, I felt <u>happy</u> when . . .

_____
_____
_____
_____

This week, I felt <u>mad</u> when . . .

_____
_____
_____
_____

This week, I felt <u>sad</u> when . . .

_____
_____
_____
_____

This week, I felt <u>worried</u> when . . .

_____
_____
_____
_____

This week, I felt <u>scared</u> when . . .

_____
_____
_____
_____

From Margaret E. Blaustein and Kristine M. Kinniburgh (2019). Copyright © 2019 The Guilford Press. Permission to photocopy this material is granted to purchasers of this book for personal use or use with clients (see copyright page for details). Purchasers can download additional copies of this material (see the box at the end of the table of contents).

What Are They Feeling?

Name: _____ Date: _____

Please look in magazines and find one picture of a person. Name all the possible emotions that you think this person/character is feeling.

Place your picture here:

Possible emotions that this person/character is feeling:

1. _____

2. _____

3. _____

4. _____

5. _____

From Margaret E. Blaustein and Kristine M. Kinniburgh (2019). Copyright © 2019 The Guilford Press. Permission to photocopy this material is granted to purchasers of this book for personal use or use with clients (see copyright page for details). Purchasers can download additional copies of this material (see the box at the end of the table of contents).

Tuning In to Feelings

Name: _____ Date: _____

Name of Emotion: _____

Rate the intensity of this feeling on the following scale:

_____

| -1 | 0 | 1 | 2 | 3 | 4 | 5 | 6 | 7 | 8 | 9 | 10 |

Shut   Low Energy/   Moderate Energy   High Energy/
Down   Calm   Intense Emotion

Did you like the feeling or not?   Why?

_____

_____

_____

_____

_____

What was going on at the time? What do you think led to this feeling?

_____

_____

_____

_____

_____

_____

_____

From Margaret E. Blaustein and Kristine M. Kinniburgh (2019). Copyright © 2019 The Guilford Press. Permission to photocopy this material is granted to purchasers of this book for personal use or use with clients (see copyright page for details). Purchasers can download additional copies of this material (see the box at the end of the table of contents).

Where Do I Feel . . . ?

Name: _____ Date: _____

Key:

Happy ☐
Sad ☐
Angry ☐
Worried ☐
Scared ☐
Excited ☐
Frustrated ☐
Proud ☐
_____ ☐

From Margaret E. Blaustein and Kristine M. Kinniburgh (2019). Copyright © 2019 The Guilford Press. Permission to photocopy this material is granted to purchasers of this book for personal use or use with clients (see copyright page for details). Purchasers can download additional copies of this material (see the box at the end of the table of contents).

Where Do I Feel . . . ?

Name: _____ Date: _____

Key:

Happy ☐
Sad ☐
Angry ☐
Worried ☐
Scared ☐
Excited ☐
Frustrated ☐
Proud ☐
_____ ☐

From Margaret E. Blaustein and Kristine M. Kinniburgh (2019). Copyright © 2019 The Guilford Press. Permission to photocopy this material is granted to purchasers of this book for personal use or use with clients (see copyright page for details). Purchasers can download additional copies of this material (see the box at the end of the table of contents).

The Feelings Bubble Technique

Staff Name: _____   Date: _____

Child Name: _____   Sup. Signature: _____

What are all of the emotions that you are having right now? Some emotions may feel good; some may feel bad; others may be confusing. Write them next to a box below. Pick a color for each emotion and color in the box. You may be feeling just a few things or you may be feeling a lot of things.

☐ _____   ☐ _____

☐ _____   ☐ _____

☐ _____   ☐ _____

We all have a lot of different emotions that we feel at the same time. Some emotions take up a lot of space and energy, and some take up less space and little energy. If you are having a big feeling, color in a big space in the bubble below; a small feeling, color in a small space in the bubble. (It can be helpful for staff members to model this exercise by creating their own bubbles. Be careful with boundaries.)

From Margaret E. Blaustein and Kristine M. Kinniburgh (2019, The Guilford Press). Copyright © 2019 by the authors. Permission to photocopy this material is granted to purchasers of this book for personal use or use with clients (see copyright page for details). Purchasers can download additional copies of this material (see the box at the end of the table of contents).

The Thought Head Technique

Staff Name: _____   Date: _____

Child Name: _____   Sup. Signature: _____

What are all of the things that you are thinking about right now? Some of the things in our
head may feel good and others may be worries we have. Write them next to a box below. Pick a
color for each and color in the box. You may be thinking about just a few things or you may be
thinking about a lot of things.

☐ _____   ☐ _____

☐ _____   ☐ _____

☐ _____   ☐ _____

We all have a lot of different things going on in our heads at the same time. Some things take
up a lot of space and energy, and some take up less space and little energy. How much space
does each thought take up in your head? If it's a big thought, color in a big space; a small
thought, color in a small space.

From Margaret E. Blaustein and Kristine M. Kinniburgh (2019, The Guilford Press). Copyright © 2019 by the authors. Permission to photocopy this material is granted to purchasers of this book for personal use or use with clients (see copyright page for details). Purchasers can download additional copies of this material (see the box at the end of the table of contents).

Noticing My Feelings

Name: _____ Date: _____

In order to cope with our feelings, we first must be aware of *what* we are feeling. This week, pick one feeling each day and complete the feelings log.

Day 1: Feeling: _____

When I felt it (what was happening?): _____

_____

Rate the intensity of the feeling: –1----0--------------5--------------10

Where in your body was the feeling held? _____

_____

Day 2: Feeling: _____

When I felt it (what was happening?): _____

_____

Rate the intensity of the feeling: –1----0--------------5--------------10

Where in your body was the feeling held? _____

_____

Day 3: Feeling: _____

When I felt it (what was happening?): _____

_____

Rate the intensity of the feeling: –1----0--------------5--------------10

Where in your body was the feeling held? _____

_____

(continued)

From Margaret E. Blaustein and Kristine M. Kinniburgh (2019). Copyright © 2019 The Guilford Press. Permission to photocopy this material is granted to purchasers of this book for personal use or use with clients (see copyright page for details). Purchasers can download additional copies of this material (see the box at the end of the table of contents).

Day 4: Feeling: _____

When I felt it (what was happening?): _____

_____

Rate the intensity of the feeling: –1----0-------------5-------------10

Where in your body was the feeling held? _____

_____

Day 5: Feeling: _____

When I felt it (what was happening?): _____

_____

Rate the intensity of the feeling: –1----0-------------5-------------10

Where in your body was the feeling held? _____

_____

Day 6: Feeling: _____

When I felt it (what was happening?): _____

_____

Rate the intensity of the feeling: –1----0-------------5-------------10

Where in your body was the feeling held? _____

_____

Day 7: Feeling: _____

When I felt it (what was happening?): _____

_____

Rate the intensity of the feeling: –1----0-------------5-------------10

Where in your body was the feeling held? _____

_____

All About Energy

- **Everyone Has Energy:** Everyone has energy in their bodies. Sometimes our energy is really low, like when we're sleepy; sometimes our energy is somewhere in the middle, like when we're feeling really focused and calm—like doing homework or playing a board game. Other times our energy can be really high, like when we're running around with friends or playing sports.

- **The Function of Energy:** Energy helps us do what we need to do, and all kinds of energy are important. Low energy is important, because sometimes we need to sleep and rest, and high energy is important, because sometimes we need to be really active or focused.

- **The Connection between Feelings and Energy:** One of the really important things that can affect our energy level is how we feel. For example, being excited or angry or scared can make our energy get really high; being sad or lonely can make our energy get really low. This is especially true for danger energy: When our brains think something is dangerous, our energy can change really quickly. Sometimes, having our energy change can be an important clue that something is going on with our feelings.

- **The Comfort Zone:** All of us have different bodies and different brains. That means that each of us feels most comfortable with different kinds of energy. Some people really, really like it when their energy is high, other people really like it when their energy stays low, and still other people like their energy to stay somewhere in the middle. The place we like our energy to stay is our "comfort zone." If our energy gets too far out of our comfort zone— like if someone who likes low energy gets too heated up—it can feel really uncomfortable. Sometimes, we try to do things to change our energy, to get it back where it's comfortable.

- **Effective Energy/Energy In Context:** Where we are and what we are doing can make a difference in whether our energy level helps us or gets in our way, and in whether our energy is safe or not safe. Having really high energy may feel really good, but there are places that high energy can get in our way. When high energy starts to get out of control, like if we're really mad or really upset, it can get in the way of getting our needs met, or make us do things that aren't safe.

- The same thing is true for low energy—low energy can be really good when we're sleepy, but can get in the way if we need to do something like chores or homework. Shutting down our energy when we're feeling scared or upset can sometimes feel safer, but can also get in the way of asking for help or doing something that feels good.

- **Using Sensory Tools or Movement to Change Energy:** There are a lot of different things we can do to change our energy when it doesn't feel comfortable or when it's getting in the way of something we want to do. We can think of these things as "energy tools." An energy tool helps us move our energy up or down. Not every tool works for every person, and not every tool works every time (just like sometimes you need a hammer, and sometimes you need a screwdriver). Because of that, we're going to practice different tools and figure out which ones you like, which ones feel good in your body, and which ones feel like they might work.

From Margaret E. Blaustein and Kristine M. Kinniburgh (2019, The Guilford Press). Copyright © 2019 by the authors. Permission to photocopy this material is granted to purchasers of this book for personal use or use with clients (see copyright page for details). Purchasers can download additional copies of this material (see the box at the end of the table of contents).

Check In

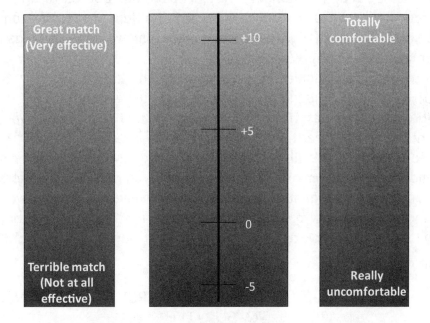

Take a moment to check in with yourself and mark the following on the scales provided below:

- Where is your energy? How high or how low?
- How comfortable does that energy feel in your body?
- How good of a match is your energy for what you are doing *right now?*

Great match (Very effective)	+10	Totally comfortable
	+5	
	0	
Terrible match (Not at all effective)	-5	Really uncomfortable

If your energy is **comfortable** *and* **a good match,** great! If not, what can you do to get it there? Identify one strategy or skill that you can use to feel more comfortable and effective.

From Margaret E. Blaustein and Kristine M. Kinniburgh (2019, The Guilford Press). Copyright © 2019 by the authors. Permission to photocopy this material is granted to purchasers of this book for personal use or use with clients (see copyright page for details). Purchasers can download additional copies of this material (see the box at the end of the table of contents).

The Body's Alarm System

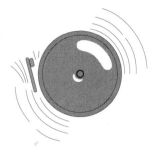 We all have a built-in alarm system that signals us when we might be in danger. One reason why human beings have been able to survive over time is because our brains recognize signals around us that tell us danger might be coming. This helps our bodies prepare to deal with danger when it comes.

THE HUMAN DANGER RESPONSE

When our brains recognize danger, they prepare our bodies to deal with it. We have four major ways to deal with something dangerous: We can **fight** it, we can get away from it **(flight)**, we can **freeze**, or we can give in as a way to keep ourselves safe **(comply/submit)**.

What we pick to do sometimes depends on the kind of danger. So, for example, if a really small squirrel is attacking you, you might fight it, because you're bigger and stronger than it is. If a car comes speeding at you, and you're standing in the street, you'd probably run, because you can't really fight it, and if you stand still, you'll get hit. If you saw a big bear or some other animal nearby, you might freeze, because you can't really fight it, and you're probably not fast enough to run away. If someone more powerful than you is trying to force you to do something, you might comply or submit—even if you don't really want to—as a way to keep that person from hurting you.

OUR BODIES GIVE US THE FUEL/ENERGY THAT WE NEED TO-SURVIVE

When it's time for our bodies to **fight**, or **run**, or **freeze**, or even **submit** we need a lot of energy to do those things. So, when the brain recognizes danger, its "action" or "doing" part sends a signal to the body to release a bunch of chemicals, like fuel for a car. Those chemicals give us the energy that we need to cope with the danger.

(continued)

From Margaret E. Blaustein and Kristine M. Kinniburgh (2019). Copyright © 2019 The Guilford Press. Permission to photocopy this material is granted to purchasers of this book for personal use or use with clients (see copyright page for details). Purchasers can download additional copies of this material (see the box at the end of the table of contents).

THE OVERACTIVE ALARM

When the danger signal goes off, the "thinking" part of our brains check out what is going on around us. If it is a false alarm, and there is no real danger, the "thinking brain" shuts off the alarm, and we can keep doing whatever we were doing. If there is danger, the "doing brain" takes over and gives the body fuel to deal with whatever is going on.

Sometimes, though, the danger alarm goes off too much. That usually happens when kids have had lots of dangerous things happen—like their parents hurting them, or someone touching them when they didn't want it, or someone yelling or fighting a lot. For kids who have had to deal with danger a lot, the "thinking brain" has gotten tired of checking things out and just assumes that the signals mean more danger. So now, when the alarm goes off, the "thinking brain" stays out of the way and lets the "doing brain" take over.

FALSE ALARMS

False alarms can happen when we hear, or see, or feel something that reminds us of bad things that used to happen or that sometimes still happen in other situations. Those reminders are called "triggers." Our brains have learned to recognize those reminders because in the past or in other situations when the reminders were around, dangerous things happened, and we had to react pretty quickly.

Different people have different reminders. So, if someone got yelled at a lot, hearing people yell might activate the alarm and make the "doing" part of the brain turn on. If someone didn't have enough attention paid to him or her when little, feeling all alone or scared might turn on the alarm.

WHAT HAPPENS WHEN THE ALARM GOES OFF?

Once our alarm turns on, our brains prep our bodies for action. When that happens, our bodies fill with "fuel" to prepare us for dealing with danger. This activation is really important if it's real danger (like a bear, or a speeding car, or a really mean squirrel), but not so helpful if it's a false

(continued)

alarm, and there isn't really any danger around. Imagine if you were in math class and something felt dangerous—suddenly, your body is filled with fuel.

Remember that the fuel gives us the energy to fight, or get away, or freeze. When our bodies have all that energy, we have to *do* something. So, some kids suddenly feel really angry or want to argue or fight with someone. Other kids just feel antsy or jumpy. Still other kids want to hide in a corner or get as far away as they can—and sometimes they don't even know why. And some kids will suddenly feel really shut down, like someone flipped a switch and turned them off. All of these are ways your body is trying to deal with something it thinks is dangerous.

Sometimes, though, what set off the alarm isn't really dangerous—it's just something that feels bad or reminds us of something bad that happens. When kids have a false alarm like that, it can be hard for other people to understand what just happened, and to help. Sometimes, kids even get into trouble.

RECOGNIZING TRIGGERS

It's important to learn about what kinds of reminders might feel dangerous to you and how your body reacts when those alarm signals are around. Everyone has different triggers and different ways to respond when the alarm goes off. If we know what sets off your alarm, and how you respond, we can get your thinking brain on board to help figure out when the danger is real and when it's a false alarm.

My Body's Alarm System

Name: _____ Date: _____

Please come up with one example of each of the ways that our bodies protect us from danger . . . fight, flight, freeze, and submit/comply.

Fight Response:

Example: A squirrel jumps out of the trash can as you are walking to school. You jump and scream at the squirrel. (high energy—fight)

Your Personal Fight Response Example:

_____

_____

_____

_____

_____

Flight Response:

Example: A car speeds toward you as you cross the street. You quickly run back to the sidewalk away from the car. (flight)

Your Personal Flight Response Example:

_____

_____

_____

_____

_____

(cont.)

From Margaret E. Blaustein and Kristine M. Kinniburgh (2019). Copyright © 2019 The Guilford Press. Permission to photocopy this material is granted to purchasers of this book for personal use or use with clients (see copyright page for details). Purchasers can download additional copies of this material (see the box at the end of the table of contents).

Freeze Response:

Example: A bear suddenly appears while you are out on a walk in the woods. You know that the bear is much bigger, stronger, and faster than you, so you stand perfectly still and quiet so the bear goes away and doesn't chase you. (freeze)

Your Personal Freeze Response Example:

_____

_____

_____

_____

_____

Comply/Submit response:

Example: A teacher who often says mean things to you and has threatened to fail you asks for volunteers to stay late and help clean the classroom. When no one responds, she looks at you and says, "I'm sure you want to help." You don't, but are scared of her, so you agree. (submit/comply)

Your personal Submit/Comply Response Example:

_____

_____

_____

_____

_____

My False Alarm Goes Off When . . .

Name: _____ Date: _____

Trigger	Reminds Me of . . .
1. Hearing people yell in loud tone of voice	Times when I was yelled at a lot
2. Feeling alone or being ignored	Times when I did not get enough attention when I was little
3. Smell of smoke	A bad fire

4. _____

_____

_____

5. _____

_____

_____

6. _____

_____

_____

7. _____

_____

_____

8. _____

_____

_____

From Margaret E. Blaustein and Kristine M. Kinniburgh (2019). Copyright © 2019 The Guilford Press. Permission to photocopy this material is granted to purchasers of this book for personal use or use with clients (see copyright page for details). Purchasers can download additional copies of this material (see the box at the end of the table of contents).

Identifying Triggers

Name: _____ Date: _____

Trigger: <u>Something that sets off our brain's alarm system and kick-starts our survival strategies: fighting, fleeing, freezing, or submitting.</u> Notice your triggers. Pay attention to a time this week (or recently) when you were triggered.

What was the situation? What do you think triggered you?

_____

What was your response? Describe as many of the following clues as you can identify.

Body: _____

Thoughts: _____

Feelings: _____

Behavior: _____

Was this a fight, flight, or freeze response? _____

Rate the intensity of your arousal:

-1	0	1	2	3	4	5	6	7	8	9	10
Shut Down		Low Energy/ Calm			Moderate Energy				High Energy/ Intense Emotion		

How did you cope with the situation or the feeling?

_____

_____

_____

_____

From Margaret E. Blaustein and Kristine M. Kinniburgh (2019). Copyright © 2019 The Guilford Press. Permission to photocopy this material is granted to purchasers of this book for personal use or use with clients (see copyright page for details). Purchasers can download additional copies of this material (see the box at the end of the table of contents).

My Nonverbal Cues

Name: _____ Date: _____

Please come up with examples of how people would know that you were _____

_____.

(Pick a feeling.)

When I'm _____, my face might look like this . . .

_____

_____

_____

When I'm _____, my body might look like this . . .

_____

_____

_____

When I'm _____, my voice might sound like . . .

_____

_____

_____

When I'm _____, people might notice that I behave
like this . . .

_____

_____

_____

From Margaret E. Blaustein and Kristine M. Kinniburgh (2019). Copyright © 2019 The Guilford Press. Permission to photocopy this material is granted to purchasers of this book for personal use or use with clients (see copyright page for details). Purchasers can download additional copies of this material (see the box at the end of the table of contents).

Emotional Intensity Meter

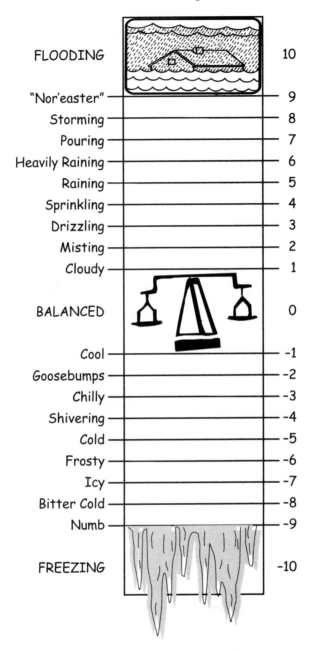

FLOODING		10
"Nor'easter"		9
Storming		8
Pouring		7
Heavily Raining		6
Raining		5
Sprinkling		4
Drizzling		3
Misting		2
Cloudy		1
BALANCED		0
Cool		−1
Goosebumps		−2
Chilly		−3
Shivering		−4
Cold		−5
Frosty		−6
Icy		−7
Bitter Cold		−8
Numb		−9
FREEZING		−10

From Margaret E. Blaustein and Kristine M. Kinniburgh (2019). Copyright © 2019 The Guilford Press. Permission to photocopy this material is granted to purchasers of this book for personal use or use with clients (see copyright page for details). Purchasers can download additional copies of this material (see the box at the end of the table of contents).

Checking My Pulse

Name: _____ Date: _____

My resting heart rate is _____ beats per minute.

After exercise my heart rate is _____ beats per minute.

After taking deep breaths my heart rate is _____ beats per minute.

Plot it! On the chart below, color in your heart rate.

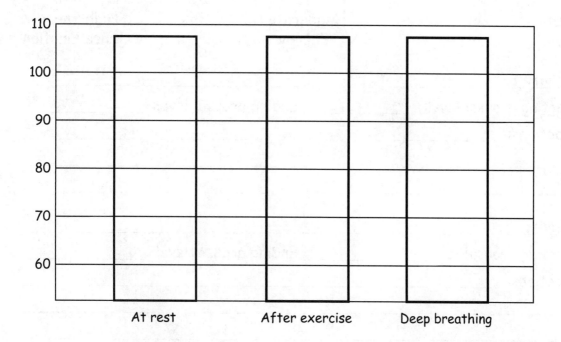

From Margaret E. Blaustein and Kristine M. Kinniburgh (2019). Copyright © 2019 The Guilford Press. Permission to photocopy this material is granted to purchasers of this book for personal use or use with clients (see copyright page for details). Purchasers can download additional copies of this material (see the box at the end of the table of contents).

Tracking My Energy

Name: _____ Date: _____

Physical activities can help you cope with emotions and manage energy. Some physical activities <u>increase</u> your body's arousal level, and some <u>decrease</u> it; all of us respond in different ways. We will be exploring different activities and their effect on your arousal—your energy level. Track your response on this sheet.

<u>Start Point:</u> How do you feel right now? What are you noticing in your body? Jot a few notes: _____

_____

_____

Rate your energy level right now on the following scale:

-1	0	1	2	3	4	5	6	7	8	9	10
Shut Down		Low Energy/ Calm				Moderate Energy				High Energy/ Intense Emotion	

<u>Activity 1:</u> _____

Starting arousal level: _____ Ending arousal level: _____

Reactions: _____

_____

_____

<u>Activity 2:</u> _____

Starting arousal level: _____ Ending arousal level: _____

Reactions: _____

_____

_____

(continued)

From Margaret E. Blaustein and Kristine M. Kinniburgh (2019). Copyright © 2019 The Guilford Press. Permission to photocopy this material is granted to purchasers of this book for personal use or use with clients (see copyright page for details). Purchasers can download additional copies of this material (see the box at the end of the table of contents).

Activity 3: _____

Starting arousal level: _____ Ending arousal level: _____

Reactions: _____

_____

_____

Activity 4: _____

Starting arousal level: _____ Ending arousal level: _____

Reactions: _____

_____

_____

Activity 5: _____

Starting arousal level: _____ Ending arousal level: _____

Reactions: _____

_____

_____

Activity 6: _____

Starting arousal level: _____ Ending arousal level: _____

Reactions: _____

_____

_____

Making My Energy Comfortable

Name: _____ Date: _____

Please practice your coping skills at least one time before our next meeting when you are calm. Try to practice ways to help your energy feel comfortable in your body.

You may want to try things like . . .
Calming activities
- Putting a weighted blanket or weights on your shoulders or lap
- Listening to soft, calming music
- Looking at pictures of sand and stones and concentrating on the details
- Squeezing a stress ball or tightening and relaxing your muscles
- Belly breathing

Energetic activities
- Listening to fun music
- Dancing
- Taking a walk
- Jumping on a small trampoline
- Jumping rope

This week I practiced . . .

_____

_____

_____

_____

_____

_____

_____ to bring my energy to a comfortable place in my body.

(continued)

From Margaret E. Blaustein and Kristine M. Kinniburgh (2019). Copyright © 2019 The Guilford Press. Permission to photocopy this material is granted to purchasers of this book for personal use or use with clients (see copyright page for details). Purchasers can download additional copies of this material (see the box at the end of the table of contents).

This is how I knew that my energy changed:

_____

_____

_____

_____

_____

_____

_____

This is how I knew that my energy felt more comfortable:

_____

_____

_____

_____

_____

_____

_____

I practiced this skill with . . .

_____   _____
Name   Caregiver (date)

Circles

Name: _____ Date: _____

Think about all of the different people in your life. Map out how close they are to you.

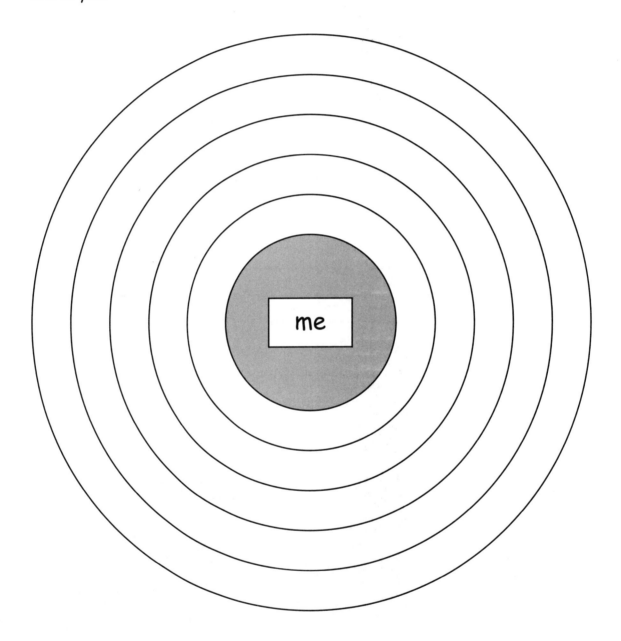

From Margaret E. Blaustein and Kristine M. Kinniburgh (2019). Copyright © 2019 The Guilford Press. Permission to photocopy this material is granted to purchasers of this book for personal use or use with clients (see copyright page for details). Purchasers can download additional copies of this material (see the box at the end of the table of contents).

Starting a Conversation

Name: _____ Date: _____

Practice starting a conversation with someone (pick who: _____)
about how you're feeling. Let _____ know ahead of time how you
will let him/her/them know that you'd like to talk (for example, by using
a hand signal, door sign, words, other?). Practice this at least one time
before our next meeting.

I practiced this with _____ (name of person)
on _____ (date/time).

Remember . . .

Comfortable state (How does your body feel?)

Effective state (Are you in control?)

Good time (What's a good and not-so-good time?)

Right person (Who can meet your needs?)

Communication style (How can you be an effective communicator?)

How did it go?

_____

_____

_____

_____

_____

_____

_____

_____

_____

_____

_____

From Margaret E. Blaustein and Kristine M. Kinniburgh (2019). Copyright © 2019 The Guilford Press. Permission to photocopy this material is granted to purchasers of this book for personal use or use with clients (see copyright page for details). Purchasers can download additional copies of this material (see the box at the end of the table of contents).

Giving Others Compliments

Name: _____ Date: _____

One thing that I like about _____ is _____

_____

_____

One thing that I like about _____ is _____

_____

_____

One thing that I like about _____ is _____

_____

_____

One thing that I like about _____ is _____

_____

_____

One thing that I like about _____ is _____

_____

_____

One thing that I like about _____ is _____

_____

_____

One thing that I like about _____ is _____

_____

_____

From Margaret E. Blaustein and Kristine M. Kinniburgh (2019). Copyright © 2019 The Guilford Press. Permission to photocopy this material is granted to purchasers of this book for personal use or use with clients (see copyright page for details). Purchasers can download additional copies of this material (see the box at the end of the table of contents).

Giving Myself Compliments

Name: _____ Date: _____

In school I'm really good at _____

_____

_____

_____

I'm really good at playing _____

_____

_____

_____ when I have free time.

I show that I'm a good friend to others by _____

_____

_____

_____

_____

One thing that I really like about myself is _____

_____

_____

_____

_____

_____

From Margaret E. Blaustein and Kristine M. Kinniburgh (2019). Copyright © 2019 The Guilford Press. Permission to photocopy this material is granted to purchasers of this book for personal use or use with clients (see copyright page for details). Purchasers can download additional copies of this material (see the box at the end of the table of contents).

What Has Influenced My Identity?

Name: _____ Date: _____

<u>Directions:</u> All of us are influenced by many different things. Below are some examples of things that might influence who you are. Pick six things that you think have had the <u>most</u> influence on you and list them. Assign a different color to each thing on your list (for example, "family" might be <u>red</u>; "peers," <u>purple</u>). Using those colors, create a sculpture (using colored Play-Doh, modeling clay, or similar) or some other art project (such as a painting, drawing, or colored tissue-paper collage) to represent some of the influences on your identity.

<u>Possible Influences:</u>

- Family
- Neighborhood
- Peers
- Religion
- Cultural background
- Role models

- Music
- Social media
- School
- Life experiences
- Other?

Your top six influences:

1.

2.

3.

4.

5.

6.

Color code:

1.

2.

3.

4.

5.

6.

From Margaret E. Blaustein and Kristine M. Kinniburgh (2019). Copyright © 2019 The Guilford Press. Permission to photocopy this material is granted to purchasers of this book for personal use or use with clients (see copyright page for details). Purchasers can download additional copies of this material (see the box at the end of the table of contents).

Quality of Influence Pyramid

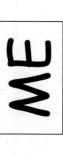

Negative Quality of Influence

Positive Quality of Influence

In the box write the name of a person you know who has influenced you in some way.

On the line next to the box, write the quality he/she has that has influenced you.

For instance, one person might write "Grandma" in one of the left-side boxes, and on the line next to it, write "caring," because her caring was a positive influence. Someone else might write "my cousin" on the right side and put "hard to trust" on the line, because it always felt like the cousin couldn't be counted on.

From Margaret E. Blaustein and Kristine M. Kinniburgh (2019). Copyright © 2019 The Guilford Press. Permission to photocopy this material is granted to purchasers of this book for personal use or use with clients (see copyright page for details). Purchasers can download additional copies of this material (see the box at the end of the table of contents).

Identity Shields

Directions: All of us have many different qualities—for instance, different parts of our personality, different ways we behave with various people, and things we keep on the inside and things we show on the outside. Use the shield below to create your own personal crest, or identity shield. In each section, draw or write something that symbolizes a different part of who you are.

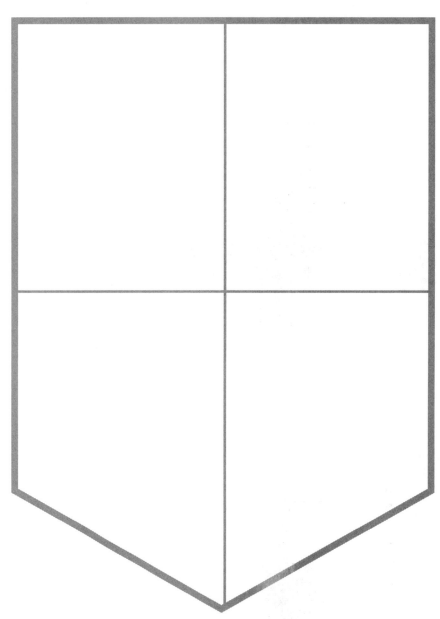

From Margaret E. Blaustein and Kristine M. Kinniburgh (2019). Copyright © 2019 The Guilford Press. Permission to photocopy this material is granted to purchasers of this book for personal use or use with clients (see copyright page for details). Purchasers can download additional copies of this material (see the box at the end of the table of contents).

Identity Shields

Directions: All of us have many different qualities—for instance, different parts of our personality, different ways we behave with various people, and things we keep on the inside and things we show on the outside. Use the shield below to create your own personal crest, or identity shield. In each section, draw or write something that symbolizes a different part of who you are.

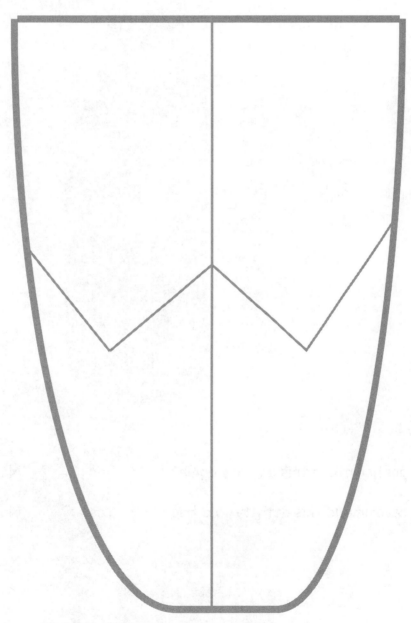

From Margaret E. Blaustein and Kristine M. Kinniburgh (2019). Copyright © 2019 The Guilford Press. Permission to photocopy this material is granted to purchasers of this book for personal use or use with clients (see copyright page for details). Purchasers can download additional copies of this material (see the box at the end of the table of contents).

Your Fun-o-meter

Name: _____

Your opinion matters: How fun is this activity?

Please circle how fun this activity was!

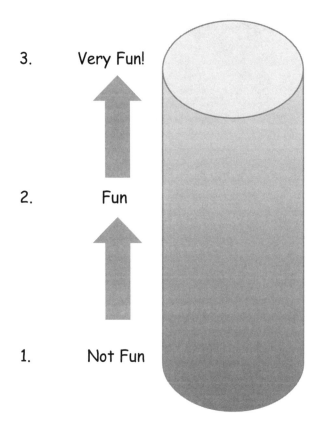

3.   Very Fun!

2.   Fun

1.   Not Fun

Would you participate in this activity again?   Yes   No

Would you recommend this activity to a friend?   Yes   No

From Margaret E. Blaustein and Kristine M. Kinniburgh (2019, The Guilford Press). Copyright © 2019 by the authors. Permission to photocopy this material is granted to purchasers of this book for personal use or use with clients (see copyright page for details). Purchasers can download additional copies of this material (see the box at the end of the table of contents).

Overarching Goal of the Week:
Learning about My Feelings and Energy
(Identification)

My selected goal this week: (For example: <u>Notice when my energy gets</u> <u>really high</u>.)

_____

_____

_____

_____

_____

Why am I choosing this goal? (Specific information that tells me why this will be helpful for me)

_____

_____

_____

_____

_____

A few examples of what I might try (what/when/how):

1. _____

_____

(Who can help me with this?) _____

2. _____

_____

(Who can help me with this?) _____

3. _____

_____

(Who can help me with this?) _____

From Margaret E. Blaustein and Kristine M. Kinniburgh (2019, The Guilford Press). Copyright © 2019 by the authors. Permission to photocopy this material is granted to purchasers of this book for personal use or use with clients (see copyright page for details). Purchasers can download additional copies of this material (see the box at the end of the table of contents).

Overarching Goal of the Week: Managing My Feelings and Behavior
(Modulation)

My selected goal this week: (For example: <u>Practice using my calming space</u>
<u>at least once every day)</u>

_____

_____

_____

_____

_____

Why am I choosing this goal? (Specific information that tells me why this
will be helpful for me)

_____

_____

_____

_____

_____

A few examples of what I might try (what/when/how):

1. _____

_____

(Who can help me with this?) _____

2. _____

_____

(Who can help me with this?) _____

3. _____

_____

(Who can help me with this?) _____

From Margaret E. Blaustein and Kristine M. Kinniburgh (2019, The Guilford Press). Copyright © 2019 by the authors. Permission to photocopy this material is granted to purchasers of this book for personal use or use with clients (see copyright page for details). Purchasers can download additional copies of this material (see the box at the end of the table of contents).

Overarching Goal of the Week: Making Choices That Work for Me
(Executive Functions)

My selected goal this week: (For example: <u>Ask for help when problems feel too big to solve by myself)</u>

_____

_____

_____

_____

_____

Why am I choosing this goal? (Specific information that tells me why this will be helpful for me)

_____

_____

_____

_____

_____

A few examples of what I might try (what/when/how):

1. _____

_____

(Who can help me with this?) _____

2. _____

_____

(Who can help me with this?) _____

3. _____

_____

(Who can help me with this?) _____

From Margaret E. Blaustein and Kristine M. Kinniburgh (2019, The Guilford Press). Copyright © 2019 by the authors. Permission to photocopy this material is granted to purchasers of this book for personal use or use with clients (see copyright page for details). Purchasers can download additional copies of this material (see the box at the end of the table of contents).

Overarching Goal of the Week: Learning All about Myself
(Self and Identity)

My selected goal this week: (For example: <u>Do one thing I really enjoy</u> <u>every day; I might do one of these three things: . . .)</u>

_____

_____

_____

Why am I choosing this goal? (Specific information that tells me why this will be helpful for me)

_____

_____

_____

_____

A few examples of what I might try (what/when/how):

_____

_____

_____

_____

1. _____

_____

   (Who can help me with this?) _____

2. _____

_____

   (Who can help me with this?) _____

3. _____

_____

   (Who can help me with this?) _____

From Margaret E. Blaustein and Kristine M. Kinniburgh (2019, The Guilford Press). Copyright © 2019 by the authors. Permission to photocopy this material is granted to purchasers of this book for personal use or use with clients (see copyright page for details). Purchasers can download additional copies of this material (see the box at the end of the table of contents).

APPENDIX E

Milieu–Systems Materials

Processing Form

- Similar to the "Taking a Break" form, this one provides an example of a processing form to be used by staff and youth when a child/adolescent has earned a specific consequence or limit for behavior. This form supports youth in recognizing precipitating triggers for behavior, affect, energy, level of control, and specific coping strategies that will support successful reengagement with the larger group.

Processing Packet: Getting Back On Track

- This packet is designed to be used with youth after they have earned a limit for behavior and/or needed to take a break from program activities due to dysregulation. This packet should be implemented by staff members after the children/adolescents have regained control of their emotions and behavior. The packet supports youth in identifying triggers for behavior, body clues, energy/ arousal level, feelings clues, and thinking clues, and helps youth to engage in problem solving around future coping and expression skills, such as accessing resources.

Program-to-Caregiver Behavior Communication Form

Caregiver-to-Program Behavior Communication Form

- These forms may be used to support programmatic staff in communicating with caregivers about ways that behaviors are being addressed within a milieu, and/or supporting caregivers in communicating about observed behaviors with programmatic staff.

ARC-Based Milieu Program: Self-Evaluation Form

An ARC-based/ARC-informed program:

1. **Has a designated team, ideally comprised of multidisciplinary professionals, who bear the responsibility for strategic planning, ongoing development, monitoring, and adjusting their systems-based program approach to incorporate a trauma-informed practice.**

   Please rate the extent to which your program addresses this goal:

0	1	2	3	4	5
Not at all		Somewhat		A great deal	

   Identify team members:

   _____

   _____

   _____

   _____

   Describe team meetings (frequency, agenda):

   _____

   _____

   _____

   _____

2. **Supports staff knowledge and awareness of trauma through purposeful sequences of or approaches to training/consultation/supervision that are integrated into ongoing programmatic structures (i.e., beyond initial orientation).**

   Please rate the extent to which your program addresses this goal:

0	1	2	3	4	5
Not at all		Somewhat		A great deal	

   Describe: In what ways do staff members receive training in trauma that includes orientation, supervision, consultation, and ongoing didactic instruction)?

   _____

   _____

   _____

   Who is responsible for developing, monitoring, and delivering training?

   _____

   _____

   _____

(continued)

From Margaret E. Blaustein and Kristine M. Kinniburgh (2019, The Guilford Press). Copyright © 2019 by the authors. Permission to photocopy this material is granted to purchasers of this book for personal use or use with clients (see copyright page for details). Purchasers can download additional copies of this material (see the box at the end of the table of contents).

3. **Supports integration of trauma-related concepts in established program structures (e.g., meetings, client discussion, supervision), policies, and paperwork.**

Please rate the extent to which your program addresses this goal:

0	1	2	3	4	5
Not at all		Somewhat		A great deal	

Provide examples of ways trauma-related concepts (e.g., triggers, adaptive response, helpful regulatory strategies) are routinely integrated into client discussion and key paperwork:

_____

_____

_____

_____

4. **Actively targets staff and adult affect management, including reflective awareness of staff experience, awareness and development of systematic and individual support resources, and integration of adult supports into system structures, policies, and procedures.**

Please rate the extent to which your program addresses this goal:

0	1	2	3	4	5
Not at all		Somewhat		A great deal	

Describe approaches. Consider: specific training in self-awareness; availability of supervision; availability of concrete resources for staff support and regulation; explicit discussion of youth impact on staff experience; presence of "backup" in staffing; awareness and training in vicarious trauma.

_____

_____

_____

_____

(continued)

5. **Purposefully develops active staff curiosity and understanding of youth behaviors, and integrates these qualities into systematic approaches to supporting youth functioning.**

   Please rate the extent to which your program addresses this goal:

0	1	2	3	4	5
Not at all		Somewhat		A great deal	

   Describe approaches. Description should include both initial training in understanding the functions underlying youth behavior, as well as ongoing structures that support staff in exploring the possible underlying drivers of youth behavior. Consider how youth behaviors are discussed in meetings, if information regarding triggers is included, responses on behavior forms and plans, proactive approaches to observing and addressing youth behaviors, etc.

   _____

   _____

   _____.

   _____

6. **Develops behavior plans that integrate understanding of the drivers of youth behavior, and which emphasize individualized approaches to supporting success**

   Please rate the extent to which your program addresses this goal:

0	1	2	3	4	5
Not at all		Somewhat		A great deal	

   Describe system approach to behavioral response. Be specific about the ways in which understanding of youth behavior is incorporated into the response to that behavior.

   _____

   _____

   _____

   _____

7. **Has a systematic approach to reviewing staff behaviors, responses, and interactions with youth in a manner that supports positive adult–child interaction.**

   Please rate the extent to which your program addresses this goal:

0	1	2	3	4	5
Not at all		Somewhat		A great deal	

   Describe forums in which staff–youth interactions are discussed. May include supervision, small- or large-group staff meetings, and forums for integrated youth–staff community discussion. Describe forums for reparative work between staff and youth, when applicable.

   _____

   _____

   _____

   _____

(continued)

8. Actively builds and supports staff skill in mirroring youth experience/providing a reflective response and in supporting youth acquisition of problem-solving skills.

Please rate the extent to which your program addresses this goal:

0	1	2	3	4	5
Not at all		Somewhat		A great deal	

Describe approaches to staff training in these skills, and ways these are integrated into ongoing practice. Consider didactic processes such as orientation or in-service training, as well as ongoing structures such as supervision, coaching, and systematic approaches to supporting staff–youth interaction (routine reflection meetings, organized problem-solving meetings, etc.).

_____

_____

_____

_____

9. Actively targets engagement of the child's family system (if applicable), and systematically targets caregiver education about trauma, caregiver attunement, caregiver affect management, and other caregiver skills as relevant.

Please rate the extent to which your program addresses this goal:

0	1	2	3	4	5
Not at all		Somewhat		A great deal	

Describe approaches to working with the child's family system. Do formal/systematic approaches exist for initial family engagement, caregiver psychoeducation, caregiver skill building, and caregiver–child relationship building? How are these approaches monitored and adjusted? In what ways are caregivers/family systems actively collaborating in the treatment process?

_____

_____

_____

_____

10. Has a systematic approach to developing and supporting youth regulation skills in all facets of milieu functioning, with all staff members acting in an integrated way to cue, support, and reinforce these skills.

    (10a) Approaches to youth regulation actively target youth understanding of emotional and physiological experience, and acknowledge/integrate the role of historical influences on current functioning.

    (10b) Approaches to youth regulation integrate supports for youth to actively explore and identify concrete resources for managing emotion and arousal.

    (10c) Identified strategies for regulation are routinely and systematically integrated into daily procedures, and staff at all levels is trained in role-specific ways to support youth skills.

(continued)

466

Please rate the extent to which your program addresses this goal:

0	1	2	3	4	5
Not at all			Somewhat		A great deal

Describe ways that youth served by the program are taught and supported in exploration of regulation strategies.

_____

_____

Describe staff role in supporting youth regulation.

_____

_____

Describe systematic structures that facilitate regulation/coregulation (e.g., access to regulation resources, purposeful use of routines, individualized toolboxes).

_____

_____

11. **Is aware of the importance of routines and rhythms, and actively uses these to support adult and youth modulation and in service of key goals.**

Please rate the extent to which your program addresses this goal:

0	1	2	3	4	5
Not at all			Somewhat		A great deal

List and briefly describe the role of routines and rhythms in your system. Consider both daily schedule and specific targeted routines (e.g., transition times, bedtime). Describe ways these routines are made explicit to both staff and youth.

_____

_____

_____

Are routines used to support unpredictable experiences (e.g., youth or staff departures, critical incidents)? In what ways are approaches to these salient events systematic versus reactive?

_____

_____

What community-specific rituals exist?

_____

_____

(continued)

12. **Routinely and systematically assesses, identifies, and builds and supports areas of youth strength and competency.**

Please rate the extent to which your program addresses this goal:

0	1	2	3	4	5
Not at all		Somewhat		A great deal	

Describe ways that youth areas of strength and competency are actively assessed and addressed:

_____

_____

_____

_____

13. **Actively targets and builds opportunity for agency, empowerment, and active decision making by child and adolescent clients.**

Please rate the extent to which your program addresses this goal:

0	1	2	3	4	5
Not at all		Somewhat		A great deal	

Describe opportunities for youth empowerment. Consider the ways in which youth are invited (1) to provide feedback about programmatic experience, (2) to provide input into treatment goals and process, (3) to participate in community decision making, and so on.

_____

_____

_____

_____

14. **Works with youth, families, and/or collaterals to support and plan for positive functioning beyond the treatment program, and to develop a future template.**

Please rate the extent to which your program addresses this goal:

0	1	2	3	4	5
Not at all		Somewhat		A great deal	

Describe ways that youth and families are supported in developing goals and accessing concrete resources for postprogram functioning.

_____

_____

_____

_____

(continued)

15. **(If applicable) Has clinicians who are trained in the understanding and integration of traumatic experiences in a format that matches the population, timeframe, and structural limitations of the setting.**

Please rate the extent to which your program addresses this goal:

0	1	2	3	4	5
Not at all		Somewhat		A great deal	

Consider both external and internal training processes and opportunities for clinicians.

_____

_____

_____

_____

ARC-BASED/ARC-INFORMED SYSTEMS CHECKLIST SUMMARY SHEET

	Degree to which your system addresses this goal					
	Not at all/ Never		Somewhat		A great deal/ Always	
	0	1	2	3	4	5
1. Lead implementation team	0	1	2	3	4	5
2. Purposeful training approach	0	1	2	3	4	5
3. Integration of trauma-related concepts	0	1	2	3	4	5
4. Targets staff affect management	0	1	2	3	4	5
5. Staff curiosity about youth behavior	0	1	2	3	4	5
6. Behavior plans that are trauma-informed	0	1	2	3	4	5
7. Approach to supporting positive staff–child interaction	0	1	2	3	4	5
8. Actively builds staff skill	0	1	2	3	4	5
9. Targets family engagement	0	1	2	3	4	5
10. Integrated approach to youth regulation	0	1	2	3	4	5
11. Routines and rhythms	0	1	2	3	4	5
12. Targets youth competency	0	1	2	3	4	5
13. Supports youth empowerment	0	1	2	3	4	5
14. Future planning	0	1	2	3	4	5
15. Trauma-specific clinical approaches and training	0	1	2	3	4	5

Staff Self-Care Plan

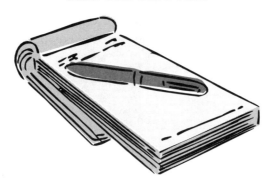

Name: _____ Date: _____

Two **in-the-moment strategies** (e.g., counting to 10, taking three deep breaths, reciting my ABC's) that I will practice when dealing with challenging youth behaviors are:

1. _____

   _____

2. _____

   _____

Two **long-term strategies** (e.g., getting together with friends, doing something I enjoy) that I will practice upon leaving work are:

1. _____

   _____

2. _____

   _____

_____   _____
Staff Signature/date of review   Supervisor Signature/date

From Margaret E. Blaustein and Kristine M. Kinniburgh (2019). Copyright © 2019 The Guilford Press. Permission to photocopy this material is granted to purchasers of this book for personal use or use with clients (see copyright page for details). Purchasers can download additional copies of this material (see the box at the end of the table of contents).

The Trauma Cycle Worksheet

Think back on an interaction between you and a child or young person. Reflect on patterns of experience notable for you and the child or young person.

Use this grid to comment on your observations.

	Youth	Staff/Caregiver
Cognitive Thinking patterns, perceptions, assumptions, attitudes		
Emotional Core feelings expressed verbally and/or nonverbally; obvious or implied		
Behavior (Coping Strategy) Core behaviors and strategies used to regulate, manage, or avoid the interactions or situation		
The Cycle Core interactions (thoughts, behaviors, communications) that keep the cycle going		

Adapted by Steve Granaham from material by Margaret E. Blaustein and Kristine M. Kinniburgh. From Margaret E. Blaustein and Kristine M. Kinniburgh (2019). Copyright © 2019 The Guilford Press. Permission to photocopy this material is granted to purchasers of this book for personal use or use with clients (see copyright page for details). Purchasers can download additional copies of this material (see the box at the end of the table of contents).vt

Sample of ARC-Informed System Orientation and Intake Packet

ABOUT US: INTRODUCTION TO ARC AND THE TRAUMA FRAME

Our program is designed to help kids who have experienced very stressful events in their lives. Kids who have been through hard things often have very big, sometimes overwhelming emotions. The way that kids deal with these big feelings is often what leads them to us. Some kids hurt themselves or others; other kids struggle with rules and relationships; still others just try to hide from the world. Many strategies are used in an attempt to manage big emotions or experiences. Our goal is to support you in learning to better understand your emotions and to work with you to build a toolbox of strategies that will help you to feel more comfortable and to reach your goals.

ABOUT YOU

This is a form to find out some things about you. Let me know if you have anything you would like to share or anything you would like to talk about as we learn more about you.

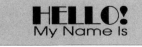

Where I'm Coming From

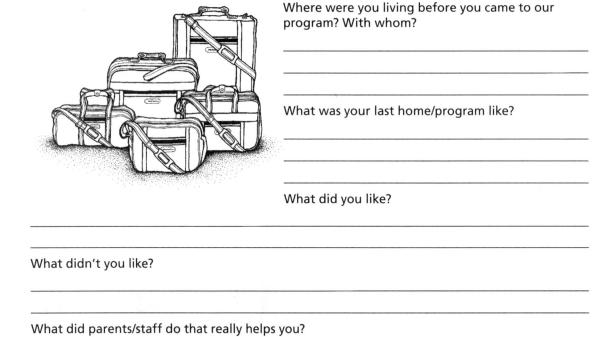

Where were you living before you came to our program? With whom?

_____

_____

_____

What was your last home/program like?

_____

_____

_____

What did you like?

_____

_____

What didn't you like?

_____

_____

What did parents/staff do that really helps you?

_____

_____

(continued)

From Margaret E. Blaustein and Kristine M. Kinniburgh (2019, The Guilford Press). Copyright © 2019 by the authors. Permission to photocopy this material is granted to purchasers of this book for personal use or use with clients (see copyright page for details). Purchasers can download additional copies of this material (see the box at the end of the table of contents).

CIRCLE OF SUPPORT

Think about people in your life who are very important to you. Using the circles below, write in the people that are close to you and ones that are far away (talk about the distance as being physical and/or emotional).

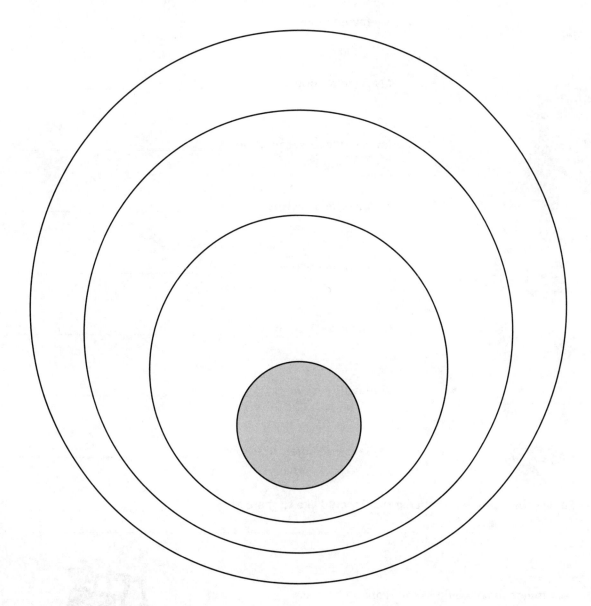

USING YOUR CIRCLES

Some of the people above are people who can help you when you may be struggling with something. We hope that you will add some people from our program to your circles as you get to know us better.

(continued)

MY FAVORITES (OR THE THINGS THAT YOU LIKE IF YOU DON'T HAVE FAVORITES)

My favorite color is _____

My favorite music is _____

My favorite food is _____

My favorite ice cream flavor is _____

My favorite activity is _____

My favorite shoes are _____

My favorite TV show is _____

My favorite movie is _____

My favorite subject in school is _____

Some other favorites about me that I would like to share are _____

_____

MY GOALS

Two things that I would like to work on here are:

1. _____

    _____

2. _____

    _____

The Comfort Zone: Sample Guidelines for Systems

The primary focus of a comfort zone is to provide a dedicated space with tools that can support children/adolescents in regulating their arousal or energy so that it feels **comfortable** for them and so that they can engage **effectively** in their daily routines. The comfort zone may be a room, a corner, or an identified area within the child or adolescent's room or residence.

The secondary benefit of this dedicated space is that it provides opportunities for one-on-one time to connect with staff. The **need for connection** is an acceptable motive for use of the room because that connection may serve a coregulatory function.

Note: although we describe this as "comfort zone" here, the system or individual child/adolescent may wish to refer to this room in some other way. It is important that the language resonate with the child and be consistent with other systemic initiatives.

The guidelines for working with children/adolescents in this space are as follows:

1. *Engage:* Children using the comfort zone should be using tools *with* staff. You are intervening in two primary ways: by modeling use of the tools for kids, and by coregulating through your own actions.

2. *Assess and Check In:* When you enter the comfort zone, your first task is assess the child/adolescent's current level of arousal and comfort. It may be helpful to collaborate with the child/adolescent in this assessment by using a specific energy-tracking tool.

3. *Use the Language of Experimentation:* After your initial assessment, engage the child/adolescent in experimentation with the tools in the room. If there are preferred tools and/or activities, then allow for choice.

4. *Match Low Energy:* If the child/adolescent's energy level is low, then it may be helpful to suggest a "low-energy" tool such as slow movement, drawing, breathing, or applying deep pressure. Suggest a low-energy tool but don't struggle if the child/adolescent gravitates toward something else. Allow for choice.

5. *Match High Energy:* If the child/adolescent's energy level is high, then it may be helpful to suggest a "high-energy" strategy such as bouncing up and down on the ball, a fast game of catch, a follow-the-leader movement activity, etc. Again, allow for choice.

6. *Model:* If the child/adolescent doesn't engage with a tool, then you can select something to "try it out" by modeling use of the tool.

7. *Attune:* It is important to be continuously monitoring the child/adolescent's changing or unchanging arousal level while he or she is using the tool. If energy appears to be increasing/decreasing to an uncomfortable/ineffective level, then reflect what you see and suggest and model a change: Consider a change in the pace of movement, the amount of pressure, the location of pressure, the tool itself, etc.

8. *Assess and Check Out:* When the allotted time is up, child/adolescent is done, or staff has assessed the session to be completed, repeat the **energy check** or assessment of the child/adolescent's level of arousal and comfort.

From Margaret E. Blaustein and Kristine M. Kinniburgh (2019, The Guilford Press). Copyright © 2019 by the authors. Permission to photocopy this material is granted to purchasers of this book for personal use or use with clients (see copyright page for details). Purchasers can download additional copies of this material (see the box at the end of the table of contents).

Supporting Regulation with Sensory Tools

Staff Name: _____ Date: _____

Student Name: _____ Sup. Signature: _____

ENERGY CHECK

First, let's figure out where your energy is right now. Color in the number of squares that best tells us about your energy.

Low   Medium   High

Are you feeling comfortable or uncomfortable? _____

_____

SKILL CHOICE

OK. Now we are going to pick a skill or two that we can practice to see what happens to your energy. The skill/s that we practiced was/were _____

_____

_____

_____

RECHECK ENERGY

After practicing the skill where is your energy now? Color in the number of squares that best tells us about your energy.

Low   Medium   High

Are you feeling comfortable or uncomfortable? _____

_____

(continued)

From Margaret E. Blaustein and Kristine M. Kinniburgh (2019, The Guilford Press). Copyright © 2019 by the authors. Permission to photocopy this material is granted to purchasers of this book for personal use or use with clients (see copyright page for details). Purchasers can download additional copies of this material (see the box at the end of the table of contents).

STAFF OBSERVATIONS

For staff: Please describe what you noticed about:

Energy:		
Emotions:		
Facial Expressions:		
Tone of Voice:		
Rate of Speech (fast, slow):		
Activity Level		

Other observations: _____
_____
_____
_____
_____
_____
_____
_____

Developing Systematic Approaches to Regulation: Agency Worksheet

PART 1: WHAT ARE YOU DOING NOW, AND WHAT ARE YOUR GOALS?

Primary Facets of a Systematic Approach	Current Approaches (What do you already do?)	Obstacles to Addressing This Area (What gets in the way of this?)	Agency-Specific Goal(s) (Broadly, what do you want to be doing?)
Systematic approaches to supporting baseline or routine modulation *(In what ways do youth routinely have opportunities to engage in modulating/ regulating activities? How are these built into daily structures?)*			
Routine opportunities to build capacity to identify internal experience (both proactively and during challenging experience) *(In what ways do you create opportunities for youth to reflect upon and identify internal experience? This should occur routinely as well as systematically during more challenging time periods.)*			
Child-specific experimentation with and identification of targeted modulation strategies *(Where and how can youth practice more targeted modulation strategies? Consider opportunities for youth to identify, practice, and engage with various approaches to managing experience.)*			

(continued)

From Margaret E. Blaustein and Kristine M. Kinniburgh (2019, The Guilford Press). Copyright © 2019 by the authors. Permission to photocopy this material is granted to purchasers of this book for personal use or use with clients (see copyright page for details). Purchasers can download additional copies of this material (see the box at the end of the table of contents).

Primary Facets of a Systematic Approach	Current Approaches (What do you already do?)	Obstacles to Addressing This Area (What gets in the way of this?)	Agency-Specific Goal(s) (Broadly, what do you want to be doing?)
Systematic approaches to supporting/cuing modulation strategies, including staff/caregiver training *(In what ways are identified strategies supported and integrated into ongoing routine and child-specific regulation plans? How are staff/caregivers educated about youth needs and ways to support those?)*			

PART 2: BRAINSTORM AND PLANNING: IDEAS FOR BUILDING BOTH PROGRAM-LEVEL AND TARGETED (CHILD-SPECIFIC) APPROACHES

Primary Facets of a Systematic Approach	Possible Strategies
Systematic approaches to supporting baseline or routine modulation *(Where are there opportunities to support youth in routinely engaging in modulating/regulating activities? How might these be built and sustained in daily structures?)*	
Routine opportunities to build capacity to identify internal experience (both proactively and during challenging experience) *(Where in your schedule and structure can you create opportunities for youth to reflect upon and identify internal experience? This should occur routinely as well as systematically during more challenging time periods.)*	

(continued)

Primary Facets of a Systematic Approach	Possible Strategies
Child-specific experimentation with and identification of targeted modulation strategies *(Where and how can youth practice more targeted modulation strategies? How will these opportunities be provided and supported? How will you track those tools which are found to be successful?)*	
Systematic approaches to supporting/cuing modulation strategies, including staff/caregiver training *(How can you build structures that will integrate identified strategies into ongoing routine and child-specific regulation plans? How will you work with staff/caregivers to educate them about youth needs and ways to support those?)*	

Client Support Planning Tool

What are some of your triggers that staff should be aware of?

☐ Being alone	☐ Lack of privacy	☐ Feeling pressured
☐ Feeling lonely	☐ Darkness	☐ Not being listened to
☐ Loud noise	☐ Arguments	☐ People yelling
☐ Being touched	☐ Not enough room	☐ Being in a large group of people
☐ Humor/jokes	☐ Being stared at	
☐ Being asked questions	☐ Being around men	☐ Being told to be quiet
☐ Not having control/input	☐ Being ignored	☐ Being around women
☐ Contact with family	☐ Having a limit set on your behavior	☐ Being teased or picked on

☐ Time of day: _____   ☐ Specific person: _____

☐ Anniversaries/time of year: _____

☐ Other triggers not listed above: _____

How would other people know that you were upset or having a hard time?

☐ Sweating	☐ Red face	☐ Breathing hard	☐ Act rude/ disrespectful
☐ Heart racing	☐ Clenched teeth	☐ Clenched fists	☐ Poor hygiene
☐ Wringing hands	☐ Bouncing legs	☐ Rocking	☐ Stop following rules
☐ Pacing	☐ Can't sit still	☐ Swearing	☐ Can't pay attention
☐ Loud voice	☐ Singing inappropriate songs	☐ Crying	☐ Hide things
☐ Hiding/wandering	☐ Silly	☐ Eat less/more	☐ Look spaced out
☐ Can't sleep	☐ Sleep during the day	☐ Stay away from people	
☐ Argue with peers	☐ Talk about sex/ relationships	☐ Give stuff away	
☐ Messy room	☐ Stop taking medications	☐ Break or throw stuff	
☐ Talk about dying			

☐ Other: _____

Do you ask for help if you need it to stay safe?   ☐ Yes   ☐ No   ☐ Sometimes

(continued)

From Margaret E. Blaustein and Kristine M. Kinniburgh (2019, The Guilford Press). Copyright © 2019 by the authors. Permission to photocopy this material is granted to purchasers of this book for personal use or use with clients (see copyright page for details). Purchasers can download additional copies of this material (see the box at the end of the table of contents).

Five Steps to in-the-Moment Safety

1. **Reflect:** "Your behavior is telling me that you are having a hard time right now because you're having a hard time listening [jumping up and down in your seat, sitting by yourself, etc.]. Your energy looks really high [low] right now. Is there something that you need from me [staff, your therapist] right now?"

2. **Validate:** "It makes sense that you're having a hard time because it's been a long day."

3. **Comfort/Support Regulation:** "You're letting me know that you need a break right now. Let's go to your comfort zone."

4. **Engage:** "I would really like to help you by tossing the ball [singing, dancing, sitting here quietly, reading a story, etc.] with you."

   ■ *If a child wants to be alone, then honor his or her request as long as safety is not an issue.*

5. **Praise:** Praise the decision to use strategies or go to a calming space.

   ■ *If a child refuses to go to a calming space or use strategies, then try to offer him or her other quiet alternatives.*

   ■ *If that doesn't work then assert the need for safety and use this counting technique:* "I am going to quietly count to 5. If you do not choose to go to the comfort zone/your room [language is optional], then you are going to [insert appropriate consequence here]."

From Margaret E. Blaustein and Kristine M. Kinniburgh (2019, The Guilford Press). Copyright © 2019 by the authors. Permission to photocopy this material is granted to purchasers of this book for personal use or use with clients (see copyright page for details). Purchasers can download additional copies of this material (see the box at the end of the table of contents).

Taking a Break

Name of Student: _____ Date: _____

Procedure: This form should be completed by staff in discussion with student when a **break or time-out** from the group has been earned due to minor misbehaviors, such as being disrespectful or failing to follow directions.

I understand that I earned a break because I was:

_____

_____

I think that I was feeling: Happy   Sad   Mad   Worried   Other _____

(circle all that apply) when I earned a break.

Happy	Sad	Mad	Worried

I earned a break from the group because I was not fully in control of my emotions/behavior. I can learn about how much control I have right now by checking the following:
(Use these questions as a guide to help assess student's experience in the moment.)

_____ Where's my energy level?   Low   Medium   High

_____ How does my body feel?: breathing (fast or slow); heartbeat (fast or slow); muscles (tense like uncooked spaghetti or loose like cooked spaghetti) _____

_____ What am I thinking right now? _____

_____ What am I feeling right now? _____

_____ What are my triggers right now? _____

On a scale from 1 to 5, my self-control is:

1	2	3	4	5
No control	Little control	Not sure	Okay control	Good control

(Give examples of no control and good control: an engine overheating and exploding versus an engine that is running smoothly; a train running off the tracks versus a train running at a comfortable speed for its passengers.)

(continued)

From Margaret E. Blaustein and Kristine M. Kinniburgh (2019). Copyright © 2019 The Guilford Press. Permission to photocopy this material is granted to purchasers of this book for personal use or use with clients (see copyright page for details). Purchasers can download additional copies of this material (see the box at the end of the table of contents).

Staff will know I am in control when I am able to:

_____ Stay in the designated break area until staff gives me permission to leave.

_____ Talk with staff in a safe, respectful way.

_____ Focus on myself, not my peers.

_____ Listen to staff.

_____ Follow staff directions.

_____ Practice a sensory skill of my choice right now *(for at least 1 minute and make note of which skill used).*

_____ Join routines when staff and I agree I am ready.

_____ Other _____

How will I show staff I am ready to join community routines? _____

_____

_____

_____

I would like staff to help me stay on track by *[try to encourage student input here and note any observations you think are important; consider check-ins, reminders, playing a game during quiet time, etc.]:*

_____

_____

_____

When I return to the community, I will do the following in order to help myself stay on track:

_____

_____

_____

Follow up with supervisor/clinician to review student response to this discussion and finalize any decisions regarding repair work, safety agreement, or precaution status.

_____

Staff member/date and time

Processing Form

Name of student: _____

"How Do I Know When I Am in Control
and Ready to Be Part of the Community Again?"

Procedure: This form should be completed by staff in discussion with student when a consequence or time-out has been earned. It should be completed away from the group.

I understand that I earned a consequence/time-out because I was:

_____

_____

_____

This is what happened right before I earned a consequence (*check all that apply*):

_____ Someone said something to me.

_____ I was asked to do something I did not want to do.

_____ Something happened that scared me.

_____ I could not do something that I wanted to do.

_____ I heard bad news.

_____ I was feeling something I did not like.

_____ I was thinking about something I DO LIKE to think about.

_____ My body felt uncomfortable.

_____ I was thinking about something I DO NOT LIKE to think about.

_____ I had an unpleasant memory.

_____ I felt unsafe because _____

_____ Other _____

I think that I was feeling: Happy   Sad   Mad   Worried

   Other _____ *(circle all that apply)* when I earned
   a consequence.

   Happy   Sad   Mad   Worried

(continued)

From Margaret E. Blaustein and Kristine M. Kinniburgh (2019). Copyright © 2019 The Guilford Press. Permission to photocopy this material is granted to purchasers of this book for personal use or use with clients (see copyright page for details). Purchasers can download additional copies of this material (see the box at the end of the table of contents).

Processing Packet: Getting Back On Track

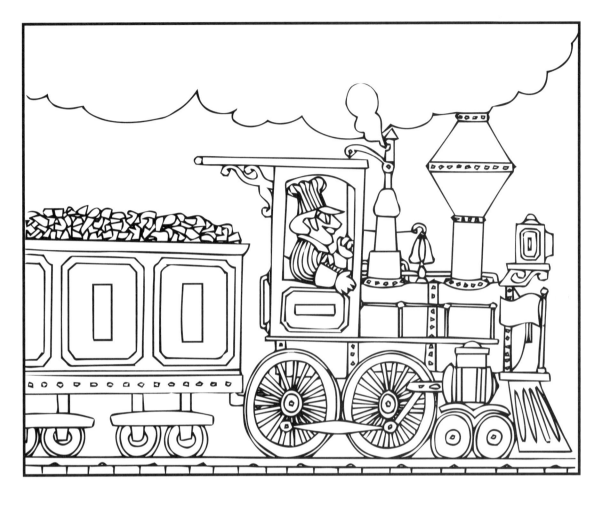

Name: _____

Date: _____

Staff: _____

(continued)

From Margaret E. Blaustein and Kristine M. Kinniburgh (2019, The Guilford Press). Copyright © 2019 by the authors. Permission to photocopy this material is granted to purchasers of this book for personal use or use with clients (see copyright page for details). Purchasers can download additional copies of this material (see the box at the end of the table of contents).

STATION 1: REGULATE: ENERGY CHECK ☑

Low energy   Medium energy   High energy

Comfortable   Uncomfortable

Body scan: Circle the item that best describes your current body clues:

1. Breathing: Fast, medium, or slow

2. Heart rate: Fast, medium, or slow

3. Muscles: Tense or loose

4. Body temperature: Hot, okay, cold

Attune: Please describe your observations of the student's energy and emotion, including any cues that you observed (facial expression, voice tone, etc.):

_____

_____

_____

_____

_____

_____

(continued)

491

STATION 2: REGULATE: PRACTICE A COPING SKILL

Please write down at least one skill that you practiced *with* the student. Here are some ideas of things that you can do together:

Drawing

Playing with a ball

Using a sensory tool

Dancing

Jumping

Singing a song

Listening to a song

Playing cards

Blowing bubbles or taking deep breaths

Writing

Doing puzzle or hidden picture

Playing cards

Attune: Which skill(s) did the student practice?

_____

_____

_____

_____

_____

Please describe your observations of the student's energy and emotions, including any clues that you observed (voice tone, facial expression, posture, etc.):

_____

_____

_____

_____

_____

(continued)

492

STATION 3: REGULATE: ENERGY CHECK ☑

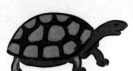 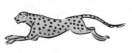

Low energy   Medium energy   High energy

Comfortable   Uncomfortable

Body scan: Circle the item that best describes your current body clues:

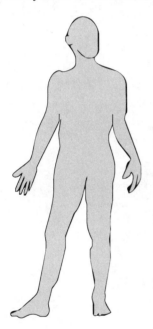

1. Breathing: Fast, medium, or slow

2. Heart rate: Fast, medium, or slow

3. Muscles: Tense or loose

4. Body temperature: Hot, okay, cold

Attune: Please describe your observations of the student's energy and emotion, including any cues that you observed (facial expression, voice tone, etc.):

_____

_____

_____

_____

_____

_____

(continued)

493

STATION 4: REGULATE: THOUGHT HEAD, PART 1

What are all of the things that you are thinking about right now? Some of the things in our head may feel good and other things may be worries that we have. Write down all of the things in your head next to each of the blocks below. You may need just a few boxes because you are not thinking about a lot of things. You may use all the boxes that are there or you may need to add boxes because you have a lot of things on your mind.

After you write your thoughts down, choose a color for each of the boxes below and color them in.

Attune: Please describe your observations of the student's energy and emotion, including any cues that you observed (facial expression, voice tone, etc.):

_____

_____

_____

_____

(continued)

494

STATION 4: REGULATE: THOUGHT HEAD, PART 2

We all have a lot of different things that we are thinking about in our head at the same time. Some things take up a lot of space and energy, and some things take up a little bit of space and energy. How much space does each of the thoughts that you put on the last page take up in your head? If it's a big thought, then color in a big space on the head below. If it's a little thought, then color in a small space on the head below.

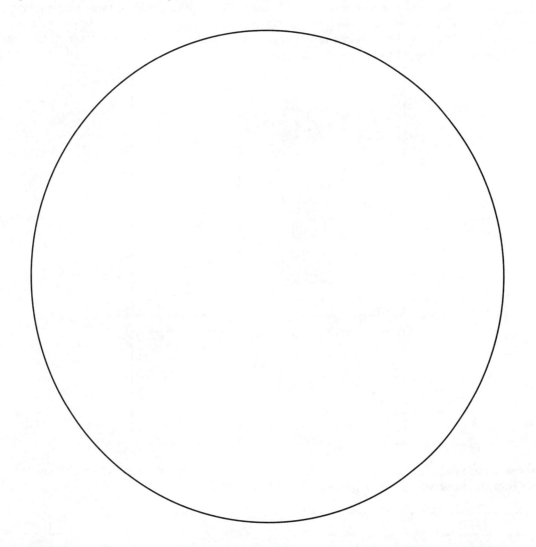

Attune: Please describe your observations of the student's energy and emotion, including any cues that you observed (facial expression, voice tone, etc.):

_____

_____

_____

_____

(continued)

STATION 5: REGULATE: FEELINGS BUBBLE, PART 1

What are all of the different emotions that you are feeling right now after talking about what happened? Some emotions may feel good, some bad, and some may be confusing. They are not right or wrong. You may be feeling a few things or a lot of things. Write all of the emotions that you are feeling next to a box below. Pick a color for each box and color it in.

Attune: Please describe your observations of the student's energy and emotion including any cues that you observed (facial expression, voice tone, etc.):

_____

_____

_____

_____

_____

_____

_____

_____

(continued)

STATION 5: REGULATE: FEELINGS BUBBLE, PART 2

We all have different emotions that we feel sometimes. Some emotions take up a lot of space and energy; other emotions take up a little bit of space and energy. If you are having a big feeling, then color in a big space in the bubble below. If you are having a small feeling, then color in a small space in the bubble below.

Attune: Please describe your observations of the student's energy and emotion, including any cues that you observed (facial expression, voice tone, etc.):

_____

_____

_____

_____

(continued)

STATION 6: PLAN OR PROBLEM-SOLVE:
WHAT CAN I DO TO GET BACK ON TRACK?!

What can I do the next time that this happens to feel more comfortable?

_____

_____

_____

How will staff know you are back on track?

List three positive behaviors that you have
when you are on track.

1. _____

_____

2. _____

_____

3. _____

_____

List three coping skills that you can use when your buttons are pushed
or when you start to feel uncomfortable.

1. _____

_____

2. _____

_____

3. _____

_____

(continued)

STATION 7: REGULATE: PRACTICE A COPING SKILL

Please write down at least one skill that you practiced *with* the student. Here are some ideas of things that you can do together:

Drawing

Playing with a ball

Using a sensory tool

Dancing

Jumping

Singing a song

Listening to a song

Playing cards

Blowing bubbles or taking deep breaths

Writing

Doing puzzle or hidden picture

Playing cards

Attune: Which skill(s) did the student practice?

_____

_____

_____

_____

_____

Please describe your observations of the student's energy and emotions, including any clues that you observed (voice tone, facial expression, posture, etc.):

_____

_____

_____

_____

_____

(continued)

STATION 8: REGULATE: FINAL ENERGY

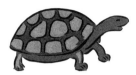 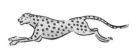

Low energy   Medium energy   High energy

Comfortable   Uncomfortable

Body scan: Circle the item that best describes your current body clues:

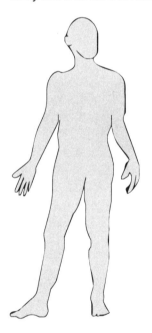

1. Breathing: Fast, medium, or slow

2. Heart rate: Fast, medium, or slow

3. Muscles: Tense or loose

4. Body temperature: Hot, okay, cold

Attune: Please describe your observations of the student's energy and emotion, including any cues that you observed (facial expression, voice tone, etc.):

_____

_____

_____

_____

_____

_____

(continued)

STAFF COMMENTS AND OBSERVATIONS

_____
_____
_____
_____
_____
_____
_____
_____
_____
_____
_____
_____
_____
_____
_____
_____
_____
_____
_____
_____
_____
_____
_____
_____
_____
_____
_____
_____
_____
_____

Program-to-Caregiver Behavior Communication Form

Target/behavior we are addressing: _____

_____

_____

Possible triggers (what makes the behavior more likely to happen?): _____

_____

_____

_____

_____

Possible function/child need (behaviors happen for a reason; why do we think your child may be showing this behavior?):

    Surface reason(s) (what are the immediate triggers?): _____

    _____

    _____

    Hidden reason(s) (what else might be leading to this behavior?): _____

    _____

    _____

Helpful adult responses (what decreases the behavior and/or helps your child reregulate/feel safe again?): _____

_____

_____

_____

Less helpful adult responses (what makes things worse?): _____

_____

_____

_____

What structures/routines/interventions have we used in the program that seem helpful?: _____

_____

_____

_____

Other information we would like to communicate: _____

_____

_____

From Margaret E. Blaustein and Kristine M. Kinniburgh (2019, The Guilford Press). Copyright © 2019 by the authors. Permission to photocopy this material is granted to purchasers of this book for personal use or use with clients (see copyright page for details). Purchasers can download additional copies of this material (see the box at the end of the table of contents).

Caregiver-to-Program Behavior Communication Form

Target/behavior we are addressing: _____

_____

_____

Possible triggers (what makes the behavior more likely to happen?): _____

_____

_____

_____

_____

Possible function/child need (behaviors happen for a reason; why do I think my child may be showing this behavior?):

    Surface reason(s) (what are the immediate triggers?): _____

    _____

    _____

    Hidden reason(s) (what else might be leading to this behavior?): _____

    _____

    _____

Helpful adult responses (what decreases the behavior and/or helps my child reregulate/feel safe again?): _____

_____

_____

_____

Less helpful adult responses (what makes things worse?): _____

_____

_____

_____

What structures/routines/interventions have we used at home or in other settings that seem helpful?: _____

_____

_____

_____

Other information I would like to communicate: _____

_____

_____

From Margaret E. Blaustein and Kristine M. Kinniburgh (2019, The Guilford Press). Copyright © 2019 by the authors. Permission to photocopy this material is granted to purchasers of this book for personal use or use with clients (see copyright page for details). Purchasers can download additional copies of this material (see the box at the end of the table of contents).

References

Abitz, M., Nielsen, R. D., Jones, E. G., Laursen, H., Graem, N., & Pakkenberg, B. (2007). Excess of neurons in the human newborn mediodorsal thalamus compared with that of the adult. *Cerebral Cortex, 17*(11), 2573–2578.

Ainsworth, M. D. S., & Bowlby, J. (1991). An ethological approach to personality development. *American Psychologist, 46,* 331–341.

Alink, L., Cicchetti, D., Kim, J., & Rogosch, F. (2009). Mediating and moderating processes in the relation between maltreatment and psychopathology: Mother–child relationship quality and emotion regulation. *Journal of Abnormal Child Psychology, 37*(6), 831–843.

American Psychiatric Association. (2013). *Diagnostic and statistical manual of mental disorders* (5th ed.). Arlington, VA: Author.

Anda, R. F., Croft, J. B., Felitti, V. J., Nordenberg, D., Giles, W. H., Williamson, D. F., et al. (1999). Adverse childhood experiences and smoking during adolescence and adulthood. *Journal of the American Medical Association, 282*(17), 1652–1658.

Anda, R. F., Felitti, V. J., Bremner, J. D., Walker, J. D., Whitfield, C., Perry, B. D., et al. (2006). The enduring effects of abuse and related adverse experiences in childhood: A convergence of evidence from neurobiology and epidemiology. *European Archives of Psychiatry and Clinical Neuroscience, 256*(3), 174–186.

Anthonysamy, A., & Zimmer-Gembeck, M. (2007). Peer status and behaviors of maltreated children and their classmates in the early years of school. *Child Abuse and Neglect, 31*(9), 971–991.

Appleyard, K., Egeland, B., van Dulmen, M., & Sroufe, A. (2005). When more is not better: The role of cumulative risk in child behavior outcomes. *Journal of Child Psychology and Psychiatry, 46*(3), 235–245.

Auslander, W., Tlapek, S. M., Threlfall, J., Edmond, T., & Dunn, J. (2015). Mental health pathways linking childhood maltreatment to interpersonal revictimization during adolescence for girls in the child welfare system. *Journal of Interpersonal Violence, 33*(7), 1169–1191.

Ballard, E. D., Van Eck, K., Musci, R. J., Hart, S. R., Storr, C. L., Breslau, N., et al. (2015). Latent classes of childhood trauma exposure predict the development of behavioral health outcomes in adolescence and young adulthood. *Psychological Medicine, 45*(15), 3305–3316.

Barnes, J., Noll, J., Putnam, F., & Trickett, P. (2009). Sexual and physical revictimization among victims of severe childhood sexual abuse. *Child Abuse and Neglect, 33,* 412–420.

Beers, S., & De Bellis, M. D. (2002). Neuropsychological function in children with maltreatment-related posttraumatic stress disorder. *American Journal of Psychiatry, 159,* 483–486.

Benoit, D., & Parker, K. (1994). Stability and transmission of attachment across three generations. *Child Development, 65*(5), 1444–1456.

Blaustein, M., & Kinniburgh, K. (2007). Intervening beyond the child: The intertwining nature of attachment and trauma. *British Psychological Society, Briefing Paper, 26,* 48–53.

Bolger, K. E., Patterson, C. J., & Kupersmidt, J. B. (1998). Peer relationships and self-esteem among children who have been maltreated. *Child Development, 69*(4), 1171–1197.

Bowlby, J. (1958). The nature of the child's tie to his mother. *International Journal of PsychoAnalysis, 39,* 1–23.

Bremner, J. D. (1999). Does stress damage the brain? *Biological Psychiatry, 45,* 797–805.

Bremner, J. D., Randall, P., Scott, T. M., Capelli, S., Delaney, R., McCarthy, G., et al. (1995). Deficits in short-term memory in adult survivors of childhood abuse. *Psychiatry Research, 59,* 97–107.

Breslau, N. (2001). The epidemiology of posttraumatic stress disorder: What is the extent of the problem? *Journal of Clinical Psychiatry, 62*(17, Suppl.), 16–22.

Briere, J., & Scott, C. (2015). Complex trauma in adolescents and adults: Effects and treatment. *Psychiatric Clinics of North America, 38*(3), 515–527.

Brock, K., Pearlman, L. A., & Varra, E. (2006). Child maltreatment, self capacities and trauma symptoms: Psychometric properties of the Inner Experience Questionnaire. *Journal of Emotional Abuse, 6*(1), 103–125.

Campbell-Sills, L., Cohan, S., & Stein, M. (2006). Relationship of resilience to personality, coping, and psychiatric symptoms in young adults. *Behaviour Research and Therapy, 44,* 585–599.

Carrion, V. G., & Wong, S. S. (2012). Can traumatic stress alter the brain?: Understanding the implications of early trauma on brain development and learning. *Journal of Adolescent Health, 51*(2), S23–S28.

Centers for Disease Control and Prevention. (2005). Adverse Childhood Experience study: Prevalence of individual adverse childhood experiences. Retrieved July 10, 2008, from *www.cdc.gov/nccdphp/ACE/ prevalence.htm.*

Chandy, J. M., Blum, R. W., & Resnick, M. D. (1996). Female adolescents with a history of sexual abuse: Risk outcome and protective factors. *Journal of Interpersonal Violence, 11*(4), 503–518.

Choi, J. Y., Choi, Y. M., Gim, M. S., Park, J. H., & Park, S. H. (2014). The effects of childhood abuse on symptom complexity in a clinical sample: Mediating effects of emotion regulation difficulties. *Child Abuse and Neglect, 38*(8), 1313–1319.

Cicchetti, D., & Curtis, W. J. (2007). Multilevel perspectives on pathways to resilient functioning. *Development and Psychopathology, 19*(3), 627–629.

Cicchetti, D., & Rogosch, F. A. (2009). Adaptive coping under conditions of extreme stress: Multilevel influences on the determinants of resilience in maltreated children. *New Directions in Child and Adolescent Development, 124,* 47–59.

Cicchetti, D., Rogosch, F. A., Lynch, M., & Holt, K. D. (1993). Resilience in maltreated children: Processes leading to adaptive outcome. *Development and Psychopathology, 5,* 629–647.

Cicchetti, D., Rogosch, F. A., & Toth, S. L. (2006). Fostering secure attachment in infants in maltreating families through preventive interventions. *Development and Psychopathology, 18*(3), 623–649.

Cicchetti, D., & Toth, S. (1995). A developmental psychopathology perspective on child abuse and neglect. *Journal of the American Academy of Child and Adolescent Psychiatry, 34*(5), 541–565.

Cicchetti, D., & Toth, S. (2005). Child maltreatment. *Annual Review of Clinical Psychology, 1*(1), 409–438.

Cicchetti, D., & Toth, S. L. (2015). Multilevel developmental perspectives on child maltreatment. *Development and Psychopathology, 27*(4, Pt. 2), 1385–1386.

Cohen, J. A., & Mannarino, A. P. (2000). Predictors of treatment outcome in sexually abused children. *Child Abuse and Neglect, 24,* 983–994.

Cook, A., Spinazzola, J., Ford, J. D., Lanktree, C., Blaustein, M., Cloitre, M., et al. (2005). Complex trauma in children and adolescents. *Psychiatric Annals, 35*(5), 390–398.

Coster, W., Gersten, M., Beeghly, M., & Cicchetti, D. (1989). Communicative functioning in maltreated toddlers. *Developmental Psychology, 25*(6), 1020–1029.

Crittenden, P. M. (1995). Attachment and psychopathology. In S. Goldberg, R. Muir, & J. Kerr (Eds.), *Attachment theory: Social, developmental, and clinical perspectives* (pp. 367–406). New York: Analytic Press.

Crittenden, P. M., & DiLalla, D. L. (1988). Compulsive compliance: The development of an inhibitory coping strategy in infancy. *Journal of Abnormal Child Psychology, 16,* 585–599.

de Bellis, M. D. (2001). Developmental traumatology: The psychobiological development of maltreated children and its implications for research, treatment, and policy. *Development and Psychopathology, 13,* 539–564.

Dexheimer Pharris, M., Resnick, M. D., & Blum, R. W. (1997). Protecting against hopelessness and suicidality in sexually abused American Indian adolescents. *Journal of Adolescent Health, 21*(6), 400–406.

Dinero, R., Conger, R., Shaver, P., Widaman, K., & Larsen-Rife, D. (2008). Influence of family-of-origin and adult romantic partners on adult romantic attachment security. *Journal of Family Psychology, 22*(4), 622–632.

Dvir, Y., Ford, J. D., Hill, M., & Frazier, J. A. (2014). Childhood maltreatment, emotional dysregulation, and psychiatric comorbidities. *Harvard Review of Psychiatry, 22*(3), 149.

D'Zurilla, T., & Goldfried, M. (1971). Problem solving and behavior modification. *Journal of Abnormal Psychology, 78,* 107–126.

D'Zurilla, T., & Nezu, A. (2007). *Problem-solving therapy: A positive approach to clinical intervention* (3rd ed.). New York: Springer.

Egeland, B., Sroufe, A., & Erickson, M. F. (1983). The developmental consequences of different patterns of maltreatment. *Child Abuse and Neglect, 7,* 459–469.

Erickson, M. F., Sroufe, L. A., & Egeland, B. (1985). The relationship between quality of attachment and behavior problems in preschool in a high-risk sample. *Monographs of the Society for Research in Child Development, 50*(1–2, Serial No. 209), 147–166.

Felitti, V. J., Anda, R. F., Nordenberg, D. F., Williamson, D. F., Spitz, A. M., Edwards, V., et al. (1998). Relationship of childhood abuse and household dysfunction to many of the leading causes of death in adults: The Adverse Childhood Experiences (ACE) study. *American Journal of Preventative Medicine, 14*(4), 245–258.

Flores, E., Cicchetti, D., & Rogosch, F. (2005). Predictors of resilience in maltreated and nonmaltreated Latino children. *Developmental Psychology, 41,* 338–351.

Ford, J. (2005). Treatment implications of altered affect regulation and information processing following child maltreatment. *Psychiatric Annals, 35*(5), 410–419.

Ford, J., Racusin, R., Daviss, W. B., Ellis, C. G., Thomas, J., Rogers, K., et al. (1999). Trauma exposure among children with oppositional defiant disorder and attention deficit-hyperactivity disorder. *Journal of Consulting and Clinical Psychology, 67,* 786–789.

Ford, J., Stockton, P., Kaltman, S., & Green, B. (2006). Disorders of extreme stress (DESNOS) symptoms are associated with type and severity of interpersonal trauma exposure in a sample of healthy young women. *Journal of Interpersonal Violence, 21*(11), 1399–1416.

Fortier, M., DiLillo, D., Messman-Moore, T., Peugh, J., DeNardi, K., & Gaffey, K. (2009). Severity of child sexual abuse and revictimization: The mediating role of coping and trauma symptoms. *Psychology of Women Quarterly, 33,* 308–320.

Gil, E. (1991). *The healing power of play: Working with abused children.* New York: Guilford Press.

Greene, R., & Ablon, S. (2005). *Treating explosive kids: The collaborative problem-solving approach.* New York: Guilford Press.

Guber, T., Kalish, L., & Fatus, S. (2005). *Yoga pretzels.* Cambridge, MA: Barefoot Books.

Haggerty, R., Sherrod, L., Garmezy, N., & Rutter, M. (1996). *Stress, risk, and resilience in children and adolescents: Processes, mechanisms, and interventions.* New York: Cambridge University Press.

Haugaard, J. (2004). Recognizing and treating uncommon behavioral and emotional disorders in children and adolescents who have been severely maltreated: Dissociative disorders. *Child Maltreatment, 9,* 146–153.

Hebert, M., Parent, N., Daignault, I., & Tourigny, M. (2006). A typological analysis of behavioral profiles of sexually abused children. *Child Maltreatment, 11*(3), 203–216.

Ingoldsby, E. (2010). Review of interventions to improve family engagement and retention in parent and child mental health programs. *Journal of Child and Family Studies, 19,* 629–645.

Jaffee, S., Caspi, A., Moffitt, T., Polo-Tomás, M., & Taylor, A. (2007). Individual, family, and neighborhood factors distinguish resilient from non-resilient maltreated children: A cumulative stressors model. *Child Abuse and Neglect, 31,* 231–253.

Kazdin, A. (1985). *Treatment of antisocial behavior in children and adolescents.* Homewood, IL: Dorsey Press.

Kazdin, A., Esveldt-Dawson, K., French, N., & Unis, A. (1987). Problem-solving skills training and relationship therapy in the treatment of antisocial child behavior. *Journal of Consulting and Clinical Psychology, 55,* 76–85.

Kazdin, A., Siegel, T., & Bass, D. (1992). Cognitive problem-solving skills training and parent management training in the treatment of antisocial behavior in children. *Journal of Consulting and Clinical Psychology, 60,* 733–747.

Kelly, J. F., Morisset, C. E., Barnard, K. E., Hammond, M. A., & Booth, C. L. (1996). The influence of early mother–child interaction on preschool cognitive/linguistic outcomes in a high-social-risk group. *Infant Mental Health Journal, 17,* 310–321.

Kilpatrick, D., Ruggiero, K., Acierno, R., Saunders, B., Resnick, H., & Best, C. (2003). Violence and risk of PTSD, major depression, substance abuse/dependence, and comorbidity: Results from the National Survey of Adolescents. *Journal of Consulting and Clinical Psychology, 71*(4), 692–700.

Kim, J., & Cicchetti, D. (2003). Social self-efficacy and behavior problems in maltreated children. *Journal of Clinical Child and Adolescent Psychology, 32*(1), 106–117.

Kim, J., & Cicchetti, D. (2004). A longitudinal study of child maltreatment, mother–child relationship quality and maladjustment: The role of self-esteem and social competence. *Journal of Abnormal Child Psychology, 32*(4), 341–354.

Kim, J., & Cicchetti, D. (2006). Longitudinal trajectories of self-system processes and depressive symptoms among maltreated and nonmaltreated children. *Child Development, 77*(3), 624–639.

Kim, J., & Cicchetti, D. (2010). Longitudinal pathways linking child maltreatment, emotion regulation, peer relations, and psychopathology. *Journal of Child Psychology and Psychiatry, 51*(6), 706–716.

Kinniburgh, K., & Blaustein, M. (2005). *Attachment, self-regulation, and competency: A comprehensive framework for intervention with complexly traumatized youth—a treatment manual.* Unpublished manuscript.

Kinniburgh, K., Blaustein, M., Spinazzola, J., & van der Kolk, B. (2005). Attachment, self-regulation, and competency: A comprehensive intervention framework for children with complex trauma. *Psychiatric Annals, 35*(5), 424–430.

Lanius, R. A., Vermetten, E., Loewenstein, R. J., Brand, B., Schmahl, C., Bremner, J. D., et al. (2010). Emotion modulation in PTSD: Clinical and neurobiological evidence for a dissociative subtype. *American Journal of Psychiatry, 167*(6), 640–647.

Lansford, J. E., Dodge, K. A., Pettit, G. S., Crozier, J., & Kaplow, J. (2002). A 12-year prospective study of the long-term effects of early child physical maltreatment on psychological, behavioral, and academic problems in adolescence. *Archives of Pediatrics and Adolescent Medicine, 156,* 824–830.

Layne, C. M., Greeson, J. K., Ostrowski, S. A., Kim, S., Reading, S., Vivrette, R. L., et al. (2014). Cumulative trauma exposure and high risk behavior in adolescence: Findings from the National Child Traumatic Stress Network Core Data Set. *Psychological Trauma: Theory, Research, Practice, and Policy, 6*(Suppl. 1), S40.

Lieberman, A. F., & van Horn, P. (2008). *Psychotherapy with infants and young children: Repairing the effects of stress and trauma on early attachment.* New York: Guilford Press.

Liem, J., & Boudewyn, A. (1999). Contextualizing the effects of childhood sexual abuse on adult self- and social functioning: An attachment theory perspective. *Child Abuse and Neglect, 23,* 1141–1157.

Linehan, M. M. (1993). *Skills training manual for treating borderline personality disorder.* New York: Guilford Press.

Lipschitz-Elhawi, R., & Itzhaky, H. (2005). Social support, mastery, self-esteem and individual adjustment among at-risk youth. *Child and Youth Care Forum, 34*(5), 329–346.

Lynch, M., & Cicchetti, D. (1991). Patterns of relatedness in maltreated and nonmaltreated children: Connections among multiple representational models. *Development and Psychopathology, 3,* 207–226.

Lyons-Ruth, K., Dutra, L., Schuder, M., & Bianchi, I. (2006). From infant attachment disorganization to adult dissociation: Relational adaptations or traumatic experiences? *Psychiatric Clinics of North America, 29,* 63–86.

Lyons-Ruth, K., Yellin, C., Melnick, S., & Atwood, G. (2005). Expanding the concept of unresolved mental states: Hostile/helpless states of mind on the Adult Attachment Interview are associated with disrupted mother–infant communication and infant disorganization. *Development and Psychopathology, 17*(1), 1–23.

Main, M., & Cassidy, J. (1988). Categories of response to reunion with the parent at age 6: Predicted from infant attachment classifications and stable over a 1-month period. *Developmental Psychology, 24,* 415–426.

Main, M., & Goldwyn, R. (1984). Predicting rejection of her infant from mother's representation of her own experience: Implications for the abused–abusing intergenerational cycle. *Child Abuse and Neglect, 8,* 203–217.

Masten, A. S. (2001). Ordinary magic: Resilience processes in development. *American Psychologist, 56,* 227–238.

Masten, A. S., Best, K. M., & Garmezy, N. (1990). Resilience and development: Contributions from the study of children who overcome adversity. *Development and Psychopathology, 2*(4), 425–444.

Masten, A. S., & Coatsworth, J. D. (1998). The development in competence in favorable and unfavorable environments. *American Psychologist, 53*(2), 205–220.

Masten, A. S., & Labella, M. H. (2016). Risk and resilience in child development. In L. Balter & C. S. Tamis-LeMonda (Eds.), *Child psychology: A handbook of contemporary issues* (pp. 423–450). New York: Routledge.

Matthews, W. (1999). Brief therapy: A problem-solving model of change. *The Counselor, 17*(4), 29–32.

McCann, I. L., & Pearlman, L. A. (1990). Vicarious traumatization: A framework for understanding the psychological effects of working with victims. *Journal of Traumatic Stress, 3,* 131–149.

McElwain, N., Cox, M., Burchinal, M., & Macfie, J. (2003). Differentiating among insecure mother–infant attachment classifications: A focus on child–friend interaction and exploration during solitary play at 36 months. *Attachment and Human Development, 5*(2), 136–164.

Mendez, J., Fantuzzo, J., & Cicchetti, D. (2002). Profiles of social competence among low-income African American preschool children. *Child Development, 73,* 1085–1100.

Mezzacappa, E., Kindlon, D., & Earls, F. (2001). Child abuse and performance task assessments of executive functions in boys. *Journal of Child Psychology and Psychiatry, 42*(8), 1041–1048.

Miller, A. L., Rathus, J. H., & Linehan, M. M. (2006). *Dialectical behavior therapy with suicidal adolescents.* New York: Guilford Press.

Min, M., Farkas, K., Minnes, S., & Singer, L. (2007). Impact of childhood abuse and neglect on substance abuse and psychological distress in adulthood. *Journal of Traumatic Stress, 20,* 833–844.

Mischel, W., Shoda, Y., & Rodriguez, M. L. (1989). Delay of gratification in children. *Science, 244,* 933–938.

Naughton, A. M., Maguire, S. A., Mann, M. K., Lumb, R. C., Tempest, V., Gracias, S., et al. (2013). Emotional, behavioral, and developmental features indicative of neglect or emotional abuse in preschool children: A systematic review. *JAMA Pediatrics, 167*(8), 769–775.

Navalta, C., Polcari, A., Webster, D., Boghossian, A., & Teicher, M. (2006). Effects of childhood sexual abuse on neuropsychological and cognitive function in college women. *Journal of Neuropsychiatry and Clinical Neurosciences, 18,* 45–53.

Nikulina, V., & Widom, C. S. (2013). Child maltreatment and executive functioning in middle adulthood: A prospective examination. *Neuropsychology, 27*(4), 417.

Noll, J. G., Shenk, C. E., Barnes, J. E., & Haralson, K. J. (2013). Association of maltreatment with high-risk internet behaviors and offline encounters. *Pediatrics, 131*(2), e510–e517.

Noll, J. G., Trickett, P., Harris, W., & Putnam, F. (2009). The cumulative burden borne by offspring whose mothers were sexually abused as children: Descriptive results from a multigenerational study. *Journal of Interpersonal Violence, 24*(3), 424–449.

Ogawa, J., Sroufe, A., Weinfield, N., Carlson, E., & Egeland, B. (1997). Development and the fragmented self: Longitudinal study of dissociative symptomatology in a nonclinical sample. *Development and Psychopathology, 9*(4), 855–879.

Ostby, Y., Tamnes, C. K., Fjell, A. M., Westlye, L. T., Due-Tonnessen, P., & Walhovd, K. B. (2009). Heterogeneity in subcortical brain development: A structural magnetic resonance imaging study of brain maturation from 8 to 30 years. *Journal of Neuroscience, 29,* 11772–11782.

Pearlman, L., & Saakvitne, K. (1995). *Trauma and the therapist: Counter-transference and vicarious traumatisation in psychotherapy with incest survivors.* New York: Norton.

Perry, B. D., Pollard, R. A., Blakley, T. L., Baker, W. L., & Vigilante, D. (1995). Childhood trauma, the neurobiology of adaptation, and "use-dependent" development of the brain: How "states" become "traits." *Infant Mental Health Journal, 16*(4), 271–291.

Philip, N. S., Sweet, L. H., Tyrka, A. R., Carpenter, S. L., Albright, S. E., Price, L. H., et al. (2016). Exposure to childhood trauma is associated with altered *n*-back activation and performance in healthy adults: Implications for a commonly used working memory task. *Brain Imaging and Behavior, 10*(1), 124.

Piaget, J. (1952). *The origins of intelligence in children* (M. Cook, Trans.). New York: Norton.

Piaget, J. (2003). Part I: Cognitive development in children—development and learning. *Journal of Research in Science Teaching, 40*(Suppl.), S8–S18.

Piaget, J. (2008). Intellectual evolution from adolescence to adulthood. *Human Development, 51*(1), 40–47.

Piaget, J., Garcia, R., Davidson, P. M., & Easley, J. (1991). *Toward a logic of meanings.* Hillsdale, NJ: Erlbaum.

Piaget, J., & Inhelder, R. (1991). The construction of reality. In J. Oates & R. Sheldon (Eds.), *Cognitive development in infancy* (pp. 165–169). East Sussex, UK: Erlbaum.

Putnam, F. W. (1997). *Dissociation in children and adolescents: A developmental perspective.* New York: Guilford Press.

Pynoos, R., Steinberg, A., & Wraith, R. (1995). A developmental model of childhood traumatic stress. In D. Cicchetti & D. Cohen (Eds.), *Manual of developmental psychopathology: Vol. 2. Risk, disorder, and adaptation* (pp. 72–95). New York: Wiley.

Resnick, M., Bearman, P., Blum, R. W., Bauman, K., Harris, K., Jones, J., et al. (1997). Protecting adolescents from harm: Findings from the National Longitudinal Study on Adolescent Health. *Journal of the American Medical Association, 278,* 823–832.

Reviere, S., & Bakeman, R. (2001). The effects of early trauma on autobiographical memory and schematic self-representation. *Applied Cognitive Psychology, 15*(7), S89–S100.

Rogers, C. (1951). *Client-centered therapy: Its current practice, implications, and theory.* Boston: Houghton Mifflin.

Rothbart, M. K., Ahadi, S. A., & Evans, D. E. (2000). Temperament and personality: Origins and outcomes. *Journal of Personality and Social Psychology, 78,* 122–135.

Runyon, M., & Kenny, M. (2002). Relationship of attributional style, depression, and posttrauma distress among children who suffered physical or sexual abuse. *Child Maltreatment, 7,* 254–264.

Saakvitne, K., Gamble, S., Pearlman, L., & Lev, B. (2000). *Risking connection: A training curriculum for working with survivors of child abuse.* Baltimore: Sidran Institute Press.

Scheeringa, M. S., & Zeanah, C. H. (2001). A relational perspective on PTSD in early childhood. *Journal of Traumatic Stress, 14,* 799–815.

Schimmenti, A., & Caretti, V. (2016). Linking the overwhelming with the unbearable: Developmental trauma, dissociation, and the disconnected self. *Psychoanalytic Psychology, 33*(1), 106.

Schore, A. (2001a). The effects of early relational trauma on right brain development, affect regulation, and infant mental health development. *Infant Mental Health Journal, 22,* 201–269.

Schore, A. (2001b). Effects of a secure attachment on right brain development, affect regulation, and infant mental health. *Infant Mental Health Journal, 22,* 7–66.

Schore, A. (2013). Relational trauma, brain development, and dissociation. In In J. D. Ford & C. A. Courtois (Ed.), *Treating complex traumatic stress disorders in children: An evidence-based guide*. New York: Guilford Press.

Schore, A. N. (2014). Dysregulation of the right brain: A fundamental mechanism of traumatic attachment and the psychopathogenesis of PTSD. In G. Leo (Ed.), *Neuroscience and psychoanalysis*. Lecce, Italy: Frenis Zero Press.

Schuder, M., & Lyons-Ruth, K. (2004). "Hidden trauma" in infancy: Attachment, fearful arousal, and early dysfunction on the stress response system. In J. Osofsky (Ed.), *Trauma in infancy and early childhood* (pp. 69–104). New York: Guilford Press.

Shields, A., Ryan, R., & Cicchetti, D. (2001). Narrative representations of caregivers and emotion dysregulation as predictors of maltreated children's rejection by peers. *Developmental Psychology, 37,* 321–337.

Shoda, Y., Mischel, W., & Peake, P. K. (1990). Predicting adolescent cognitive and self-regulatory competencies from preschool delay of gratification: Identifying diagnostic conditions. *Developmental Psychology, 26*(6), 978–986.

Shonk, S. M., & Cicchetti, D. (2001). Maltreatment, competency deficits, and risk for academic and behavioral maladjustment. *Developmental Psychology, 37,* 3–17.

Simpson, J. A., Collins, W. A., Tran, S., & Haydon, K. C. (2007). Attachment and the experience and expression of emotions in romantic relationships: A developmental perspective. *Journal of Personality and Social Psychology, 92,* 355–367.

Smith, J., & Prior, M. (1995). Temperament and stress resilience in school-age children: A within-families study. *Journal of the American Academy of Child and Adolescent Psychiatry, 34,* 168–179.

Solomon, S. D., & Davidson, J. R. T. (1997). Trauma: Prevalence, impairment, service use, and cost. *Journal of Clinical Psychiatry, 58*(Suppl. 9), 5–11.

Spinazzola, J., Blaustein, M., & van der Kolk, B. (2005). Posttraumatic stress disorder treatment outcome research: The study of unrepresentative samples. *Journal of Traumatic Stress, 18*(5), 425–436.

Spinazzola, J., Hodgdon, H., Liang, L. J., Ford, J. D., Layne, C. M., Pynoos, R., et al. (2014). Unseen wounds: The contribution of psychological maltreatment to child and adolescent mental health and risk outcomes. *Psychological Trauma: Theory, Research, Practice, and Policy, 6*(Suppl. 1), S18.

Spiraling Hearts. (n.d.). Yoga bingo. Available at *www.spiralinghearts.com*.

Stamm, B. H. (Ed.). (1999). *Secondary traumatic stress: Self-care issues for clinicians, researchers, and educators* (2nd ed.). Baltimore: Sidran Institute Press.

Strand, V., Hansen, S. & Courtney, D. (2013). Common elements across evidence-based trauma treatment: Discovery and implications. *Advances in Social Work, 14*(2), 334–354.

Streeck-Fischer, A., & van der Kolk, B. (2000). Down will come baby, cradle and all: Diagnostic and therapeutic implications of chronic trauma on child development. *Australian and New Zealand Journal of Psychiatry, 34,* 903–918.

Stronach, E. P., Toth, S. L., Rogosch, F., & Cicchetti, D. (2013). Preventive interventions and sustained attachment security in maltreated children. *Development and Psychopathology, 25*(4, Pt. 1), 919–930.

Tamnes, C. K., Ostby, Y., Fjell, A. M., Westlye, L. T., Due-Tonnessen, P., & Walhovd, K. B. (2010). Brain maturation in adolescence and young adulthood: Regional age-related changes in cortical thickness and white matter volume and microstructure. *Cerebral Cortex, 20*(3), 534–548.

Tarren-Sweeney, M. (2013). An investigation of complex attachment and trauma-related symptomatology among children in foster and kinship care. *Child Psychiatry and Human Development, 44*(6), 727–741.

Terr, L. (1990). *Too scared to cry: Psychic trauma in childhood*. New York: HarperCollins.

Toth, S., & Cicchetti, D. (1996). Patterns of relatedness, depressive symptomatology, and perceived competence in maltreated children. *Journal of Consulting and Clinical Psychology, 64*(1), 32–41.

Tronick, E. (2007). *The neurobehavioral and social–emotional development of infants and children*. New York: Norton.

Urban, J., Carlson, E., Egeland, B., & Sroufe, A. (1991). Patterns of individual adaptation across childhood. *Development and Psychopathology, 3,* 445–460.

van der Kolk, B. (2005). Developmental trauma disorder: Toward a rational diagnosis for children with complex trauma histories. *Psychiatric Annals, 35*(5), 401–408.

van der Kolk, B. A. (2015). *The body keeps the score: Brain, mind, and body in the healing of trauma.* New York: Penguin Books.

van der Kolk, B. A., & d'Andrea, W. (2010). Towards a developmental trauma disorder diagnosis for childhood interpersonal trauma. In R. A. Lanius, E. Vermetten, & C. Pain (Eds.), *The impact of early life trauma on health and disease: The hidden epidemic* (pp. 57–68). Cambridge, UK: Cambridge University Press

van der Kolk, B., Roth, S., Pelcovitz, D., & Mandel, F. S. (1994). *Disorders of extreme stress: Results from the DSM-IV field trial for PTSD.* Unpublished manuscript.

van IJzendoorn, M. H. (1995). Adult attachment representations, parental responsiveness, and infant attachment: A meta-analysis on the predictive validity of the Adult Attachment Interview. *Psychological Bulletin, 117,* 387–403.

Verhage, M. L., Schuengel, C., Madigan, S., Fearon, R. M., Oosterman, M., Cassibba, R., et al. (2016). Narrowing the transmission gap: A synthesis of three decades of research on intergenerational transmission of attachment. *Psychological Bulletin, 142*(4), 337–366.

Vondra, J., Barnett, D., & Cicchetti, D. (1989). Perceived and actual competence among maltreated and comparison school children. *Development and Psychopathology, 1,* 237–255.

Vondra, J., Barnett, D., & Cicchetti, D. (1990). Self-concept, motivation, and competence among preschoolers from maltreating and comparison families. *Child Abuse and Neglect, 14,* 525–540.

Wakschlag, L., & Hans, S. (1999). Relation of maternal responsiveness during infancy to the development of behavior problems in high-risk youths. *Developmental Psychology, 35,* 569–579.

Werker, J. F., & Tees, R. C. (1984). Cross-language speech perception: Evidence for perceptual reorganization during the first year of life. *Infant Behavior and Development, 7,* 49–63.

Werner, E. E., & Smith, R. S. (1980). An epidemiologic perspective on some antecedents and consequences of childhood mental health problems and learning disabilities. *Annual Progress in Child Psychiatry and Child Development,* pp. 133–147.

Werner, E. E., & Smith, R. S. (2001). *Journeys from childhood to midlife: Risk, resilience, and recovery.* Ithaca, NY: Cornell University Press.

Wolff, A., & Ratner, P. (1999). Stress, social support, and sense of coherence. *Western Journal of Nursing Research, 21*(2), 182–197.

Wyman, P. A., Cowen, E. L., Work, W. C., Hoyt-Meyers, L., Magnus, K. B., & Fagen, D. B. (1999). Caregiving and developmental factors differentiating young at-risk urban children showing resilient versus stress-affected outcomes: A replication and extension. *Child Development, 70,* 645–659.

Wyman, P. A., Cowen, E. L., Work, W. C., & Parker, G. R. (1991). Developmental and family milieu correlates of resilience in urban children who have experienced major life-stress. *American Journal of Community Psychology, 19,* 405–426.

Yoon, S., Steigerwald, S., Holmes, M. R., & Perzynski, A. T. (2016). Children's exposure to violence: The underlying effect of posttraumatic stress symptoms on behavior problems. *Journal of Traumatic Stress, 29*(1), 72–79.

Zelazo, P. D. (2001). Self-reflection and the development of consciously controlled processing. In P. Mitchell & K. J. Riggs (Eds.), *Children's reasoning and the mind* (pp. 169–189). London: Psychology Press.

Additional Resources

There are many, many excellent authors, researchers, and practitioners who have made significant contributions to the field of traumatic stress, and who have influenced our own thinking and our practice. Although there are far too many for us to be able to provide a comprehensive list here, we include below some of those who have most influenced us. Some are specifically referenced in this book, while others, though not directly referenced, have impacted our thinking about and approach toward the treatment of children who have experienced trauma. We are lucky enough to consider a number of the authors below to be both our colleagues and our teachers, and we are appreciative of the transmission of knowledge we have received from those we have not yet been fortunate enough to work with directly. We highly recommend these resources to other professionals.

Bloom, S. (2013). *Creating sanctuary: Toward the evolution of sane societies* (rev. ed.). New York: Routledge.

Briere, J., & Lanktree, C. (2008). *Integrative treatment of complex trauma for adolescents (ITCT-A): A guide for the treatment of multiply traumatized youth*. Long Beach, CA: MCAVIC-USC, National Child Traumatic Stress Network.

Briere, J., & Scott, C. (2006). *Principles of trauma therapy: A guide to symptoms, evaluation, and treatment*. Thousand Oaks, CA: SAGE.

Brom, D., Pat-Horenczyk, R., & Ford, J. (2009). *Treating traumatized children: Risk, resilience and recovery*. New York: Routledge.

Cohen, J. A., Mannarino, A. P., & Deblinger, E. (2017). *Treating trauma and traumatic grief in children and adolescents* (2nd ed.). New York: Guilford Press.

Courtois, C. A., & Ford, J. D. (Eds.). (2009). *Treating complex traumatic stress disorders: Scientific foundations and therapeutic models*. New York: Guilford Press.

Courtois, C. A., & Ford, J. D. (2013). *Treatment of complex trauma: A sequenced, relationship-based approach*. New York: Guilford Press.

Damasio, A. (1999). *The feeling of what happens*. San Diego, CA: Harcourt.

DeRosa, R., Habib, M., Pelcovitz, D., Rathus, J., Sonnenklar, J., Ford, J., et al. (2006). *Structured psychotherapy for adolescents responding to chronic stress*. Unpublished manual.

Ford, J. D., & Russo, E. (2006). Trauma-focused, present-centered, emotional self-regulation approach to integrated treatment for posttraumatic stress and addiction: Trauma Adaptive Recovery Group Education and Therapy (TARGET). *American Journal of Psychotherapy, 60*, 335–355.

Gil, E. (1991). *The healing power of play: Working with abused children*. New York: Guilford Press.

Gil, E. (2006). *Helping abused and traumatized children: Integrating directive and nondirective approaches*. New York: Guilford Press.

Greenwald, R. (1999). *Eye movement desensitization and reprocessing (EMDR) in child and adolescent psychotherapy*. Northvale, NJ: Jason Aronson.

Habib, M., Labruna, V., & Newman, J. (2013). Complex histories and complex presentations: Implementation of a manually guided group treatment for traumatized adolescents. *Journal of Family Violence, 28,* 717–728.

Herman, J. L. (1992). *Trauma and recovery.* New York: Basic Books.

Hughes, D. (2006). *Building the bonds of attachment: Awakening love in deeply troubled children.* Lanham, MD: Jason Aronson.

Hughes, D. (2007). *Attachment-focused family therapy.* New York: Norton.

James, B. (1989). *Treating traumatized children.* New York: Free Press.

James, B. (1994). *Handbook for treatment of attachment-trauma problems in children.* New York: Free Press.

Kagan, R. (2007a). *Real life heroes: A life storybook for children* (2nd ed.). Binghamton, NY: Haworth Press.

Kagan, R. (2007b). *Real life heroes: Practitioner's manual.* Binghamton, NY: Haworth Press.

Landolt, M., Schnyder, U., & Cloitre, M. (Eds.). (2017). *Evidence-based treatments for trauma-related disorders in children and adolescents.* New York: Springer.

Lanktree, C., & Briere, J. (2016). *Treating complex trauma in children and their families: An integrative approach.* Thousand Oaks, CA: SAGE.

Lieberman, A. F., Ghosh Ippen, C., & Van Horn, P. (2015). *Don't hit my mommy!: A manual for child–parent psychotherapy with young children exposed to violence and other trauma* (2nd ed.). Washington, DC: Zero to Three Press.

Lieberman, A. F., & Van Horn, P. (2008). *Psychotherapy with infants and young children: Repairing the effects of stress and trauma on early attachment.* New York: Guilford Press.

Lovett, J. (1999). *Small wonders: Healing childhood trauma with EMDR.* New York: Free Press.

Monahon, C. (1993). *Children and trauma: A guide for parents and professionals.* San Francisco: Jossey-Bass.

Perry, B., & Szalavitz, M. (2007). *The boy who was raised as a dog, and other stories from a child psychiatrist's notebook: What traumatized children can teach us about loss, love, and healing.* New York: Basic Books.

Putnam, F. W. (1997). *Dissociation in children and adolescents: A developmental perspective.* New York: Guilford Press.

Saxe, G. N., Ellis, B. H., & Brown, A. D. (2015). *Collaborative treatment of traumatized children and teens: The Trauma Systems Therapy approach* (2nd ed.). New York: Guilford Press.

Schore, A. (1994). *Affect regulation and the origin of the self: The neurobiology of emotional development.* Hillsdale, NJ: Erlbaum.

Shapiro, F. (2001). *Eye movement desensitization and reprocessing (EMDR): Basic principles, protocols, and procedures* (2nd ed.). New York: Guilford Press.

Sunderland, M. (2006). *The science of parenting: Practical guidelines on sleep, crying, play, and building emotional well-being for life.* New York: Dorling Kindersley.

Terr, L. (1990). *Too scared to cry: Psychic trauma in childhood.* New York: HarperCollins.

van der Kolk, B. (1987). *Psychological trauma.* Washington, DC: American Psychiatric Press.

van der Kolk, B. A. (2014). *The body keeps the score: Brain, mind and body in the healing of trauma.* New York: Viking Press.

van der Kolk, B. A., McFarlane, A. C., & Weisaeth, L. (Eds.). (1996). *Traumatic stress: The effects of overwhelming experience on mind, body, and society.* New York: Guilford Press.

Warner, E., Cook, A., Westcott, A., & Koomar, J. (2014). *Sensory Motor Arousal Regulation Treatment (SMART) Manual: A "bottom up" approach to treatment of complex trauma for children and adolescents, Version 2.* Brookline, MA: Trauma Center at JRI.

Webb, N. B. (Ed.). (2017). *Play therapy with children and adolescents in crisis* (4th ed.). New York: Guilford Press.

Index

Note. *f* following a page number indicates a figure.